Functional Anatomy
of the Spine

JEAN OLIVER MCSP
Founder, Back Care Service; Director, Back Education Programme, Cambridge;

Mary's Univ... ...ehampt...
...egist... ...tion T... ...apists...

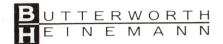

B UTTERWORTH
H EINEMANN

Butterworth-Heinemann
Linacre House, Jordan Hill, Oxford OX2 8DP
A division of Reed Educational and Professional Publishing Ltd

ℛ   *A member of the Reed Elsevier plc group*

OXFORD   BOSTON
MELBOURNE   NEW DELHI   SINGAPORE

First published 1991
Reprinted 1995, 1996

British Library Cataloguing in Publication Data
Oliver, Jean.
   Functional anatomy of the spine.
   I. Title   II. Middleditch, Alison
   616.7

ISBN 0 7506 0052 7

Library of Congress Cataloguing in Publication Data
Oliver, Jean
   Functional anatomy of the spine/Jean Oliver, Alison Middleditch.
   p.   cm.
   Includes bibliographical references and index.
   ISBN 0–7506–0052–7
   1. Spine—Anatomy.   I. Middleditch, Alison.   II. Title.
   [QM111.O55 1991]
   611′.9—dc20   91–21762
                                                           CIP

Typeset by Latimer Trend Ltd, Plymouth
Printed and bound in Great Britain by Clays Ltd, St Ives plc

11450819

Contents

10   Posture

Preface

The need for a book on functional anatomy of the whole spine became obvious to us when we ourselves were studying for our diplomas in spinal manipulation. Up-to-date literature on the subject was only to be found by ploughing through books and journals which had to be specially ordered for us. More recently, while teaching spinal mobilization on postregistration physiotherapy courses, we found that the course participants were going through the same time-consuming process. Much excellent research on spinal function has been carried out over the last few decades but, for our purposes, it needed to be brought together in a book that would be directly relevant to therapists involved in assessing and treating spinal dysfunction. This we have attempted to do, and in the process our own approach to the management of spinal disorders has changed considerably.

As research continues, and much exciting and relevant work is still being carried out, for example in the field of adverse mechanical tension in the neuromeningeal structures, we hope to be able to keep this book up-to-date to enable therapists to expand on their knowledge of the anatomy, 'normal' biomechanics and the normal ageing process that occurs in the spine. Only then can we begin to comprehend spinal *dys*function. Inevitably as our understanding increases, the spinal assessments and treatments we carry out on patients will have deeper meaning; techniques can be used logically and can be adapted as necessary to suit the individual patient; advice can be given to the patient in a specific and appropriate way rather than at random. First and foremost, our attention should be directed to the field of prevention of back injuries, starting in schools, as we believe that much suffering and loss of working hours can be avoided.

The examination and treatment of any peripheral joint inevitably includes a consideration of the anatomy of that joint together with its pathological condition. As far as spinal lesions are concerned, however, this has not been general practice, and the tendency to treat solely signs and symptoms without due regard to the clinical diagnosis is fraught with danger. The spine is often regarded as being far too complex to attempt to form a specific diagnosis unless the lesion is overtly apparent, such as a prolapsed intervertebral disc with nerve root involvement. We hope that this text will go some way towards helping therapists form a clinical diagnosis before treating spinal lesions. This saves both patient and therapist time, as treatment is applied intelligently; signs and symptoms are not in any way disregarded but the interpretation of them is clearer. An accurate diagnosis will also prevent over-zealous manipulation of joints in the presence of, for example, instability or vertebral artery disease.

In concentrating on the functional anatomy of the spine, there is no suggestion that it should ever be considered as a separate entity from the remainder of the body. Our difficulty has been in deciding what to exclude from the text rather than what to include. The format of the book has been devised to help the reader use it for reference and study purposes; some repetition is, therefore, inevitable.

We are indebted to all those whose research has helped us to write this book, in particular M. A. Adams PhD; N. Bogduk DipAnat BSc(Med) MBBS PhD; J. R. Taylor MD PhD and L. T. Twomey BApp Sc(Hons) PhD. Our grateful thanks are also due to P. Dolan PhD, J. P. G. Urban PhD and our colleagues listed below who painstakingly helped us with research or read various chapters and offered constructive advice:

Jacky Balfour MCSP
Marilyn Berry MCSP
Sally Cassar MCSP Dip TP
Anna Edwards BSc MCSP Dip TP
Elizabeth Grieve MSc MCSP Dip TP
Anne-Marie Hassenkamp MSc MCSP
Ros Heron MCSP
Raymond Pinder CEng, MI Struct E
Sally Radmore MCSP
Ann Thomson MSc BA MCSP Dip TP

We also express gratitude for the use of the Library and Physiotherapy Department at the Royal National Orthopaedic Hospital, Bolsover Street, London and for the use of Cambridge University Medical Library.

We would also like to thank Jean Horn for her assistance in typing some of the manuscript and Richard Ledwidge, who with much patience and skill produced the fine illustrations which are an essential part of the book. Lastly, we would like to thank our husbands, Peter Oliver and John Middleditch, for their support and encouragement during the undertaking of this project.

July, 1991   Jean Oliver
                                                  Alison Middleditch

1

Structure of the Vertebral Column

The vertebral column consists of 24 separate bony vertebrae (Fig. 1.1), together with 5 fused vertebrae which form the sacrum, and usually 4 fused vertebrae which form the coccyx.

Anteriorly there is an intervertebral disc between adjacent vertebral bodies, with the exception of the first and second cervical vertebrae. Posteriorly, the apophyseal joints are formed by the articular facets on the articular processes.

The vertebral column has three principal functions:

- It supports the human in the upright posture
- It allows movement and locomotion
- It protects the spinal cord

When viewed from the side, the vertebral column displays five curves in the upright posture – two cervical, and one each thoracic, lumbar and sacral. The shape of these curves varies in normal spines, and it is frequently altered by pathological changes.

The cervical curves. There are two normally-occurring curves in the cervical spine: the upper cervical curve extending from the occiput to the axis, and the longer lordotic curve of the lower cervical spine extending from the axis to the second thoracic vertebra. The lower cervical curve is convex forwards and is the reverse of the upper cervical curve.

The thoracic curve is concave forwards, extending from T2 to T12. The concavity is due to the greater depth of the posterior parts of the vertebral bodies in this region. In the upper part there is often a slight lateral curve with the convexity directed to either the right or left (*see* pp. 23–4).

The lumbar curve is convex forwards and extends from T12 to the lumbosacral junction.

The sacral curve extends from the lumbosacral junction to the coccyx. Its anterior concavity faces downwards and forwards.

In utero the vertebral column is in total flexion. The upper cervical, thoracic and sacral curves which are concave anteriorly during fetal

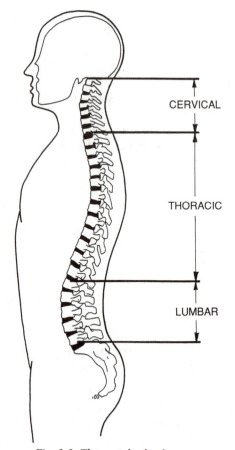

Fig. 1.1 The vertebral column.

life retain the same curvature after birth and are therefore called *primary* curves.

The lower cervical curve begins to develop in the third month of intrauterine life and is accentuated as the child starts to hold its head upright at 3 months and as it sits upright at 6–9 months. Development of the lumbar curve occurs as the child learns to stand and walk. The lower cervical and lumbar curves are *secondary* or *compensatory* curves.

These curves help to dissipate vertical compressive forces, thereby providing the spine with an important shock-absorbing capacity. If the vertebral column were straight, vertical compressive forces would be transferred through the vertebral bodies to the intervertebral discs alone. The curves of the spine thus ensure that some of the compressive forces are absorbed by the ligaments of the spine.

When the column is viewed from the back, a lateral curvature of the spine, termed a scoliosis, may be apparent in some individuals. Scoliotic curves are most common in the thoracic and lumbar regions.

Two broad divisions of scoliosis are recognized: non-structural and structural.

Non-structural curves have no underlying structural abnormality and they can be corrected temporarily with a change of posture or traction. These curves are often reduced or absent in bending forward, or in lying, where the effect of gravity is eliminated. Postural curves are examples of non-structural scoliosis.

When a *structural* scoliosis is present, there are abnormalities of the vertebrae and ribs. The vertebral bodies are rotated towards the convexity of the curve, while the spinous processes deviate towards the concavity of the curvature. During forward flexion, rib and vertebral rotation occur towards the convexity of the structural curve. In some cases, the deformity may be three-dimensional, consisting of a flexion component in addition to a lateral flexion and rotational abnormality.

Scoliosis is more common in the white than the black population and is found more frequently in females than males with a ratio of 5:1 (Palastanga *et al.*, 1989).

The aetiology of some of the curves is understood, but the mechanisms by which the deformity develops is still not clear. In terms of aetiology and pathology three classes of curves are recognized:

1. *Congenital* – structural, congenital abnormalities which can be readily identified;
2. *Neuromuscular* – following muscular or neurological impairment, e.g. poliomyelitis;
3. *Idiopathic* – the term given when the aetiology is unclear. There are four subgroups within this class: primary skeletal, neuromuscular, metabolic and hereditary.

Trabecular Systems within the Vertebral Bodies

The vertebral body consists of an outer thin shell of cortical bone. This would tend to fail in compression by buckling, and is prevented from doing so by its filling of cancellous bone, the trabeculae of which act as struts, without being excessively heavy (Wainwright *et al.*, 1976). There are three main systems of trabeculae: a primary vertical, a secondary oblique and a horizontal.

1. *Vertical system.* The vertical trabecular system is present throughout the entire vertebral column. Within the vertebral body there are three zones of trabeculae which run in a superoinferior direction. In the centre of the body, the trabeculae are vertically-arranged, large diameter cylinders whose walls are formed by thin, solid plates of lamellar bone. Trabeculae are also arranged in a circular arrangement around the basivertebral veins. The zones above and below this central zone are directly

adjacent to the vertebral end plates. In these areas the trabeculae are regularly-spaced longitudinally and transversely.

The vertical system sustains body weight and principally resists perpendicular compressive forces.

2. *Oblique system.* Four tracts of trabeculae form the oblique system: a superior and inferior tract on each side. The superior system extends from the superior articular process of one side, down through the pedicle to the lower surface of the vertebral body on the opposite side. Likewise, the inferior oblique system runs from the inferior articular process on one side, up through the pedicle to the upper surface of the vertebral body on the opposite side. Posterior to the articular processes, the oblique systems are continuous with the trabeculae within the spinous process.

The oblique systems do not reach the anterior margins of the vertebral body. They resist torsion and, together with the vertical system, resist bending and shear.

3. *Horizontal systems.* The trabeculae are arranged horizontally within the transverse processes and project into the vertebral body where they intersect in the midline.

These systems resist tension and the muscular pull of the powerful lumbar muscles which attach to the transverse processes.

There are less trabeculae in the anterior, superior and inferior regions of the vertebral bodies and these are, therefore, areas of mechanical weakness, collapse of which is evident in wedge-shaped compression fractures of the vertebral body.

Atrophy of the trabecular system is resisted principally by the vertical system. In osteoporosis, the secondary systems atrophy first and their disappearance makes the lines of the vertical system stand out more clearly on X-rays.

CERVICAL SPINE

The cervical spine is designed for mobility and, under normal circumstances, this is not at the expense of stability. Movements of the head and neck are principally concerned with the positioning of the eyes and hence the line of vision; therefore, the upper cervical muscles are highly innervated and enable movements to be made with a fine degree of precision (*see* pp. 104–5).

As already mentioned there are two normally-occurring curves in the cervical spine, and the region can be divided morphologically and physiologically into upper and lower segments at the second cervical vertebra. The craniovertebral region consists of the occiput, atlas and axis and forms the primary upper cervical curve. It is this region which controls the head in the neutral position in the upright posture.

If the neck is viewed from the side in the neutral position, it can be seen that the lower cervical curve is longer, but the degree of curvature is greater in the upper cervical spine. In the lower cervical spine the cervical curve is a secondary curve imposed between the primary upper cervical and thoracic curves.

Movements of the neck are influenced by the anatomical differences between the upper and lower cervical spine. It is important to note that in the sagittal plane independent movement is possible in the upper or lower cervical spine, and this must be considered when examining or treating the neck. For example, it is possible to extend the upper cervical spine and flex the lower cervical spine simultaneously. Regional and segmental movements of the neck are considered separately on pp. 166–7; 170–7.

Upper Cervical Spine

The first and second cervical vertebrae differ in structure from the lower cervical vertebrae.

The atlas

The atlas (C1) is the first cervical vertebra (Fig. 1.2). It articulates superiorly with the occiput and inferiorly with the axis (C2), the second cervical vertebra.

The atlas differs from all other vertebrae in that it does not have a

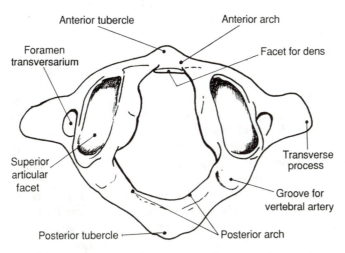

Fig. 1.2 The first cervical vertebra or atlas – superior aspect.

body, but consists of two lateral masses which are joined together by an anterior and posterior arch.

The anterior arch is curved convexly forward. It becomes slightly thickened and roughened in the midline to form the anterior tubercle. On the dorsal surface of the anterior arch there is a facet which articulates with the dens of the axis.

The posterior arch is wider than the anterior arch. It is convex posteriorly and has a tubercle at the apex. The atlas does not have a spinous process, but this is represented by the posterior tubercle, which may be palpated in some subjects (see p. 19).

The lateral masses are directed forwards and medially. On the superior surface of each lateral mass is a concave facet which articulates with the corresponding occipital condyle. These facets face upwards and medially and may be somewhat narrower in the middle. On the inferior surface of each lateral mass are small, concave, circular facets which articulate with facets on the superior surface of the axis. On the medial aspect of each lateral mass is a small rough tubercle which provides attachment for the transverse ligament of the atlas. This ligament divides the vertebral foramen into anterior and posterior cavities. The transverse ligament passes behind the dens of the axis, securing it in place in the anterior cavity of the atlas. The posterior cavity of the atlas contains the spinal cord and meninges.

Posterior to each lateral mass is a groove in the posterior arch in which the vertebral artery and first cervical spinal nerve are found. The vertebral artery is particularly susceptible to trauma at this point (see p. 152). This groove is occasionally converted into a foramen by a thin plate of bone superiorly.

The transverse processes of the atlas are longer than those of all the cervical vertebrae with the exception of C7. Their length ensures considerable leverage, which aids rotation of the head. The transverse processes of the atlas can be easily palpated between the mastoid process and the mandibular angle (see p. 19).

The axis

The axis (Fig. 1.3) provides a pivot around which the atlas and head rotate. A vertical pillar of bone projects upwards from the superior surface of the body of the axis. This is the dens (odontoid process), approximately 1.5 cm long; its tip is pointed and provides attachment for the apical ligament. On either side of the apex, the dens is flattened where the alar ligaments attach.

The dens is narrower at its base where it is grooved by the transverse ligament of the atlas. On the anterior surface of the dens is an oval articular facet, which articulates with a similar facet on the back of the anterior arch of the atlas. The dens has more compact bone than the body of the axis.

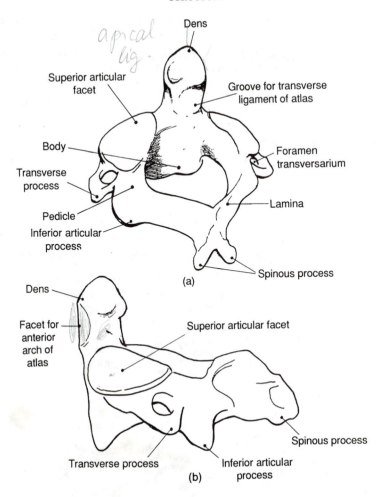

Fig. 1.3 The second cervical vertebra or axis. (a) posterolateral aspect; (b) lateral aspect.

There are large oval facets on either side at the base of the dens, which extend laterally over the body of the axis and the pedicles, and articulate with the inferior facets of the atlas. As the superior facets of the axis are somewhat anterior to the inferior facets of the axis, they do not form part of the articular pillar in the cervical spine.

At the junction of the pedicles and laminae, the inferior facets of the axis face downwards and forwards as in a typical cervical vertebra. The pedicles of the axis are stout. The laminae are thicker than in any other vertebra and provide attachment for the ligamenta flava.

The spinous process of the axis is large, usually bifid and normally provides a prominent bony landmark for palpation. The suboccipital muscles attach onto the spinous process of the axis which provides powerful leverage for the muscles' actions. Small transverse processes having a single tubercle at their tip, project laterally from the axis.

The foramina transversaria face superolaterally; this allows the vertebral arteries to pass upwards and laterally to the foramina of the atlas which are placed a little more laterally. The vertebral arteries are most prone to damage at the atlanto-axial joints (*see* p. 151).

Craniovertebral joints

Atlanto-occipital joints (Figs. 1.4; 1.5).   These joints are formed by the articulation of the concave articular facets on the lateral masses of

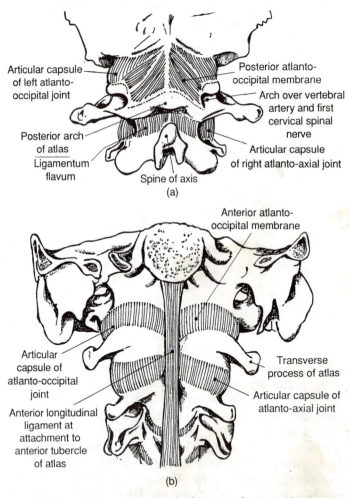

Fig. 1.4 The atlanto-occipital and atlanto-axial joints. (a) posterior aspect; (b) anterior aspect. (Adapted from P.L. Williams and R. Warwick, 1980. In *Gray's Anatomy*, 36th edn. Edinburgh: Churchill Livingstone, pp. 447, 448.)

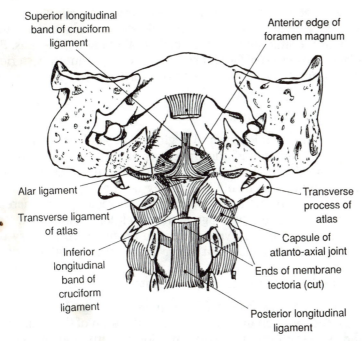

Fig. 1.5 Posterior aspect of atlanto-occipital and atlanto-axial joints after removal of posterior bony elements. (Adapted from P.L. Williams and R. Warwick, 1980. In *Gray's Anatomy*, 36th edn. Edinburgh: Churchill Livingstone, p. 449.)

the atlas with the convex facets on the occipital condyles. These joints are normally symmetrical. The lateral edges of the facets on the atlas are high and tend to restrict movements except those that occur in the sagittal plane.

Atlanto-axial joints (Figs. 1.4; 1.5).   The atlanto-axial articulation comprises three synovial joints:

1. One central atlanto-odontoid joint;
2. Two lateral atlanto-axial joints.

The atlanto-odontoid joint (median atlanto-axial joint).   This is a pivot joint, comprising:

1. The articulation of the facet on the anterior surface of the odontoid with the reciprocally-shaped facet on the posterior aspect of the anterior arch of the atlas, and
2. A synovial cavity between the posterior surface of the odontoid and the cartilage-lined anterior surface of the transverse ligament of the axis.

As this joint consists of two articulations, it may be termed a 'double joint'.

The lateral atlanto-axial joints. These are bilateral plane joints formed by the articulation of the inferior facets on the lateral masses of the atlas and the superior facets on the lateral masses of the axis. Both the inferior and superior facets are slightly convex anteroposteriorly. The facet planes lie at about 110° to the vertical.

Craniovertebral ligaments

Stability of the craniovertebral region is dependent upon the integrity of the ligaments of the upper cervical spine, and this is an important consideration when examining or treating the upper cervical spine. Ligamentous insufficiency may be the sequel to pathology such as osteoarthritis, which is common in this region. Also, increased laxity of the craniovertebral ligaments in children and adolescents should be borne in mind, even more so if an upper respiratory tract infection is present, which can cause inflammatory attenuation of these ligaments.

From anterior to posterior, the ligaments of the region are:

1. The *anterior atlanto-occipital membrane* (*see* Fig. 1.4). This connects the foramen magnum above to the arch of the atlas below, and is continuous with the anterior longitudinal ligament. It overlies the capsules of the atlanto-occipital joints laterally.
2. The *apical ligament* (*see* Fig. 1.9, p. 15). This is short, thick and attaches the tip of the dens to the anterior margin of the foramen magnum.
3. The two *alar ligaments* (Figs. 1.5; 1.6). These are symmetrically placed, arising from the posterior part of the tip of the dens. The greater portion of the fibres insert onto the occipital condyles, while some fibres attach onto the lateral masses of the atlas. Rotation to the right is limited by the left alar ligament and vice

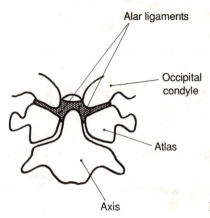

Alar ligaments

Occipital condyle

Atlas

Axis

Fig. 1.6 Coronal aspect of alar ligaments.

versa, while the contralateral ligament is relaxed. During rotation, the inferior part of the ligament is stretched initially, but with increasing rotation, the load is transferred to the superior fibres.

During lateral flexion, the occipital part of the alar ligament on the same side is relaxed while the atlantal portion is stretched. The atlas moves in the same direction of the lateral flexion, but it does not rotate. As lateral flexion increases, the contralateral occipital portion of the ligament is stretched. The stretched occipital ligament on one side and the atlantal attachment on the opposite side induce rotation of the axis in the direction of the lateral flexion, so that the spinous process of the axis moves contralaterally (Dvorak and Panjabi, 1987).

If the suboccipital muscles are relaxed, flexion of the cervical spine is limited by membrane tectoria, the longitudinal fibres of the cruciform ligament and the transverse ligament. The alar ligaments will resist flexion if these ligaments are ruptured.

Damage of the alar ligaments by impact trauma or inflammatory disease can result in increased axial rotation between the occiput and the atlas, and the atlas and axis. Excessive rotation may reduce blood flow in the vertebral artery (Fielding, 1957) – see pp. 151–4). There may also be increased lateral displacement between the atlas and axis during lateral flexion.

These ligaments are composed of collagen fibres, have limited extensibility, and are most vulnerable when the head is rotated and additionally flexed, as in a rear collision whiplash injury. Following such injury, the transverse ligament of the atlas may remain intact even if one of the alar ligaments is ruptured.

4. The *transverse ligament of the atlas* (*see* Fig. 1.5). This is a thick band which holds the odontoid in place and passes between the tubercles on the medial side of the lateral masses of the atlas. The ligament is thicker centrally, where some fibres extend up to the occiput and others pass downwards to the body of the axis. The whole ligament is in the shape of a cross and is termed the *cruciform ligament of the atlas* (*see* Fig. 1.5). If the ligament is damaged by degenerative changes or traumatic tearing, the stability of the region is compromised, and the dens may impinge upon the spinal cord.

5. The *accessory atlanto-axial ligaments*. These pass upwards and laterally from the base of the dens to the inferomedial aspect of the lateral masses of the atlas.

6. The *membrane tectoria* (*see* Fig. 1.5). Connecting the posterior surface of the body of the axis to the basiocciput, the membrane tectoria is a prolongation of the posterior longitudinal ligament.

7. The *posterior atlanto-occipital membrane* (*see* Fig. 1.4). This connects the foramen magnum above with the posterior arch of the

atlas below, and is continuous with the joint capsules laterally. It represents the ligamentum flavum in this region of the spine, and forms a channel for the vertebral artery and first cervical nerve to run between itself and the groove on the posterior arch of the atlas.

8. The *lateral atlanto-occipital ligaments*. Reinforcing the capsules of the atlanto-occipital joints, the lateral atlanto-occipital ligaments pass between the jugular processes of the occiput and lateral mass of the atlas on each side.

9. The *fibrous capsules (see* Fig. 1.4) of the craniovertebral joints. These are thin and baggy whereas those of the atlanto-axial joints are looser and permit relatively free movement to occur.

Stability between the atlas and axis is mainly provided by the transverse ligament, the alar ligaments and the accessory atlanto-axial ligaments.

Lower Cervical Spine C2–7

The 2nd to 7th cervical vertebrae are similar in structure. Together with the craniovertebral region, this region allows movements and positioning of the head. Below the second and subsequent cervical vertebrae are intervertebral discs between adjacent vertebrae. These discs contribute to more than one-quarter of the length of the cervical column and are a factor in allowing considerable movement of the neck.

Structure of a Typical Cervical Vertebra (Figs. 1.7; 1.8)

A typical cervical vertebra is composed of an anterior body and posterior arch.

Vertebral body

The vertebral body is roughly cylindrical; the superior surface is concave transversely and convex anteroposteriorly and on each side are prominent elevations which are known as the *uncinate (unciform) processes*. The inferior surface is reciprocally convex transversely and concave anteroposteriorly. Two articular facets on the inferior surface of the body articulate with the uncinate processes of the subjacent vertebra. These articulations are known as the *joints of Luschka* or the *uncovertebral joints*.

Considerable flexion and extension are possible in this region due to the convexity and concavity of the vertebral body, but lateral flexion is partially restricted by the uncinate processes.

The anterior surface of the vertebral body is convex transversely. At

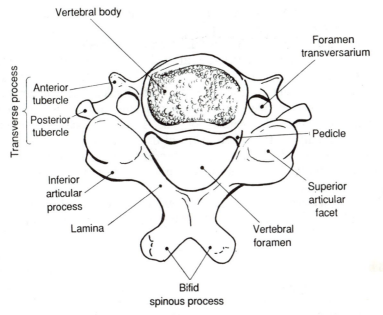

Fig. 1.7 A typical cervical vertebra – superior aspect.

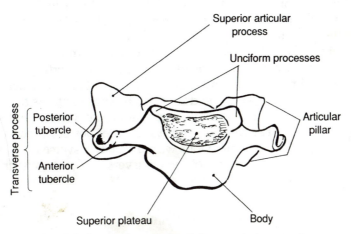

Fig. 1.8 A typical cervical vertebra – anterior aspect.

the superior and inferior margins it is marked by the fibres of the anterior longitudinal ligament. The posterior surface of the body is flattened and has foramina for two or more basivertebral veins.

Posterior arch

The posterior arch is formed by the pedicles, articular processes, laminae and spinous processes.

The *pedicles* are short and thick, projecting backwards and slightly laterally from the vertebral body.

The articular processes. At the junction of the pedicles and laminae there are superior and inferior articular processes which form an *articular pillar*. These articular processes contain the *articular facets*. The *superior* facets are oval, flat and face backwards and upwards, while the *inferior* facets correspondingly face forwards and downwards. The articular pillars of C3, 4 and 5 may be grooved anterolaterally by the dorsal rami of the cervical spinal nerves.

The *laminae* are long and thin, extending backwards and medially from the pedicles to meet in the midline, thereby completing the posterior arch.

The *spinous processes* project backwards from the junction of the laminae; they are short, bifid and often unequal in size (*see* palpation on p. 20).

The *vertebral foramen* is bounded by the vertebral body anteriorly, the pedicles laterally and the laminae laterally and posteriorly. In the cervical spine, the foramen is comparatively large and triangular. It is occupied by the spinal cord, meninges and associated vessels.

The *transverse processes* arise from two roots. Anteriorly, they arise from the vertebral body and posteriorly from the articular processes. They project anterolaterally and are at an angle of 45° to the vertical. Laterally, the transverse processes are bifid, with anterior and posterior tubercles that give attachment to the scalene muscles. The *carotid tubercle* is the anterior tubercle of the 6th cervical vertebra. It is very large and is immediately posterior to the carotid artery which can be compressed at this point. The transverse process contains the *foramen transversarium* in which lies the vertebral artery, venous and sympathetic plexuses. The medial section of the posterior root of the transverse process is homologous with a true transverse process, as in a thoracic vertebra. The rest of the transverse process constitutes the homologue of a rib.

Ligaments of the Lower Cervical Spine

The *anterior longitudinal* ligament (Fig. 1.9) is a strong band which lies anterior to the vertebral body. It is attached to the basilar part of the occipital bone from which it extends to the tubercle of the atlas, and it then attaches to the front of the vertebral bodies.

It consists of several layers of fibres fixed to the superior and inferior margins of the vertebral bodies and the intervertebral disc. The superficial fibres are long and extend over three or four vertebrae; the middle fibres extend over two or three vertebrae, while the deepest fibres are attached to adjacent vertebrae.

This ligament is thicker and narrower opposite the vertebral bodies,

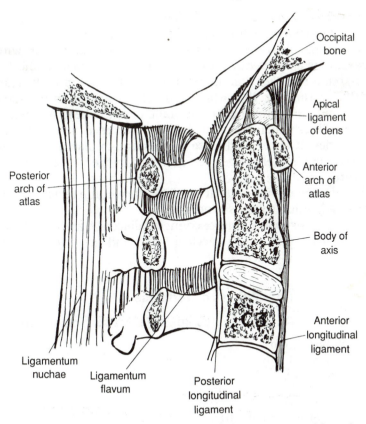

Fig. 1.9 Additional ligaments of the cervical spine. Sectional lateral aspect of the upper three segments.

and thinner opposite the intervertebral discs. It is relaxed in flexion and taut in extension.

The *posterior longitudinal* ligament is posterior to the vertebral body, lies inside the vertebral canal, and is attached to the body of the axis, and then to the margins of the vertebral bodies and the intervertebral discs. It consists of superficial fibres extending over three or four vertebrae and deep fibres which extend between adjacent vertebrae. This ligament is broad and uniform in width in the cervical spine. It is stretched on neck flexion and relaxed in extension.

The *articular capsules* of the apophyseal joints are attached to the margins of the articular facets. They are loose in the cervical spine and, therefore, allow considerable mobility.

The *ligamenta flava* are predominantly yellow elastic tissue and connect the laminae of adjacent vertebrae. These ligaments, which are broad and long in the neck, allow flexion to occur, but prevent hyperflexion by braking the movement so that the end of range is not reached abruptly.

The *ligamentum nuchae* is a fibroelastic membrane which extends from the external occipital protuberance and external occipital crest to the spines of all the cervical vertebrae. It is homologous with the supraspinous and interspinous ligaments in the thoracic and lumbar spines, but is stronger than in other parts of the column. The ligament forms a septum for the attachment of the trapezius and splenius muscles, and it contributes to the stability of the head and neck with its strong fibres which are of particular importance in flexion-acceleration injuries. If an applied force is sufficient to tear the ligamentum nuchae, there is likely to be even greater damage to the intrinsic joint structures.

The *interspinous ligaments* are rudimentary in the cervical spine and connect adjoining spinous processes.

The *intertransverse ligaments* connect adjacent transverse processes. They are irregular in the cervical spine and are reinforced by the intertransverse muscles.

Joints between Typical Cervical Vertebrae

Three different types of joints link adjacent cervical vertebrae:

- Interbody joints
- Apophyseal joints
- Joints of Luschka

Interbody joints (Fig. 1.10)

Below C2, adjacent cervical vertebrae are linked by an intervertebral disc at the interbody joint which is termed a *symphysis*. As mentioned earlier, in the cervical spine the discs contribute more than one-quarter of the length of the column. One of the functions of the intervertebral disc is to allow and restrain movement, and in the cervical region the discs allow considerable mobility. The joints between the vertebral bodies and discs are saddle articulations; they are concave in the frontal and convex in the sagittal plane. They are reinforced anteriorly by the anterior longitudinal ligament and posteriorly by the posterior longitudinal ligament.

Apophyseal joints (*see* Fig. 1.10)

The paired cervical apophyseal joints are plane joints formed by the articulation of the inferior facets of one cervical vertebra with the superior facets of the subjacent vertebra. Direction and range of movement at these joints is determined by the orientation of the articular facets. The inferior facets of a typical cervical vertebra face forwards and downwards, articulating with the superior facets of the vertebra below, which face upwards and backwards. These joints

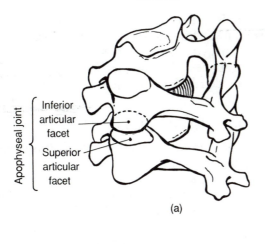

(a)

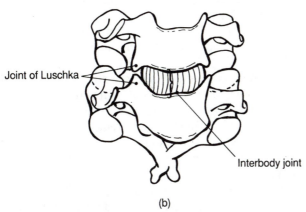

(b)

Fig. 1.10 Apophyseal joint. (a) posterolateral aspect of typical cervical vertebra; (b) anterolateral aspect of cervical interbody joint and joint of Luschka.

allow flexion, extension, rotation and lateral flexion to occur (*see* pp. 174–5). The facet planes lie at approximately 45° to the vertical, the upper joints being more horizontally placed, lying at approximately 55° to the vertical, while the facet planes of the lower joints lie at approximately 25° to the vertical.

The joint surfaces are reciprocally concave and convex. Articular cartilage lines the apophyseal joints and is subjected to weight-bearing stresses, as the apophyseal joints share the weight of the head with the vertebral bodies and discs. Degenerative changes at the cervical apophyseal joints are very common due to their weight-bearing function.

A long, loose capsule, which has a degree of elasticity, surrounds the joints, thereby allowing the relatively large amount of movement in this area. Apophyseal joint capsules are highly innervated and may, therefore, be a primary source of pain (*see* p. 230).

There are small meniscoid structures which project into the joint space. These are semilunar fringes of synovium which resemble the alar folds of the knee. Subsynovial tissue has a particularly rich nerve supply, and it has been suggested that it may be this structure which is 'trapped' during the sudden locking of a joint (Kos and Wolf, 1972).

Joints of Luschka (uncovertebral joints) (see Fig. 1.10)

The uncinate processes project upwards from the superior, lateral border of the vertebral bodies of C3–6 and correspond with reciprocally-shaped cavities on the lower border of the vertebra above. Corresponding surfaces are covered with hyaline cartilage and these clefts are lined with synovium which sends small meniscoid fringes into the cleft space (Penning, 1968). These clefts are bound medially by the intervertebral disc and posterolaterally by an extension of the annulus fibrosus. They provide some protection against posterolateral herniations of the disc. The joints become apparent in the first or second decade of life, but can be seen microscopically much earlier (Hirsch et al., 1967).

Opinion is divided as to whether these structures are indeed joints. They have been described as synovial articulations (von Luschka, 1858; Boreadis and Gershon Cohen, 1956), while others believe that they are a degenerative phenomenon (Hadley, 1957; Orofino et al., 1960; Hirsch et al., 1967), and some have suggested that these clefts undergo metaplasia to synovial 'joints' secondary to hypermobility (Silberstein, 1965).

The clinical significance of these structures is in their tendency to develop marked degenerative changes and form bony exostoses which may impinge the vertebral artery or cervical nerve roots. Degenerative changes in the uncovertebral joints have been shown to be twice as common as in the apophyseal joints.

During flexion and extension, shearing movements occur in these joints, but the uncinate processes limit lateral flexion of the neck.

Movement between adjacent cervical vertebrae involves movement at all of the above three joints. Movement cannot occur at one joint alone. Any lesion affecting one of the joints (e.g. osteoarthritis) will affect movement of the other two joints at that motion segment.

PALPATION OF THE CERVICAL SPINE (Figs. 1.11; 1.12)

In the cervical spine the following bony points may be palpated:

- Posterior tubercle of the atlas
- Posterolateral arch of the atlas
- Transverse process of the atlas

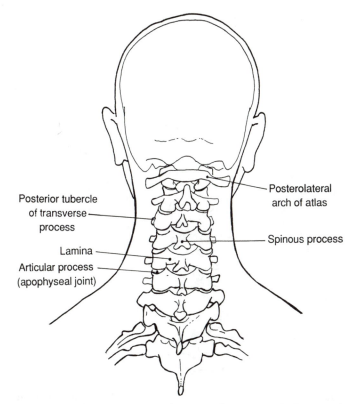

Posterior tubercle
of transverse
process

Posterolateral
arch of atlas

Lamina

Spinous process

Articular process
(apophyseal joint)

Fig. 1.11 Palpation points in the cervical spine – posterior aspect.

- Spinous processes C2–7
- Laminae C2–7
- Articular pillar/processes C2–7
- Transverse processes C1–7

Most of the bony landmarks may be easily palpated with the subject in prone-lying with the forehead supported.

The surface mark of the *posterior tubercle* of the atlas (C1) is in the soft tissue sulcus between the base of the occiput and the large spinous process of C2. This is not palpable in everyone, but in many people the bony tubercle may be identified.

The *posterolateral arches* of the atlas can be palpated just below the base of the occiput on either side.

Between the angle of the jaw and the mastoid process, the lateral tip of the *transverse process* of the atlas can be palpated. The tip of the transverse process is frequently tender to even gentle palpation. In some individuals, it is easier to palpate the transverse process if the head is placed in slight extension. It may be best palpated with the person in side-lying.

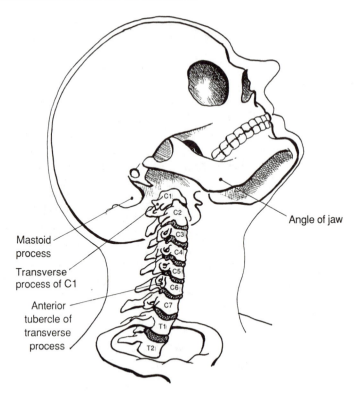

Fig. 1.12 Palpation points in the cervical spine – anterolateral aspect.

The *spinous process* of C2 is large and is felt as the first prominent bony landmark below the base of the occiput. The spinous process of C3 is smaller and tucked under the larger process of C2, while those of C4 and 5 are slightly larger. Palpation of the spinous process of C3 is often difficult as it is tucked under the larger process of C2; it may be easier to feel if the direction of the palpating thumb is angled slightly cranially as well as anteriorly. The spinous processes of C3–5 are usually bifid and may feel asymmetrical on palpation.

The spinous processes of C6 and 7 are not usually bifid and that of C7 is particularly prominent. In order to differentiate between C6 and 7, both spinous processes are palpated, the person is asked to extend the neck and the process of C7 remains palpable while that of C6 glides away.

The tip of the spinous processes of C2–6 are at the level of the inferior articular facet. Hence, the spinous process of C5 is at the same level as the inferior margin of the C5/6 apophyseal joint.

Deeper and lateral to the spinous process, the *laminae* may be palpated on either side. Palpation of the laminae may give a good indication of symmetry of the vertebra if the spinous process is asymmetrically bifid.

The posterior surface of the inferior *articular processes* of C2–7 may be palpated bilaterally 2–3 cm from the midline. The processes of C2–4 are easier to find than those of the lower cervical spine. Because the lateral atlanto-axial joints lie anterior to the articular pillar, they are easier to palpate anteriorly.

In supine lying, the anterior aspect of the *transverse processes* can be palpated and it may be necessary to lift the musculature gently to one side in order to make bony contact. This palpation must be performed with great care, as it is frequently uncomfortable and may produce neck and arm pain in a normal spine. In the long, slim-necked person, it has been reported (Grieve, 1986) that it is possible to palpate from C1 to T3.

Considerable differences may be felt between individuals. This may be due to congenital anomalies or as a result of degenerative changes. People who have even minor degenerative changes may develop tightening of the overlying soft tissues, which may make palpation of some bony landmarks more difficult. The bars and osteophytes which develop as part of the degenerative process may often be palpated, particularly over the articular processes.

CERVICO-THORACIC JUNCTION

At the cervico-thoracic junction, where the relatively mobile lower cervical spine articulates with the stiff thoracic spine, the intervertebral discs and apophyseal joints are particularly subject to stress and strain. Degenerative changes commonly occur at C6/7 and C7/T1 segments. In cervical spondylosis, the spinous processes of C7 and T1 may become unduly prominent with an overlying fatty tissue pad. These spinous processes are often tender to palpation, and the characteristic stiffness that develops is frequently the source of pain in this area.

Cervical ribs

Cervical ribs are the most common bony anomaly associated with the cervicothoracic region. Although cervical ribs have been reported as high as C4, they most frequently originate from the body and transverse process of the seventh cervical vertebra (Brain *et al.*, 1967). A true cervical rib has a head and neck, articulating with the transverse process and body of a cervical vertebra in a similar fashion to the articulation of a true rib with a thoracic vertebra. Cervical ribs may be long or short, unilateral or bilateral, symmetrical or asymmetrical. Soft tissue and nervous tissue anomalies are often associated with cervical ribs, e.g. supernumerary fascial bands, anomalies of the scalene muscles, a pre- or postfixed brachial plexus.

Vascular and neurological symptoms may arise from trespass of the cervical ribs on the brachial plexus and subclavian/axillary vessels (the neurovascular bundle), although it has been reported that less than 10% of those with cervical ribs have symptoms arising from their presence (Brown, 1983).

Thoracic Outlet (or Inlet)

As the neurovascular bundle passes from the thorax into the upper extremity, it courses through the thoracic outlet. The neurovascular bundle is particularly susceptible to trespass at four sites within the thoracic outlet (Pratt, 1986).

1. *Superior thoracic outlet*

The boundaries of this space are the manubrium anteriorly, first and second thoracic vertebrae posteriorly and the first rib laterally. The inferior contributions of the brachial plexus (ventral rami C8 and T1) and the subclavian vessels pass through this space and are vulnerable here to space-occupying lesions, e.g. thyroid gland, pancoast tumour. The anterior portion of the first rib is lower than the posterior portion, and the neurovascular structures pass over it at its lowest point. If the first rib is elevated as in, for example, chronic respiratory disease, or if there is an alteration in the obliquity of the rib, the neurovascular bundle may be subject to traction or entrapment.

2. *Scalene triangle*

This is formed by the anterior and middle scalene muscles which attach superiorly to the transverse processes of the upper and middle cervical spine and inferiorly to the first rib, where the attachments are approximately 2 cm apart. The ventral rami of C5–T1 occupy the vertical dimensions of the triangle, while the subclavian artery lies in the scalene groove at the base of the triangle. The dimensions of the triangle are affected by cervical spine movement. During extension or rotation to the ipsilateral side, dimensions of the triangle, particularly anteroposteriorly, are reduced (Pratt, 1986).

Other factors which alter the size of the triangle include cervical ribs, variations in the scalene muscles, e.g. extra slips of muscle, hypertrophy of the scalene muscles and supernumerary fascial bands. Any decrease in the size of the scalene triangle may put the neurovascular bundle at risk.

3. *Costoclavicular interval*

Trunks or divisions of the brachial plexus and subclavian/axillary vessels course through the bony interval between the clavicle and the first rib. During depression and retraction of the shoulder girdle, the two bones are approximated so that the neurovascular structures may be embarrassed. Symptoms arising from this area are associated with poor posture, carrying heavy objects or using a shoulder bag. Fractures, dislocations or exostosis of either bone may predispose to this type of entrapment.

4. *Coracoid pectoralis minor loop*

Cords of the brachial plexus surround the axillary artery as they pass the coracoid process and the nervous and vascular structures are bound together by a tight fascial sheath. As the arm is abducted and laterally rotated, the bundle passes around the coracoid process which acts as a fulcrum, pectoralis minor ensuring that the bundle does not slip over the coracoid process. Hyperabduction and lateral rotation of the shoulder may place excessive stretch on the neurovascular structures, thereby giving rise to neurological and vascular symptoms in the arm (Daskalakis, 1983).

THORACIC SPINE AND RIBS

The thoracic region is the least mobile area of the spine. Individual components of the thorax are flexible, but the stability of the area is due to:

1. Costotransverse, costovertebral and sternocostal joints;
2. Rib cage and sternum;
3. Increased moment of inertia which stiffens the spine when rotatory forces are sustained.

An important function of the thoracic spine and rib cage is to prevent compression of the heart, lungs and major vessels. Protection of these structures is at the expense of mobility in this region. In addition to increasing stiffness, the rib case has an energy-absorbing capacity, so that the load-bearing capacity of the thoracic spine is increased threefold (Andriacchi *et al.*, 1974). Stability of the thoracic spine is also increased by rises in intrathoracic pressure which convert the thorax into a solid unit capable of transmitting large forces (Morris *et al.*, 1961).

The thoracic curve is a primary curve, the apex of which is normally at T7/8. This kyphotic curve results from the shorter vertical height of the anterior thoracic vertebral bodies, differing from the cervical and lumbar spines where the intervertebral discs have a major influence on the shape of the curve. A slight lateral curve is often noticeable in the thoracic spine, and it has been suggested that this may be due to the dominance of either hand (e.g. in a right-handed individual there may be a slight curve convex to the right and vice versa) or the position of the aorta may influence this curve.

Women under 40 tend to have a straighter thoracic spine than men (Loebl, 1967). However, after 40 the female thoracic kyphosis is the same as the male's and, in later years, the female thoracic spine becomes more flexed as the familiar 'dowager's hump' develops. It has been hypothesized that this may occur due to the biomechanical changes, weight alteration and soft tissue extensibility that are a feature of pregnancy which is later perpetuated by the demands of nursing, feeding and carrying children (Grieve, 1988).

As the kyphosis increases, intervertebral joint movements decrease and the developing stiffness is frequently found to be a significant factor in thoracic musculoskeletal disorders.

Gravitational forces tend to increase the thoracic kyphosis; however, this is resisted by the posterior ligaments of the neural arch and muscular activity in the paravertebral back muscles. In the transverse plane the intervertebral disc fibres resist translation (particularly anteriorly) and shear deformation. Anterior displacement of the vertebral body is also resisted by the planes of the apophyseal joints. Rotational stresses in the transverse plane are restricted by the intervertebral disc fibres and the articular facets.

The intervertebral discs form one-seventh of the length of the thoracic spine. The nucleus pulposus is situated more centrally than in the cervical and lumbar regions, but it is smaller and has less capacity to swell (Koeller et al., 1984).

Although the rib cage contributes to the stiffness of the thoracic spine, the most restricting element is the intervertebral disc. Thoracic discs behave in a more viscous manner than lumbar discs and this may be due to the difference in structure of the collagen network or their framework (Koeller et al., 1984).

Thoracic disc height is less than lumbar disc height. A larger disc height tends to decrease stiffness, whereas a larger cross-sectional area increases it. Flexibility of thoracic and lumbar discs is the same in flexion, extension and lateral flexion and this may be because the effect of the greater cross-sectional area of the lumbar disc is neutralized by the shorter height of the thoracic disc. The ratio of disc diameter to height results in fewer circumferential stresses in thoracic discs, and is one of the reasons why fewer prolapsed discs occur in the thoracic than the lumbar spine.

The ribs which attach to the thoracic vertebrae and sternum present increased resistance to torsion whereas, in the lumbar spine, the apophyseal joints resist torsional stresses. The discs in intermediate segments are subject to relatively greater torsional stresses and represent a site of weakness (Markolf, 1972).

Structure of a Typical Thoracic Vertebra (Fig. 1.13)

Vertebral body

This is more or less cyclindrical and 'heart'-shaped, with its antero-posterior and transverse dimensions almost equal. The vertebral bodies diminish in size from T1 to T3 and then progressively increase in size to T12. On the vertebral body's upper and lower lateral borders are the demifacets for articulation with the heads of the ribs. The two superior facets are usually larger and are near the root of the pedicle, while the two inferior facets lie anterior to the inferior vertebral notch.

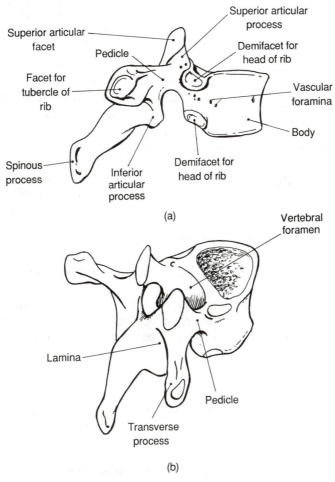

(a)

(b)

Fig. 1.13 A typical thoracic vertebra. (a) lateral aspect; (b) postero-lateral aspect.

Posterior arch

The *vertebral foramen* is circular in shape and relatively small. The spinal canal is narrowest at T6, although a narrow zone extends from T4 to T9. In this region the spinal cord is particularly vulnerable to any degenerative changes or space-occupying lesions that further decrease the size of the vertebral foramen.

The *pedicles* are short, stout processes passing directly posteriorly from the posterolateral parts of the body. The two *superior articular processes* arise from the superior borders of the laminae near their respective pedicles. They are thin plates of bone projecting superiorly and bearing articular facets, which are almost flat and oval, and face posteriorly, slightly laterally and slightly superiorly. The *inferior articular processes* are fused to the lateral ends of the laminae. They have a facet on their anterior surfaces which faces anteriorly, slightly inferiorly and slightly medially. These facets on the articular processes form the *apophyseal joints*.

The *spinous process* is long. It arises from the junction of the laminae and is directed inferiorly and posteriorly. In the mid-thoracic region, the inferior angulation is particularly marked, the tip of the spinous process lying at the level of the subjacent vertebral body. In the upper and lower thoracic spine, however, the spinous processes face more posteriorly. This is relevant when performing mobilizing techniques on the spinous processes; 'posteroanterior' techniques usually need some modification, and transverse pressures on the spinous processes in the mid-thoracic region will have a different effect on the apophyseal joints, due to longer leverage, than those performed in the upper and lower thoracic spine.

The two *transverse processes* project laterally and slightly posteriorly from the junction of the pedicles and laminae. In the upper thoracic spine, they may extend laterally for 4–5 cm but they progressively decrease in size downwards.

The *costal facets* which articulate with the tubercle of the rib are found anteriorly on the transverse processes of T1–6 while the costal facets of T7–12 are placed more superiorly on the transverse processes.

Particular Features of Thoracic Vertebrae

T1

The superior costal facets lie on the sides of the body and are circular, as they alone articulate with the first rib. The lower facets are much smaller and semilunar in shape.

T10, T11 and T12

These usually articulate with the head of their numerically corresponding rib alone and so only bear one circular costal facet on each side. The transverse processes of T11 and 12 are small and do not bear articular facets.

The Ribs

There are usually 12 ribs on each side except where a cervical (or lumbar) rib has developed. Cervical ribs have been found as high as C4 (*see* p. 21). Nomenclature of R1–12 is as follows:

R1–7:   *true* ribs. These are connected via the costal cartilages to the sternum.

R8–12:   *false* ribs. The costal cartilages of R8–10 are joined to that of the rib above.

R11–12: *floating* ribs, so called as they are not connected anteriorly to the sternum.

The direction of the ribs varies, the upper ones being more horizontal. They increase in obliquity down to R9 and then become more horizontal again, with the breadth of the ribs decreasing caudally.

The spaces between the ribs are termed *intercostal* spaces.

Typical ribs (Fig. 1.14)

R3–9. Each rib consists of a shaft, an anterior and a posterior end. The *shaft* is thin and flattened with a superior and inferior border and an internal concave and external convex surface. The internal surface is marked along its inferior border by the *costal groove*. It is gently curved and twisted in its long axis. The *rib angle*, where the rib is more bent, lies approximately 5–6 cm from the tubercle and provides useful leverage for performing mobilizing techniques aimed at the spinal joints.

At the *anterior end* there is a small, cup-shaped depression for connection with the costal cartilage. The *posterior end* has a head, neck and tubercle. The *head* of the rib bears an upper smaller and lower larger facet separated by a crest, which lies opposite the intervertebral disc. The upper facet articulates with the vertebra above and the lower facet articulates with the body of the numerically corresponding vertebra. The *neck* is flattened and lies between the head and tubercle of the rib. The *tubercle* is situated on the external surface of the posterior part of the rib at the junction of the neck with the shaft. It has a roughened lateral non-articular part for ligamentous attachment, and a medial articular part with a small, oval facet for articulation with the transverse process of the numerically corresponding vertebra.

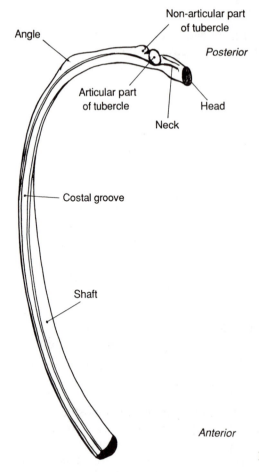

Fig. 1.14 A typical rib.

Atypical ribs

R1. The first rib (Fig. 1.15) is usually the shortest one, but has the largest curvature. Its flattened surfaces face superiorly and inferiorly, and its borders internally and externally. It is higher at its posterior end, sloping downwards towards its anterior end. The *head* has only one facet for articulation with the first thoracic vertebra. The *neck* is rounded and is directed superiorly, posteriorly and laterally. Angulation of the rib occurs at the *tubercle*, which has an oval facet for articulation with the transverse process of the first thoracic vertebra. Two shallow grooves for the subclavian artery and vein cross the upper surface of the shaft. Any changes in obliquity of the rib may cause traction or entrapment of the inferior portions of the brachial plexus and subclavian vessels (*see* p. 22). A small ridge and scalene tubercle lie between the grooves on its internal border.

R2. The second rib is much longer than the first, its angle being near the tubercle. The shaft is not twisted and the rib has a convex

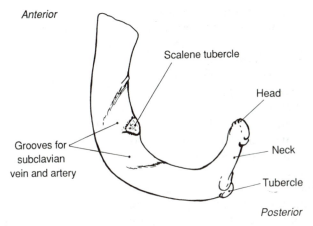

Fig. 1.15 The first rib – superior aspect.

external surface facing superiorly and slightly externally, and a concave internal surface facing inferiorly and slightly internally.

R10.   The *head* has a single facet for articulation with the upper border of the 10th thoracic vertebra and also the T9/10 disc.

R11, R12.   Each *head* bears a large articulating facet, but these ribs do not have necks or tubercles. R11 has a slight angle, but R12 does not and is much shorter, sometimes being almost insignificant. Their anterior ends are pointed and are covered with cartilage.

Ligaments of the Thoracic Spine

In the thoracic region, the *anterior longitudinal ligament* is thicker and narrower than the cervical and lumbar portions of the ligament. It consists of several layers of longitudinally orientated fibres. Superficial fibres extend over three or four vertebrae, intermediate fibres extend over two or three vertebrae, while the deep layers connect adjacent vertebrae. The ligament is relatively taut in extension and relaxed in flexion.

The *posterior longitudinal ligament* is broad and almost uniform in width in the upper thoracic spine, but in the lower thoracic and lumbar regions it has a denticulated appearance, being narrower over the vertebral bodies and wider over the discs. Fibres are attached to the vertebral bodies and intervertebral discs, and are arranged in superficial layers, which extend over three or four vertebrae and deeper layers where fibres connect adjacent vertebrae.

Articular capsules of the thoracic apophyseal joints attach to the margins of the articular processes of adjacent vertebrae. They are reinforced anteriorly by ligamenta flava and posteriorly by a posterior ligament.

The ligamenta flava connect adjacent laminae and are thicker in the thoracic spine than in any other region. Each ligament extends along the length of the lamina, forming the posterior boundary of the intervertebral foramen. It is composed mainly of elastic fibres with a 2:1 ratio of elastic to collagen fibres. This elastic property gives considerable static compression to the vertebral segment (Nachemson and Evans, 1968).

The ligamenta flava help to brake the movement of flexion and assist the paravertebral muscles in restoring the trunk to the upright posture. As the vertebral column moves from a flexed to an upright position, the elastic property of ligamenta flava prevents them from forming folds. If such folds were to occur, they could be trapped between adjacent laminae or press upon the dura mater. Fibrosis of these ligaments occurs with increasing age and, as the elasticity decreases, the ligaments have a tendency to buckle, thereby decreasing the neural space of the intervertebral foramen.

Adjacent spinous processes are connected by the *supraspinous* and *interspinous* ligaments. The interspinous ligaments blend posteriorly with the supraspinous ligaments and anteriorly with the articular capsules. *Intertransverse* ligaments connect adjacent transverse processes.

Joints of the Thoracic Spine

Thoracic apophyseal joints (Fig. 1.16)

A typical thoracic apophyseal joint is formed by the articulation of the inferior articular facets of one thoracic vertebra with the superior articular facets of the vertebra below. The superior articular facets are flat and face posteriorly, superiorly and slightly laterally, while the

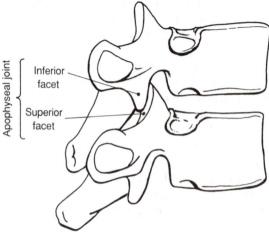

Apophyseal joint

Inferior facet

Superior facet

Fig. 1.16 A typical thoracic apophyseal articulation – lateral aspect.

inferior articular facets face predominantly anteriorly, slightly medially and downwards. In the horizontal plane, the combined plane of these facets forms the arc of a circle. The position of the centre of this arc varies according to the individual level. In the first and second thoracic vertebrae, the centre of the arc lies in front of the vertebral body, in the mid-thoracic spine it lies in the vertebral body, whilst in the lower thoracic spine it once again lies in front of the anterior border of the vertebral body. This difference is due to the change in medial orientation of the facets at various levels of the thoracic spine (Davis, 1959).

The planes of the apophyseal joints are orientated backward and upward. In the upper thoracic spine the angle between the planes of the joints and the horizontal is approximately 60°. In the mid-thoracic spine the angle becomes closer to the vertical, while the lower thoracic segments have characteristics of the lumbar spine and the joints lie more in the sagittal plane.

In the thoracic region, the vertebral bodies and intervertebral discs take most of the weight-bearing forces in the upright position. However, when the column is flexed and rotated, the apophyseal joints are stressed by compression forces and the upward-facing superior facets then contribute to weight-bearing. If a thoracic spine deformity develops, e.g. kyphoscoliosis, the superior facets will be subject to greater weight-bearing forces and, hence, they may be more likely to undergo degenerative changes.

The backward-facing superior facets contribute to the stability of the motion segment by preventing forward translation of the superior vertebra on the inferior vertebra. In the horizontal plane the facets are orientated to allow axial rotation to occur.

The joint surfaces are covered with hyaline cartilage and they contain the meniscoid structures (*see* p. 49).

THORACO-LUMBAR JUNCTION

The transition from the thoracic-type vertebra to the lumbar type does not always occur at T12/L1. It can occur anywhere between T10/11 and T12/L1. Most frequently it occurs between T11/12 where T11 has superior articular facets with thoracic characteristics (i.e. facing backwards, upwards and slightly outwards) and lower articular facets with lumbar characteristics (facing laterally and forwards). When this level is fully extended, the upper vertebra forms a bony block with the subjacent lumbar-type vertebra, preventing any lateral flexion or rotation; only flexion is then possible.

The practical significance of this is that, when the transitional level is in full extension, it is impossible to gain any other movement than flexion, and in treatment it is dangerous to attempt it.

Costovertebral and Costotransverse Joints (Fig. 1.17)

Each rib is connected to the thoracic vertebral column at two joints:

1. The costovertebral joint between the head of a rib, the bodies of two adjacent vertebrae and the intervening disc;
2. The costotransverse joint between the tubercle of the rib and the transverse process of the numerically corresponding vertebra.

R1, 10, 11 and 12 articulate with their own numerically corresponding vertebral body, but the 11th and 12th ribs do not articulate with their transverse process.

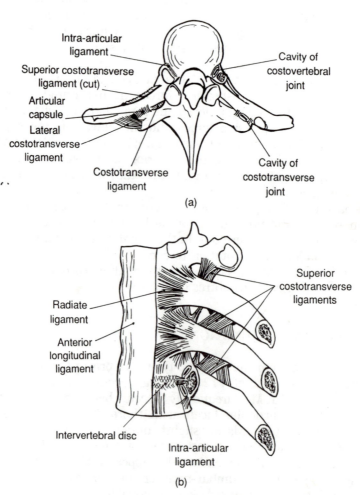

Fig. 1.17 Costovertebral and costotransverse joints. (a) superior aspect; (b) lateral aspect. (Adapted from P.L. Williams and R. Warwick, 1980. In *Gray's Anatomy*, 36th edn. Edinburgh: Churchill Livingstone, pp. 450, 451.)

Costovertebral joints

These joints are synovial, 'plane' joints. The two slightly convex facets on the head of a typical rib fit into the concavity formed by two costal facets on adjacent vertebrae and the intervertebral discs inbetween. The costal facets lie one on the inferior border of the vertebra above, and the other on the superior border of the subjacent vertebra to which the rib numerically corresponds. A single loose fibrous capsule surrounds the joint, the surfaces of which are covered with hyaline cartilage.

The joint cavity is divided into two by an *intra-articular* ligament which is attached laterally to the crest on the head of a typical rib and passes inside the joint to be attached medially to the intervertebral disc. The *radiate* ligament reinforces the joint anteriorly, and is attached laterally to the anterior part of the head of the rib. It has three sets of fibres: the superior fibres are attached to the body of the vertebra above; the inferior fibres to the body below; and the horizontal fibres to the intervertebral disc. As the 1st, 10th, 11th and 12th ribs articulate with their own vertebral body only, they have a single joint cavity, no intra-articular ligament and a poorly developed radiate ligament.

Costotransverse joints

These are also synovial joints and are formed by the articulation of the facet on the front of the transverse process with the oval facet on the posteromedial aspect of the tubercle of the rib. In the upper costotransverse joints, the facet on the rib is convex and that on the transverse process is reciprocally concave. In the lower costotransverse joints, the facets of the rib and transverse processes become flatter. This change in shape of the facets is one of the factors responsible for the different movements of the upper and lower ribs during respiration. The joint has a thin fibrous capsule lined with synovium.

The ligaments of the joint are strong, so that movements are markedly limited to small gliding motions.

The *superior costotransverse ligament* has two layers: (1) the anterior fibres are attached below to the crest of the neck of the rib and pass upwards and laterally to the lower border of the transverse process above; (2) the posterior fibres are attached below to the posterior surface of the neck of the rib and pass upwards and medially behind the anterior fibres to the transverse process above. The two bands are separated by the external intercostal membrane, and fibres of the anterior band blend laterally with the internal intercostal membrane.

The *costotransverse ligament* attaches the posterior part of the neck of the rib to the anterior surface of the transverse process.

The *lateral costotransverse ligament* attaches the tip of the transverse process to the roughened articular portion of the tubercle of the rib. This ligament strengthens the posterolateral aspect of the joint capsule.

Sternocostal Joints

These joints are formed by the articulation of the medial end of the costal cartilages of the 1st–7th ribs and the sternum. The joint between the 1st costal cartilage and the sternum is a primary cartilaginous joint (synchondrosis) where the cartilage unites with the upper lateral border of the manubrium sterni. Movement does not occur at this joint – this is a relevant factor during respiration (*see* p. 180). The 2nd–7th joints are synovial and surrounded by a fibrous capsule.

An *intra-articular ligament* divides the joint cavity into two although, with increasing age, these joint cavities (except that of the 2nd costal cartilage) become obliterated. Movement at the sternocostal joints is restricted by the intra-articular ligament.

Anterior and posterior radiate ligaments pass from the medial end of the costal cartilage to the anterior and posterior aspects of the sternum. Anteriorly, from the costal cartilage, the superior fibres pass upwards and medially, the middle fibres horizontally and the lower fibres medially and downwards. The fibres interlace with those from the joints above and below. Tendinous fibres of pectoralis major fuse with the anterior radiate ligaments. The posterior radiate ligaments have a similar arrangement on the posterior aspect of the sternum.

Interchondral Joints

These joints are formed by the tips of the costal cartilages of the 8th, 9th and 10th ribs with the lower border of the cartilage above. The 8th and 9th interchondral joints are synovial, while the 10th is more fibrous. Small synovial joints also occur between the adjacent margins of the 5th–9th costal cartilages. A fibrous capsule surrounds these joints and they are strengthened anteriorly and posteriorly by the oblique interchondral ligaments.

The costochondral and interchondral joints may give rise to symptoms of local pain, tenderness, localized swelling (Tietze, 1921), or they may simulate disease of the thoracic viscera or mimic the anterior reference of pain from vertebral joint problems. This condition may arise from torsion of the rib secondary to a segmental vertebral lesion of fixation (Patriquin, 1983).

PALPATION OF THE THORACIC SPINE (Fig. 1.18)

The following bony points can be palpated:

Spinous processes

The tips of the spinous processes are slightly bulbous and sometimes deviate from the midline. Palpation of the levels of the *laminae* will clarify whether or not the vertebra is rotated. The tip of the spinous process of T1 is usually prominent (as is C7). The spinous processes project downwards more in the mid-thoracic spine, a fact which merits consideration when performing treatment techniques on them. The position of their tips relative to that of the apophyseal joints,

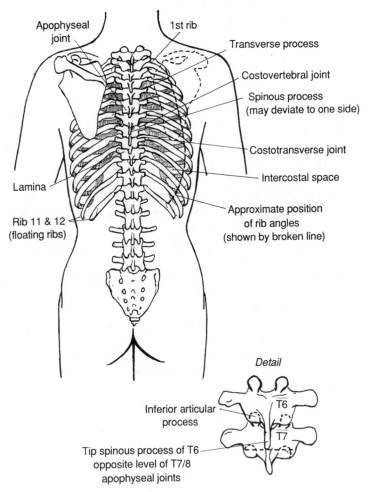

Fig. 1.18 Palpation points in the thoracic spine – posterior aspect.

therefore, varies from being more level in the upper and lower thoracic spine than in the mid-thoracic spine, where they may project downwards as far as the subjacent apophyseal joints.

TO CLARIFY: the tip of T6's spinous process lies approximately level with the T7/8 apophyseal joints.

Dorsal aspects of apophyseal joints (inferior articular processes)

These lie in the paravertebral sulci and can be felt in slim patients.

Transverse processes

The transverse processes (overlying the costotransverse joints) lie in a more posterior plane than the articular processes, approximately 3 cm from the midline, reducing to 2 cm in the lower thorax. Their tips lie more or less level with the tip of the spinous process of the vertebra above.

Ribs

Due to the obliquity of the direction of the ribs posteriorly, the *intercostal spaces* are narrower behind than in front. The *rib angles* are roughly level with their corresponding transverse process and with the tip of the spinous process of the vertebra above, and lie at a varying distance from the midline, the furthest away being that of R8. Caudally and cranially from this rib angle, they become progressively closer to the midline. They provide useful leverage for mobilizing the costotransverse and costovertebral joints. R12 is small and sometimes difficult to palpate. The flattened tendons of the erector spinae muscle arise and insert into the rib angles and local soft tissue lesions here are not uncommon.

With the person in prone-lying, R1 may be felt by lifting up the upper fibres of trapezius with the thumbs directed caudally; its upper surface faces superiorly and is often tender on palpation. Anteriorly, R1 is covered mainly by the clavicle, its costal cartilage lying just under the sternal end. The narrow posterior border of R1 may also be palpated with the person in prone-lying. The sternocostal and interchondral joints can normally be palpated depending on the individual's build.

Osteoporosis affecting the ribs in the elderly is common and warrants particular care.

LUMBAR SPINE

The lumbar vertebral column comprises five vertebrae and the intervening intervertebral discs. When an upright normal lumbar spine is viewed from the side, it can be seen that the lumbar column has a curve that is concave posteriorly. This curve is known as the lumbar lordosis. (Fig. 1.19).

In the standing position, the sacrum is tilted forwards so that its upper surface is inclined forwards and downwards forming an angle between the top of the sacrum and the horizontal, which varies between 50–53° (Hellems and Keates, 1971). If the lumbar spine articulated in a straight line with the sacrum, the trunk would be inclined forwards. In order to compensate for the inclination of the sacrum and to allow the upright standing position to be achieved, the lumbar spine curves posteriorly.

Several factors contribute to the normal shape of the lumbar lordosis:

1. The L5 vertebral body is wedge-shaped: the anterior body wall is 3 mm higher than the posterior body wall (Gilad and Nissan, 1985). This brings the upper surface of the L5 body closer to the horizontal plane than the upper surface of the sacrum.
2. In addition, the L5/S1 disc is also wedge-shaped and its anterior vertical height is 6–7 mm greater than its posterior height. As a result of the wedge-shape of the disc, the lower surface of the L5 vertebral body is not parallel to the upper surface of the sacrum, so that the angle formed between the two surfaces may vary between 6–29° and has an average size of 16° (Schmorl and Junghanns, 1971).
3. Each vertebra above L5 is inclined slightly backwards in relation to the vertebra below.
4. In 75% of adults the centre of gravity lies anterior to the vertebral column. In these individuals there is constant slight activity in the erector spinae muscles, which work to prevent the

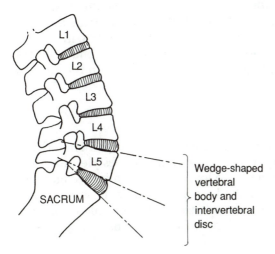

Wedge-shaped vertebral body and intervertebral disc

Fig. 1.19 The lumbar lordosis – lateral aspect.

trunk from falling forwards and hence assist in maintaining the lumbar lordosis.

In a normal spine in the upright posture, the body of L5 lies directly vertically above the sacrum (Bogduk and Twomey, 1987). Various attempts have been made to measure the lumbar lordosis, but as investigators have used different parameters the results differ substantially (Torgerson and Dotter, 1976; Ferdinand and Fox, 1985; Hansson *et al.*, 1985a). In the standing position, measurement from radiographs of the angle between the top of L1 and the sacrum have been recorded as 67° (±3° standard deviation) in children and 74° (±7° standard deviation) in young males (Hansson *et al.*, 1985a).

Development of the lumbar lordosis begins as an infant starts to stand, usually between 12–18 months of age, and it continues to develop until the completion of spinal growth, normally between 13–18 years. In old age, the lumbar column usually becomes flattened.

Factors Affecting the Lumbar Lordosis

The degree of curvature of the lumbar lordosis varies considerably between individuals, and in each individual it alters in different postures and positions. The following influence lumbar lordosis:

Sex

It has been shown that the L5/S1 angle of the lordosis is greater in women during childbearing years than in men (Twomey and Taylor, 1987), and it has been speculated that this difference may be, in part, due to hormones – and to one in particular, known as relaxin. Relaxin is secreted by the ovary and has been shown to relax the spinal ligaments, symphysis pubis and the sacroiliac joints. During pregnancy, large amounts of this hormone are present in the blood, but it is also found in small amounts in the blood of non-pregnant women (Hytten and Leitch, 1971) and the level of relaxin present between adolescence and middle-age may be responsible for a relaxing of the spinal ligaments and an increase in lumbar lordosis in women. Before adolescence and after middle-age, there is no difference in the lordosis of the two sexes.

Age

In most individuals the lumbar spine flattens with age (Schmorl and Junghanns, 1971) due in part, at least, to a flexed lifestyle. However, some individuals have an increase in lordosis which may become very pronounced in some instances. An increased lordosis is often accompanied by an increase in weight and size of the abdomen, together with a decrease in the strength of the abdominal muscles.

Prolonged static standing position

If the lumbar spine is in an upright static position for a long period, the trunk muscles begin to fatigue and intervertebral disc height is reduced due to 'creep' (*see* p. 76), so that the natural tendency of the lumbar spine towards extension becomes exaggerated.

Pathology

Studies investigating the relationship between lumbar lordosis and the presence or absence of back-pain symptoms have failed to find any correlation between the two (Torgerson and Dotter, 1976; Hansson *et al.*, 1985b;). However, the causes of back pain are often multifactorial and the shape of the lumbar curve is but one factor. In clinical practice, it will be noted that in some individuals the presence of a mechanical joint lesion, muscle spasm or pain may affect the normal lumbar curvature.

Compression

Compression or vertical loading of the spine tends to increase the lordosis. If a weight is held in front of the spine, activity of the erector spinae rises to prevent the trunk falling forwards, and there is a subsequent increase in the lordosis.

Footwear

When high-heeled shoes are worn, the body's centre of gravity is displaced forward, and it is associated with an increase in pelvic tilt and thereby an increase in lordosis.

Lordosis and Stability

As the sacrum tilts forwards, there is a tendency in the erect posture for L5 to slip forward on the sacrum, and to a lesser extent for L4 to slide forward on L5. This tendency to forward displacement is resisted by:

1. *Orientation of the apophyseal joints.* The superior facets of the sacrum face backwards and form a bony locking mechanism with the inferior facets on L5 which face forward (*see* pp. 51, 54). The orientation of the L4/5 apophyseal joints also prevents forward displacement, but above L4 the vertebral bodies are inclined slightly back and there is no tendency, at rest, for the upper lumbar vertebrae to slide forwards.
2. *Ligamentous support:*
   a. The *ligaments connecting the bony arches of the vertebrae* prevent forward displacement. Under normal circumstances, in the

upright position, the posterolateral annulus fibrosus is not under strain and does not prevent forward displacement of the vertebral body. If there is a breakdown of the bony mechanism or if the joints are affected by disease or injury as, for example, in spondylolisthesis (*see* p. 277), the annular fibres may then be placed under strain.

b. The strong *ilio-lumbar ligaments* attach the thick transverse processes of L5 to the ilium. They help to prevent L5 from sliding forwards.

c. The *anterior longitudinal ligament* and *anterior annulus fibrosus*. When compression forces are applied to the lumbar spine, the lordosis tends to increase so that the posterior ends of the intervertebral discs are compressed, while the anterior ends of the vertebral bodies tend to separate. In so doing, the anterior longitudinal ligaments and anterior annulus fibrosus are placed under tension to resist the tendency of the vertebral bodies to separate. Eventually, a state of equilibrium is achieved so that the force tending to separate the vertebral bodies is balanced exactly by the anterior ligaments. Any further increase in force is resisted by tension in these ligaments (Bogduk and Twomey, 1987).

The curve of the lumbar spine gives it a certain resilience and helps to protect the spine from compressive forces. If the spine were straight, compressive forces would be transferred through the vertebral bodies to the intervertebral discs alone. In the curved lumbar spine, some of the compressive force is taken by the anterior longitudinal ligaments.

Pelvic tilt

As the lumbar spine articulates directly with the sacrum, any alteration in the angle of the pelvis inevitably affects the lordosis. If the pelvis is tilted forwards, the lumbar lordosis increases; when the pelvis is tilted backwards, the lordosis becomes flattened. Pelvic tilt is to a great extent determined by muscle action. The erectores spinae act to increase the lordosis, while the abdominal muscles, glutei and hamstrings flatten the lordosis through their action on the pelvis. Psoas muscle also acts to increase the lordosis when the legs are extended. In some individuals, an accentuated lordosis is associated with tightness of the psoas major and hamstrings. Shortened hamstrings would tend to tilt the pelvis backwards, thereby flattening the lumbar spine and are, therefore, unlikely to be the cause of an increased lordosis.

Lateral pelvic tilt and leg length inequality

A scoliosis in the lumbar spine may be (1) an idiopathic structural scoliosis, or (2) a functional or postural scoliosis.

A structural scoliosis is most common in teenage girls and develops during the growth period. A postural scoliosis often occurs as a result of another factor such as leg-length inequality, muscle spasm, degenerative changes of the intervertebral discs and apophyseal joints and osteoarthritic changes of the hip and knee. The commonest cause of a postural scoliosis is leg-length inequality. In some individuals with a short leg, there is a dipping down of the pelvis on the short side, and necessarily a compensatory lumbar curve convex to the short side will be present, with a corresponding thoracic convexity to the long-leg side. However, in some individuals the convexities and concavities may be reversed (Grieve, 1989).

Minor structural changes are associated with the postural scoliosis of leg-length inequality. On the convex side, early attenuation of the lateral annulus fibrosis may occur, while the joints of that side have thicker subchondral bone plates and thinner articular cartilage than the concave side, suggesting that greater loading occurs on the convex side of the curve (Giles and Taylor, 1984). It is thought that this may be related to the greater effect of the forces of the postural muscles on the convex side, which act to prevent the scoliotic column giving way under axial loading.

Although some investigators have demonstrated a correlation between leg-length inequality and low back pain (Giles and Taylor, 1981), other investigators have not found any conclusive evidence of a relationship between back pain and unequal leg length (Farfan, 1973; Troup, 1975).

Structure of a Typical Lumbar Vertebra (L1–4) (Fig. 1.20)

The five lumbar vertebrae are the largest moveable vertebrae, their large bodies taking more weight and their vertebral arches being more developed than in other regions to sustain greater stresses.

Vertebral body

This is large and kidney-shaped. It is wider transversely than anteroposteriorly, and is slightly deeper in front than behind. Its outer surface is somewhat concave from above downwards, except posteriorly, where it is flatter.

Posterior arch

With the body, the posterior arch encloses the *vertebral foramen* which is normally triangular in this region. It is larger than in the

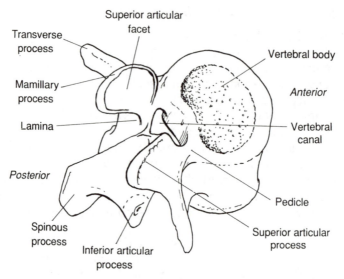

Fig. 1.20 A typical lumbar vertebra.

thoracic region, but smaller than in the cervical. Collectively, the vertebral foramina constitute the vertebral canal in which lies the spinal cord/cauda equina.

Stenosis (narrowing) of the foramen, which is more pronounced in men, can be a congenital abnormality or acquired through degenerative changes such as bony or ligamentous hypertrophy or disc bulging/herniation. This can result in signs and symptoms arising from cauda equina compression, which may not otherwise have manifested in a normal, more spacious foramen.

The posterior arch is formed by the pedicles, laminae and articular processes.

The *pedicles* are short, stout processes projecting backwards from the posterolateral aspect of the vertebral body just below its upper border. The superior border of each pedicle forms the shallow *superior vertebral notch*; the inferior border forms the more pronounced *inferior vertebral notch*. These notches form the inferior and superior boundaries of the *intervertebral foramen*.

The two *laminae* are broad, strong plates of bone which run posteromedially. They meet in the midline to form the *spinous process* which projects posteriorly and is broad and quadrangular. Its tip is bulbous and is sometimes slightly indented. At the junction of the laminae with the pedicles lie two *superior articular processes* and these house the concave *superior articular facets* which face medially and slightly posteriorly. The posterior border of each process is reinforced by a bony elevation called the *mamillary process*. The two *inferior articular processes* arise from the junction of the laminae with the spinous process. They house the convex *inferior articular facets* which face laterally and slightly anteriorly.

The two *transverse processes* are long and thin, and project laterally and slightly posteriorly from the junctions of the superior articular processes with the laminae.

Particular Features of the 5th Lumbar Vertebra (Fig. 1.21)

This usually has the largest body, which is more wedge-shaped (deeper in front than behind). With the correspondingly wedge-shaped L5/S1 disc, this accounts for the prominence of the lumbosacral angle (*see* p. 37). The articular processes are wider apart than in other vertebrae, while the transverse processes of L5 are strong and large. The latter arise from the whole of the lateral aspect of the pedicles and part of the vertebral body itself and give rise to the strong iliolumbar ligaments which assist in stabilizing the lumbar spine to the pelvis. The spinous process, however, is usually the smallest of the five, with a blunted tip.

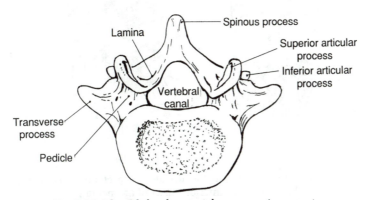

Fig. 1.21 The 5th lumbar vertebra – superior aspect.

Ligaments of the Lumbar Spine (Fig. 1.22)

On the whole, these ligaments are stronger and denser than higher in the spine.

Anterior longitudinal ligament

The anterior longitudinal ligament is a strong band lying anterior to the vertebral bodies and discs. It is firmly attached to the discs and the margins of the bodies and sacrum, and is thicker and narrower opposite the bodies, where it is loosely attached and fills in the concavities. Its longitudinal fibres have several layers – the deeper, shorter fibres joining adjacent vertebrae and the more superficial

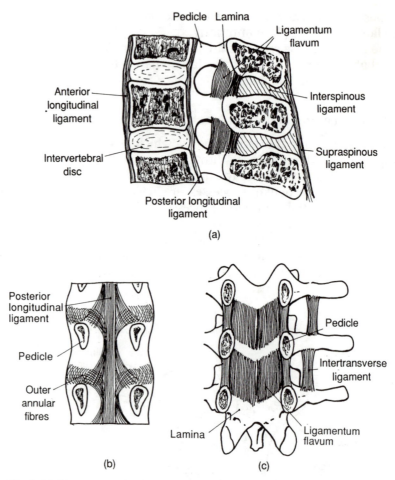

Fig. 1.22 Ligaments in lumbar region. (a) lateral aspect; (b) posterior longitudinal ligament; (c) anterior aspect of ligamenta flava.

layers extending over 2–4 vertebrae. The main function of this ligament is to prevent anterior separation of the vertebral bodies during extension. It also helps to stabilize the lumbar lordosis (*see* p. 40). Forward and backward sliding of the vertebral body is resisted principally by the annulus fibrosus, although the anterior longitudinal ligament also restricts this movement.

Posterior longitudinal ligament

Lying posterior to the vertebral bodies and discs in the vertebral canal, the posterior longitudinal ligament generally narrows towards its insertion into the sacrum. It has a denticulated appearance, being broader over the discs, to which it is attached, and narrower over the bodies. It is attached to the margins of the bodies, but is separated from the middle of them by basivertebral veins. Separation of the posterior ends of the vertebral bodies is resisted by this ligament. Due to the polysegmental arrangement of the ligament, its action is exerted over several interbody joints.

Articular capsules

Articular capsules of the apophyseal joints are attached to the margins of the articular facets; they are thin and loose, allowing freedom of movement in the sagittal plane (see pp. 182–5).

Ligamenta flava

Adjacent laminae are connected by ligamenta flava, which are short, thick ligaments fusing in the midline with the contralateral ligament. Superiorly, the ligament is attached to the lower half of the anterior surface of the lamina and the inferior aspect of the pedicle. The ligament divides into medial and lateral portions (Ramsey, 1966). The medial portion attaches to the upper, dorsal surface of the subjacent lamina, while the lateral portion passes in front of the apophyseal joint formed by the two vertebrae that the ligament connects. Fibres attach to the anterior aspects of the superior and inferior articular processes and replace the joint capsule anteriorly.

These ligaments normally have a high proportion of elastic fibres, allowing separation of the laminae in flexion. They protect the discs by graduating this movement so that an abrupt limit is not reached. Another important function is to assist, by their elasticity, the return movement from flexion to the neutral position. Especially in the young, the ligaments exert a certain pressure on the discs, which gives them more resistance to stresses.

The elasticity of these ligaments allows them to return to their normal length after they have been stretched during flexion. If these ligaments consisted principally of collagen fibres, they would tend to buckle once the laminae were approximated, although they would resist separation of the laminae during flexion. Buckling of a ligamentum flavum could compromise either the spinal cord or spinal nerve roots in the vertebral canal. Necrotic ligamenta flava in degenerative spines can, however, buckle into the vertebral canal and cause compression of neural tissue.

Interspinous ligaments

The interspinous ligaments connect adjacent spinous processes from their roots to their apices. They are continuous with the ligamenta flava anteriorly and the supraspinous ligament posteriorly.

Supraspinous ligament

A fibrous cord joining the tips of the spinous processes, the supraspinous ligament ends between L4 and 5. Below the L5 spinous process, fibres from the thoracolumbar fascia intersect.

Both the interspinous and supraspinous ligaments resist separation of the spinous processes during flexion of the vertebral column, but they do not come into play until about half full flexion. They are, therefore, slack at small angles of flexion and are only under tension for a few degrees but, as they are relatively weak, they are the first to be sprained immediately after the limit of flexion is reached (Adams *et al.*, 1980). Rissanen (1960) reported that more than 20% of adult lumbar spines had visibly ruptured interspinous ligaments and that torn attachments to the spinous processes were 'very common' after 30 years of age.

Intertransverse ligaments

Intertransverse ligaments connect adjacent transverse processes and are unlike other ligaments in the lumbar spine in that their collagen fibres are not as densely packed or as regularly orientated. These ligaments have been described as connective tissue sheets (Vallois, 1926) which separate the anterior lumbar muscles from the posterior lumbar musculature.

Laterally, the ligaments divide into two layers: the anterior layer becomes the thoracolumbar fascia, while the posterior layer blends with the aponeurosis of transversus abdominis to form the middle layer of the thoracolumbar fascia (*see* pp. 118–9). Medially, the ligament divides into ventral and dorsal portions (Lewin *et al.*, 1962). The dorsal leaf attaches to the lateral margin of the lamina of the vertebra that lies opposite the intertransverse space. Inferiorly, it blends with the capsule of the subjacent apophyseal joint. The ventral leaf passes anteriorly round the vertebral body to blend with the lateral margins of the anterior longitudinal ligament. This part of the ligament forms a connective tissue sheet that closes the outer end of the intervertebral foramen. It is pierced by nerve branches to psoas and also the ventral ramus of the spinal nerve and accompanying arteries and veins.

Between the ventral and dorsal leaves is a fat-filled space called the *superior articular recess*. The fat in this recess is continuous with the intra-articular fat of the joint below. This recess accommodates movements of the subjacent apophyseal joint and the fat acts as a displaceable space filler (*see* p. 49).

Transforaminal ligaments

Bands of fibres that cross the outer end of the intervertebral foramen have been identified and are known as transforaminal ligaments

(Golub and Silverman, 1969). They are not always present and more closely resemble bands of fascia. It is possible that, when present, they may decrease the space available for the emerging spinal nerve. Five different bands have been described:

1. *Superior corporotransverse ligament*. This connects the inferior, posterolateral aspect of a vertebral body with the transverse process of the same vertebra.
2. *Inferior corporotransverse ligament*. This connects the inferior, posterolateral aspect of a vertebral body with the transverse process of the subjacent vertebra.
3. *Superior transforaminal ligaments*. These cross the inferior vertebral notch.
4. *Inferior transforaminal ligaments*. These cross the superior vertebral notch.
5. *Mid-transforaminal ligament*. This connects the posterolateral annulus fibrosus to the joint capsule and ligamentum flavum behind.

The commonest band is the superior corporotransverse ligament which is found in 27% of individuals (Golub and Silverman, 1969). These ligaments may be thickenings of the ventral leaf of the intertransverse ligaments (Bogduk and Twomey, 1987).

Mamillo-accessory ligament

This attaches to the tips of the ipsilateral mamillary and accessory processes. In 10% of individuals it may be ossified, forming a small foramen at the mamillo-accessory notch. The ligament covers the medial branch of the dorsal ramus of the spinal nerve.

Iliolumbar ligaments

The iliolumbar ligaments connect the transverse processes of L5 to the ilium. They occur bilaterally and are only present in adults. In early life the ligament is represented by a muscle which only becomes ligamentous in the third decade (Leong *et al.*, 1985). Five parts of the iliolumbar ligament have been identified (Shellshear and Macintosh, 1949):

1. Fibres of the *anterior iliolumbar ligament* arise from the entire anteroinferior border and tip of the L5 transverse process. Passing posterolaterally, in line with the long axis of the transverse process, the fibres attach to the ilium. A thick bundle of fibres beyond the tip of the transverse process provides attachment for the lower end of the quadratus lumborum muscle.
2. Thickenings of the anterior and posterior fascia surrounding quadratus lumborum give rise to the *superior iliolumbar ligament*.

These thickenings arise from the anterior, superior border of the L5 transverse process near its tip, pass in front and behind quadratus lumborum and attach to the ilium.

3. Fibres from the tip and posterior border of the transverse process of L5 attach to the ilium behind the insertion of quadratus lumborum, forming the *posterior iliolumbar ligament.*
4. The *inferior iliolumbar ligament* arises from the lower border of the transverse process of L5 and the L5 vertebral body. The fibres pass downwards and laterally, attaching to the superior and posterior parts of the iliac fossa.
5. Fibres from the anteroinferior border of the L5 transverse process descend vertically to attach to the iliopectineal line. This is the *vertical iliolumbar ligament*, forming the lateral margin of the channel for the L5 ventral ramus in its course to the pelvis.

The powerful, complex structure of the iliolumbar ligaments provides stability at the lumbo-sacral junction, preventing the fifth lumbar vertebra from being displaced forwards.

Structure of a Typical Lumbar Apophyseal Joint (Fig. 1.23)

The lumbar apophyseal joints are true synovial joints. They are non-axial and diarthrodial, allowing small gliding movements to occur.

Joint capsule

The joint capsule surrounds the dorsal, superior and inferior margins of each apophyseal joint, attaching just beyond the margins of the cartilage. The collagen fibres pass transversely from one articular process to the other. The fibrous capsule is replaced completely anteriorly by the ligamentum flavum (Lewin *et al.*, 1962). Posteriorly,

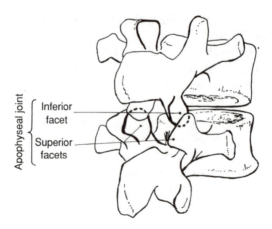

Apophyseal joint { Inferior facet / Superior facets

Fig. 1.23 A typical lumbar apophyseal joint – posterolateral aspect.

although the capsule is thick, it is reinforced by the deep fibres of multifidus.

At the superior and inferior ends of the joint, the capsule is loose and forms subcapsular pockets which contain fat. There are two tiny holes in the superior and inferior parts of the capsule, through which fat can communicate with the fat in the extracapsular space. Fat within the joint is covered externally by the capsule and, internally, it is lined with synovium.

Intra-articular structures

Three types of intra-articular structures have been identified; they are known as meniscoid structures (Engel and Bogduk, 1982).

1. *Fibroadipose meniscoids* are the largest meniscoid structures. They are leaf-like folds of synovium which project from the inner surfaces of the superior and inferior capsules. These folds enclose fat, collagen and blood vessels and may project 5 mm into the joint cavity. The fat is situated at the base of the meniscoid and it is continuous with the rest of the fat within the joint, which communicates with the extra capsular fat through the superior and inferior capsular foramina.

   It is suggested that failure of a fibroadipose meniscoid to re-enter an apophyseal joint cavity can be one of the causes of the acute locked back. The tip of the meniscoid instead enters the subcapsular recess into which it is driven further as the patient attempts to straighten from the flexed position. The patient will, therefore, tend to adopt the flexed position as this reduces the strain on the joint (Bogduk and Jull, 1985).

2. *Adipose tissue pads* are found at the superior and inferior ends of the joint; they enclose fat and blood vessels and may project into the joint capsule for about 2 mm. The fibroadipose meniscoids and the adipose tissue pads have a protective function. In flexion, the inferior articular facets slide upwards along the superior facet and, in doing so, the upper portion of the inferior facet and the lower portion of the superior facet are exposed. The fibroadipose meniscoids are well situated to protect the exposed surfaces of the articular facets (Bogduk *et al.*, 1984).

3. The *connective tissue rim* is the smallest identified structure. It is a wedge-shaped thickening of the internal surface of the capsule, filling the space left by the curved margins of the articular cartilages. This structure can increase the surface area of contact when the articular facets are impacted, thereby transmitting some loads (Lewin *et al.*, 1962).

Articular facets

Each lumbar apophyseal joint is formed by the articulation of the inferior facets of one lumbar vertebra with the superior facets of the subjacent vertebra.

The shape and orientation of the lumbar facets varies, thereby affecting the direction and range of movement of a motion segment. The orientation of these joints is an important factor in preventing forward displacement and rotatory dislocation of the intervertebral joint.

If the facets of the joints are viewed from behind, the joint surfaces appear to be straight surfaces. However, when viewed from above in the transverse plane, the facets may be seen to be curved or flat (Fig. 1.24). The curved superior articular facets have been described as depicting a 'J' shape or a 'C' shape. Horwitz and Smith (1940) found that curved joints predominated between the 1st and 2nd, 2nd and 3rd, and 3rd and 4th lumbar vertebrae, but flat joints were more common between the 4th and 5th vertebrae and at the lumbo-sacral junction.

Orientation of a lumbar apophyseal joint is defined by the angle between the average plane of the joint with respect to the sagittal plane. In joints with flat articular facets, the plane of the joint is

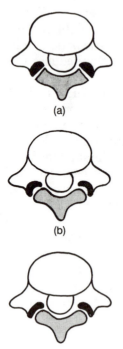

(a)

(b)

(c)

Fig. 1.24 Variations in curvature of lumbar apophyseal joints. (a) flat joints; (b) 'C' shaped joints; (c) 'J' shaped joints. (Adapted from T. Horwitz and R.M. Smith, 1940. An anatomical, pathological and roentgenological study of the intervertebral joints of the lumbar spine and of the sacroiliac joints. *Am. J. Roentgenol. Rad. Ther.*, **43**, 173–186.)

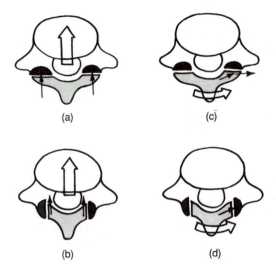

Fig. 1.25 Variations in orientation of lumbar apophyseal joints. (a) joints orientated in the frontal plane strongly resist forward displacement; (b) joints orientated in the sagittal plane are less able to resist forward displacement; (c) joints orientated in the frontal plane are less able to resist rotation; (d) joints orientated in the sagittal plane strongly resist rotation. (Adapted from N. Bogduk and L.T. Twomey, 1987. In *Clinical Anatomy of the Lumbar Spine.* Edinburgh: Churchill Livingstone, p. 27.)

parallel to the line of the facets. In curved joints, the average plane is taken as a line through the anteromedial and posterolateral ends of the joint surfaces.

The angle between the plane of the facet joints and the sagittal plane varies between individuals and in any individual it varies at different spinal levels. The larger the angle, the more the joints tend to face in the frontal plane. This is more common at the lower two lumbar levels (Fig. 1.25).

In flat (planar) apophyseal joints, where the superior articular facets face backwards and medially, the facets resist forward displacement. If the upper vertebra moves forward, its inferior facets impinge upon the superior articular facets of the vertebra below. The more the joint is orientated in the frontal plane, the more it resists forward displacement; however, these joints are less able to resist axial rotation.

The more the joint is orientated in the sagittal plane, the more it can resist rotation; however, these joints are less able to resist forward displacement.

In joints with curved articular facets, different parts of the articular surfaces resist different movements. In curved joints, the anteromedial end of the superior facet which faces backwards resists forward displacement. 'C'-shaped joints have a greater surface area and offer greater resistance to forward displacement than 'J'-shaped joints. Both 'C' and 'J'-shaped joints resist rotation well.

Load-bearing

In early studies, opinion was divided as to whether the lumbar apophyseal joints were weight-bearing. It has been reported that the apophyseal joints bear 28% (Lorenz et al., 1983) or 40% (Hakim and King, 1976) of a vertically-applied load. Other investigators report that the lumbar apophyseal joints have a very minor role in weight-bearing (Miller et al., 1983). Bogduk and Twomey (1987) state that these differences are due to variations in experimental design and differing appreciation of the anatomy of the apophyseal joints and their behaviour in axial compression. In the normal erect posture, if the articular surfaces are viewed in the sagittal and coronal planes, it is evident that the facets lie parallel to each other. During axial compression, it is suggested that the facets slide relative to each other and, as they do not impact, they are not involved in weight-bearing (Bogduk and Twomey, 1987).

If the normal alignment of the facet joints is altered, the apophyseal joints may then become involved in the weight-bearing process. This situation may occur if a vertebral body rocks backwards on the subjacent intervertebral disc without also sliding backwards, so that the tips of the inferior articular processes impact onto the superior articular facets of the vertebra below. During vertical compression, some of the load will be transferred through the area of impact – usually the inferior medial portion of the facets. Dunlop et al. (1984) demonstrated that the inferomedial portion of the facets was the site where maximal pressure is sustained when the vertebrae are loaded in extension.

When the intervertebral discs become narrowed, as may occur with severe sustained axial compression or degenerative changes, the inferior articular facets of a vertebra may impact on the lamina of the vertebra below. Impaction of the inferior facets on the laminae can also happen if the vertebrae are axially compressed when the spine is in the extended position. Hence, in those people with an increased lordosis, the apophyseal joints may be subjected to loading during axial compression. Experimentation has shown that in the lordotic spine during prolonged standing, the impacted joints at each segmental level bear an average 16% of the axial load (Adams and Hutton, 1983), but that the lower joints (L3/4, L4/5, L5/S1) take approximately 19% of the load, while the L1/2 and L2/3 joints bear around 11% of the load (Adams and Hutton, 1980).

Adams and Hutton (1983) also estimated that pathological disc space narrowing may result in up to 70% of the axial load being transmitted through the articular processes and laminae.

Joints involved in weight-bearing are more prone to degenerative changes and, therefore, if weight-bearing occurs through the apophyseal joints, there is a greater risk of a pathological condition developing.

Tropism (Fig. 1.26)

Articular tropism is asymmetrical orientation of the apophyseal

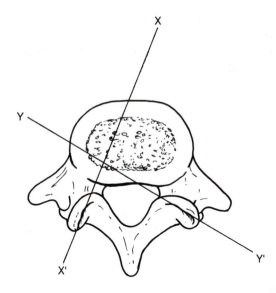

Fig. 1.26 Tropism of the 5th lumbar vertebra – superior aspect. X–X′ = plane of sagittally orientated facet; Y–Y′ = plane of coronally orientated facet.

joints so that at one vertebral level the plane of one apophyseal joint is more inclined in the frontal or sagittal plane than the plane of the contralateral apophyseal joint. It is most common at the lowest two lumbar levels (Cyron and Hutton, 1980), and it is reported to occur in up to one-quarter of human spines (Grieve, 1989). Tropism causes imbalanced movement between the facets (Kraft and Levinthal, 1951) and probably leads to altered spinal mechanics of the segment (Lippitt, 1984). Premature degenerative changes often occur at vertebral levels where tropism is present (Cyron and Hutton, 1980).

Tropism has been linked with a rotation instability which puts the ligaments of the apophyseal joint under strain (Cyron and Hutton, 1980). This may also lead to a rotation strain of the disc as more stress is placed on the intervertebral disc on the side of the more obliquely orientated apophyseal joint.

When flexion occurs in the presence of tropism it will usually do so about some oblique axis x-x′ (*see* Fig. 1.26), so that the capsular ligaments will be equidistant from the axis of rotation. Flexion about x-x′ causes maximum stretching of the posterior lateral annulus; hence, posterolateral tears will usually be at the side of the more oblique facet. In studies done by Farfan and Sullivan (1967), there was a high correlation between the side of the more oblique facet and the side of sciatica.

L5/S1 apophyseal joint

It is not surprising that this level is particularly subject to the most degenerative changes in the lumbar region: at this junction, the long mass of five fused vertebrae forming the sacrum articulate with the fifth lumbar vertebra.

In the standing position, the lordotic curve of the lumbar spine places particular stress on the L5/S1 junction. With the wedge-shaped disc and body of L5, the tendency would be for L5 to slide forward on the sacrum. The inferior articular processes of L5, instead of facing laterally and slightly anteriorly as in the typical lumbar vertebrae, may tend to face more anteriorly, thereby forming a more effective 'hook' to prevent a forward slip.

Nerve supply

Each joint receives a multiple innervation from a dorsal ramus of a spinal nerve and two medial branches of a dorsal ramus. The capsules are richly innervated with encapsulated, unencapsulated and free nerve endings, and can, therefore, transmit proprioceptive and nociceptive information.

PALPATION OF THE LUMBAR SPINE (Fig. 1.27)

In 60% of subjects, the iliac crests are level with the L4/5 interspace. In 20%, they are level with the vertebral body of L4 and in the remaining 20% they are level with the body of L5. Using the level of the iliac crests to identify a spinous process is not, therefore, always accurate.

The following bony points may be palpable:

1. *Spinous processes.* With the patient lying prone, the spinous processes may be palpated. The small, blunted tip of the L5 spinous process lies in the lumbosacral depression and the therapist's thumbs usually need to be angled slightly caudally in order to palpate its 'posteroanterior' movement. In some people the spinous process of L5 may be difficult to find and, in order to confirm palpation findings, the therapist may need to have the patient in side-lying to palpate the interspinous space between L5 and the sacrum by flexing the lumbar spine to feel if gapping occurs.

   The remaining spinous processes are larger and may be indented, so care needs to be taken to clarify whether the therapist is actually on one of these indentations rather than an interspinous space. Palpating the lateral aspect of the spinous process may help, or gapping the joints as described above.

2. *The interspinous spaces.* In a healthy spine, the interspinous spaces are easily palpable. In patients who have chronic degenerative changes in the lumbar spine, or who have performed excessive exercise over a period of time, the spinous processes may almost appear to be joined together due to chronic ligamentous thickening and the interspinous spaces are less obvious.

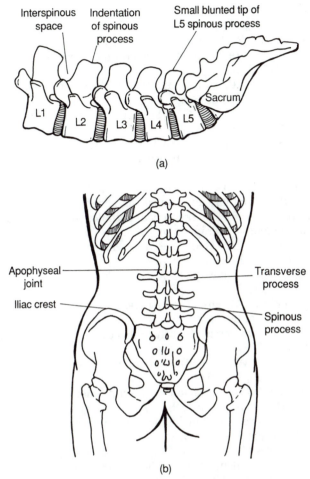

Fig. 1.27 Palpation points in the lumbar spine. (a) lateral
aspect; (b) posterior aspect.

3. *Apophyseal joints*. Except in slim patients, the apophyseal joints
   may be difficult to palpate in this region. However, if one of these
   joints has marked degenerative changes with swelling, it can be
   more easily located. They lie just lateral to the lower third of the
   spinous process, i.e. the L3/4 apophyseal joint lies level with the
   lower third of L3's spinous process. At the L5/S1 level, the joints
   lie slightly more laterally and caudally than above.
4. *Transverse processes*. Approximately 4–5 cm lateral to the spinous
   processes, the tips of the transverse processes lie level with the
   interspinous space, i.e. the tip of L3's transverse process lies level
   with the L2/3 interspinous space. The length of the transverse
   processes increases from L1 to 3, then decreases again.

REFERENCES

Adams M.A., Hutton W.C. (1980). The effect of posture on the role of the apophyseal joints in resisting intervertebral compression force. *J. Bone. Jt. Surg. (Br.)*, **62-B**, 358.

Adams M.A., Hutton W.C., Stott J.R.R. (1980). The resistance to flexion of the lumbar intervertebral joint. *Spine*, **5**, 3, 245.

Adams M.A., Hutton W.C. (1983). The mechanical function of the lumbar apophyseal joints. *Spine*, **8**, 327.

Andriacchi T., Schultz A., Belytschko T. *et al.* (1974). A model for studies of the mechanical interactions between the human spine and rib cage. *J. Biomech.*, **7**, 497.

Bogduk N., Engel R. (1984). The menisci of the lumbar zygapophyseal joints. A review of their anatomy and clinical significance. *Spine*, **9**, 454.

Bogduk N., Jull G. (1985). The theoretical pathology of acute locked back: a basis for manipulative therapy. *Man. Med.*, **1**, 78.

Bogduk N., Twomey L.T. (1987). *Clinical Anatomy of the Lumbar Spine.* Edinburgh: Churchill Livingstone, p. 43.

Boreadis A.G., Gershon-Cohen J. (1956). Luschka joints of the cervical spine. *Radiology*, 66, 181.

Brain, Lord, Wilkinson M., eds. (1967). *Cervical Spondylosis.* London: William Heinemann Medical Books.

Brown C. (1983). Compressive invasive referred pain to the shoulder. *Clin. Orthop.*, **173**, 55.

Cyron B.M., Hutton W.C. (1980). Articular tropism and stability of the lumbar spine. *Spine*, **5**, 2, 168.

Daskalakis M.K. (1983). Thoracic outlet syndrome: current concepts and surgical experience. *Int. Surg.*, **68**, 337.

Davis P.R. (1959). The medial inclination of the human thoracic intervertebral articular facets. *J. Anat*, **93**, 68.

Dunlop R.B., Adams M.A., Hutton W.C. (1984). Disc space narrowing and the lumbar facets. *J. Bone. Jt. Surg. (Br.)*, **66-B**, 706.

Dvorak J., Panjabi M.M. (1987). Functional anatomy of the alar ligaments. *Spine*, **12**, 2, 183.

Engel R., Bogduk N. (1982). The menisci of the lumbar zygapophyseal joints. *J. Anat*, **135**, 795.

Farfan H.F. (1973). *Mechanical Disorders of the Low Back.* Philadelphia: Lea and Febiger, pp. 51, 62.

Farfan H.F., Sullivan J.D. (1967). The relation of facet orientation to intervertebral disc failure. *Can. J. Surg.*, **10**, 179.

Ferdinand R., Fox D.E. (1985). Evaluation of lumbar lordosis. A prospective and retrospective study. *Spine*, **10**, 799.

Fielding J. W. (1957). Cineroentgenography of the normal cervical spine. *J. Bone Jt. Surg.*, **39A**, 1280.

Gilad I., Nissan M. (1985). Sagittal evaluation of elemental geometrical dimensions of human vertebrae. *J. Anat.*, **143**, 115.

Giles L.G.F., Taylor J.R. (1981). Low back pain associated with leg-length inequality. *Spine*, **6**, 5, 510.

Giles L.G.F., Taylor J.R. (1984). The effect of postural scoliosis on lumbar apophyseal joints. *Scand. J. Rheumatol.*, **13**, 209.

Golub B.S., Silverman B. (1969). Transforaminal ligaments of the lumbar spine. *J. Bone. Jt. Surg. (Am.)*, **51-A**, 947.

Grieve G.P., ed. (1986). *Modern Manual Therapy*. Edinburgh: Churchill Livingstone, Ch. 8.

Grieve G.P. (1989). *Common Vertebral Joint Problems*, 2nd edn. Edinburgh: Churchill Livingstone, p. 426.

Hadley L.A. (1957). The uncovertebral articulations and cervical foramen encroachment. *J. Bone Jt. Surg.*, **39-A**, 910.

Hakim N.S., King A.I. (1976). Static and dynamic facet loads. *Proceedings of the Twentieth Stapp Car Crash Conference*, pp. 607–639.

Hansson T., Bigos S., Beecher P. *et al.* (1985a). The lumbar lordosis in acute and chronic low back pain. *Spine*, **10**, 154.

Hansson T., Sandstrom J., Roos B. *et al.* (1985b). The bone mineral content of the lumbar spine in patients with chronic low back pain. *Spine*, **10**, 158.

Hellems H.K., Keates T.E. (1971). Measurement of the normal lumbosacral angle. *Am. J. Roentgenol.*, **113**, 642.

Hirsch C., Schajowicz F., Galante J. (1967). Structural changes in the cervical spine. *Acta Orthop. Scand. Suppl.*, **109**, 9.

Horwitz T., Smith R.M. (1940). An anatomical, pathological and roentgeno-logical study of the intervertebral joints of the lumbar spine and of the sacroiliac joints. *Am. J. Roentgenol.*, **43**, 173.

Hytten F.E., Leitch J. (1971). *The Physiology of Human Pregnancy*, 3rd edn. Oxford: Blackwell Scientific.

Koeller W., Meier W., Hartmann F. (1984). Biomechanical properties of the human intervertebral discs subjected to axial dynamic compression. A comparison of lumbar and thoracic discs. *Spine*, **9**, 725.

Kos von J., Wolf J. (1972). Les menisques intervertebraux et leur rôle possible dans les blockages vertebraux. *Ann. Med. Phys.*, **15**, 203.

Kraft G.L., Levinthal D. H. (1951). Facet synovial impingement. A new concept in the etiology of lumbar vertebral derangement. *Surg. Gynaecol. Obstet.*, **93**, 439.

Leong J.C.Y., Luk K.D.K., Ho H.C. (1985). The iliolumbar ligament – its anatomy, development and clinical significance. Paper presented at the Twelfth annual meeting of the International Society for the Study of the Lumbar Spine. Sydney, Australia. In Bogduk N., Twomey L.T. (1987). *Clinical Anatomy of the Lumbar Spine*. Edinburgh: Churchill Livingstone. p. 38.

Lewin T., Moffet B., Vildik A. (1962). The morphology of the lumbar synovial intervertebral joints. *Acta Morphol. Neerlando-Scand.*, **4**, 299.

Lippitt (1984). The facet joint and its role in spine pain. *Spine*, **9**, 7, 746.

Loebl W.Y. (1967). Measurement of spinal posture and range of spinal movement. *Ann. Phys. Med.*, **9**, 103.

Lorenz M., Patwardham A., Vanderby R. (1983). Load-bearing characteristics of lumbar facets in normal and surgically altered spinal segments. *Spine*, **8**, 122.

von Luschka H. (1858). *Die Halbelenke des menschlichen Korpers. Eine Monographie*. Berlin: Reimer.

Markolf K.L. (1972). Deformation of the thoracolumbar intervertebral joints in response to external loads. A biomechanical study using autopsy material. *J. Bone Jt. Surg.*, **54**, 511.

Miller J.A.A., Haderspeck K.A., Schultz A.B. (1983). Posterior element loads in lumbar motion segments. *Spine*, **8**, 327.

Morris J.M., Lucas D.B., Bresler B. (1961). Role of the trunk in stability of the spine. *J. Bone. Jt. Surg.*, **43**, 327.

Nachemson A., Evans J.H. (1968). Some mechanical properties of the third human interlaminar ligament (ligamentum flavum). *J. Biomech.*, **1**, 211.

Orofino C., Sherman M.S., Schechter D. (1960). Luschka's joint – a degenerative phenomenon. *J. Bone. Jt. Surg.*, **42-a**, 5, 853.

Palastanga N., Field D., Soames R. (1989). *Anatomy and Human Movement*. Oxford: Heinemann Medical, p. 796.

Patriquin D.A. (1983). The mechanical aetiology of Tietze's syndrome. *Br. Ass. Man. Med. Newsletter.*, 5th Nov.

Penning L. (1968). *Functional Pathology of the Cervical Spine*. Amsterdam: Excerpta Medica, p. 167.

Pratt N.E. (1986). Neurovascular entrapment in the regions of the shoulder and posterior triangle of the neck. *Phys. Ther.*, **66**, 12, 1894.

Ramsey R.H. (1966). The anatomy of the ligamenta flava. *Clin. Orthop.*, **44**, 129.

Rissanen P.M. (1960). The surgical anatomy and pathology of the supraspinous and interspinous ligaments of the lumbar spine with special reference to ligament ruptures. *Acta Orthop. Scand.*, Suppl. 46.

Schmorl G., Junghanns H. (1971). *The Human Spine in Health and Disease* 2nd American edn. New York: Grune and Stratton.

Shellshear J.L., Macintosh N.W.G. (1949). The transverse process of the fifth lumbar vertebra. In *Surveys of Anatomical Fields* (Shellshear J.L., Macintosh N.W.G eds.) Sydney: Grahame, pp. 21–32.

Silberstein C.E. (1965). The evolution of degenerative changes in the cervical spine and an investigation into the 'joints of Luschka'. *Clin. Orthop.*, **40**, 184.

Tietze A. (1921). Uber eine Eigenarige Haufung von Fallen mit Dystrophie der Rippenknorpel. *Berlin Klin. Woch.*, **58**, 829.

Torgerson W.R., Dotter W.E. (1976). Comparative roentgenographic study of the asymptomatic and symptomatic lumbar spine. *J. Bone. Jt. Surg. (Am.)*, **58-A**. 850.

Troup J.D.G. (1975). The biology of back pain. *New Sci.*, **65**, 17.

Twomey L.T., Taylor J.R., eds. (1987). *Physical Therapy of the Low Back*. Edinburgh: Churchill Livingstone. Ch. 2, p. 55.

Vallois H.V. (1926). Arthologie. In *Poirier and Charpy's Traité d'Anatomie Humaine*, (Nicolas A., ed.) Vol. 1. Paris: Masson, p. 68.

2

Intervertebral Discs

The intervertebral discs play a vital role in the functioning of the spine, yet their importance in relation to spinal pathology was highlighted only as recently as 1934 by Mixter and Barr.

Adjacent vertebrae from the 2nd cervical to the sacrum are linked by the annular fibres of the discs and, in this respect, they may be likened to sophisticated ligaments, the joints that they form being the interbody joints. Both the gross and microscopic structures of the discs reflect how they fulfil their two main functions, which are to allow and restrain movements at the interbody joints, and to act as the prime component in the transmission of loads from one vertebral body to the next.

GROSS STRUCTURE OF THE INTERVERTEBRAL DISC

The two basic components of the disc are the annulus fibrosus (outer part) and the nucleus pulposus (inner part).

Annulus Fibrosus (Figs. 2.1; 2.2; 2.3)

The annulus fibrosus is a composite structure consisting of concentric layers or lamellae of collagen fibres, encapsulating the nucleus pulposus, and a proteoglycan gel, which binds the collagen fibres and lamellae firmly together to prevent them from buckling. The fibres are parallel to each other and the majority of them run obliquely between the two vertebrae, lying in opposite directions in adjacent lamellae. This laminated arrangement is essential for the biomechanical properties of the fibres and function of the disc: it permits angular movements (flexion-extension, lateral flexion), while providing stability against shear and torsion. Each fibre extends for approximately half of the circumference of the disc, providing some control over rotatory movements. At the end of rotation to one side, half of the total number of annular fibres are stressed – those angled in the direction of the movement – while the other half are relaxed. The results of a study done on lumbar discs by Marchand and Ahmed (1990) suggest that the laminated structure of the annulus is more complex than hitherto

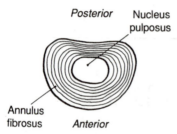

Posterior   Nucleus pulposus

Annulus fibrosus   Anterior

Fig. 2.1 Concentric bands of annular fibres.

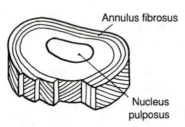

Annulus fibrosus

Nucleus pulposus

Fig. 2.2 Horizontal section through a disc.

assumed. At any 20° sector of the annulus, at least 40% of the annular layers were found to be incomplete, the posterolateral area containing the maximum percentage of incomplete layers.

The angle of the annular fibres in relation to the horizontal can vary between 40–70° depending on their position in the annulus. This angle changes on loading (Pearcy and Tibrewal, 1984) and becomes more acute (*see* Fig. 2.11, p. 75), providing the annulus with an elasticity in compression.

Increased collagen concentration has been found in the outer lamellae (Eyre, 1979). This is thought to provide additional strength in torsion as well as in flexion, extension and lateral flexion, as during these movements more stress falls on the outer lamellae than on the inner.

In the posterior part of the disc, the fibres differ from the rest of the annulus in that they have a more parallel arrangement. Here also the lamellae are thinner, more tightly packed and have less binding gel. In addition, in the lumbar spine, the anterior and lateral portions of the annulus are approximately twice as thick as the posterior portion. These factors combine to make the posterior annulus a weak area which, therefore, predisposes it to degenerative change and trauma. Greater protection is afforded to the discs in the upper lumbar spine than in the lower, because the posterior annulus there tends to be thicker and stronger.

The annulus fibrosus is anchored peripherally to the periosteum of adjacent vertebrae just beyond the epiphyseal ring of cortical bone and to the epiphyseal rings themselves, while the inner lamellae merge into the end plates above and below (Macnab, 1977; Fig. 2.3).

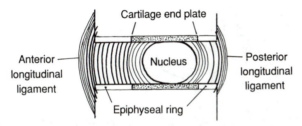

Fig. 2.3 Attachment of annular fibres.

Attached to the surface of the annulus are the anterior and posterior longitudinal ligaments (*see* pp. 14–5, 29, 43–4), the latter of which is thinner in the lumbar region than in other spinal regions.

Nucleus Pulposus (*see* Fig. 2.3)

The nucleus pulposus is a semifluid gel comprising 40–60% of the disc. At birth, the gel consists of mucoid material with a few notochordal cells and is distinct from the surrounding annulus. After the first decade, the mucoid material is gradually replaced by fibrocartilage (Sylvén, 1951) and there is less distinction between it and the annulus.

Being a fluid, the nucleus can be deformed under pressure without a reduction in volume. This essential property enables it to both accommodate to movement and to transmit some of the compressive load from one vertebra to the next.

The position of the nucleus varies in the different regions of the spine. In the thoracic region, it lies centrally within the disc, whereas in the cervical and lumbar regions, it is positioned more posteriorly.

Vertebral End Plates (Fig. 2.4)

Thin end plates separate the discs from their adjacent vertebral bodies. In the young, these consist of both hyaline cartilage and fibrocartilage. Histologically they are considered to be part of the disc, although, during the growth period, they are responsible for the growth in depth of the vertebral body. The disc side of the end plate, to which the inner annular fibres are firmly anchored, is fibrocartilage, the vertebral body side being hyaline cartilage in young discs.

The end plates have two other important functions. The first is related to the nutrition of the disc: they form a permeable barrier through which water and nutrients can pass between the nucleus pulposus and the cancellous bone of the vertebral bodies. Secondly, they play a mechanical role in preventing the nucleus bulging into the vertebral body (Urban, 1989).

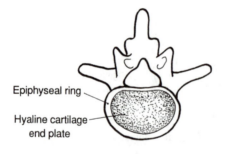

Epiphyseal ring

Hyaline cartilage
end plate

Fig. 2.4 Horizontal section showing epiphyseal ring which is wider anteriorly.

During fetal life, the end plates are well vascularized. These blood vessels gradually involute during the first 10–15 years of postnatal life (Taylor and Twomey, 1985), leaving small, weakened areas which make the vertebral body vulnerable to *intra*vertebral disc prolapses from the nucleus – called Schmorl's nodes (*see* pp. 266–7).

Under high compressive loading, the end plates are the most common site of failure and are, therefore, considered to be the weakest part of the disc.

Shape and Height of Intervertebral Discs

Cross-sections through a disc and its adjacent vertebral bodies show that the shape of the disc corresponds to that of the vertebral bodies. It is more or less elliptical with the anteroposterior axis being the minor axis, and this particular shape provides some protection against annular failure in flexion, indicating the potential danger of this movement. Were the disc to be circular in cross-section, it would then have fewer posterior annular fibres to resist flexion.

The shape of the posterior surface of the disc is variable and can be flat, rounded or re-entrant (concave, Fig. 2.5). Flattened and re-entrant discs have a greater number of posterior fibres than discs with a rounded posterior surface and are, therefore, better able to withstand the posterior stretch that occurs in flexion (Hickey and Hukins, 1980). They are, however, more easily damaged by torsional stresses as these tend to be concentrated at the points of maximum curvature. The shape of the posterior surface of the disc is an important factor in determining the pattern of radial fissure formation (*see* p. 279), particularly in the lower lumbar spine. In a study performed on 71 cadaveric discs taken from the lower two lumbar levels, the posterior surfaces of 49 were flat, 21 were rounded and 1 was re-entrant (Farfan *et al.*, 1972).

Disc height varies in the different regions of the spine, and it may also vary in different parts of the same disc. In the cervical and lumbar regions, the discs are wedge-shaped, being deeper anteriorly than posteriorly, thus helping to form their lordotic curves. The lumbosacral disc shows greater wedging, with an anterior height approximately

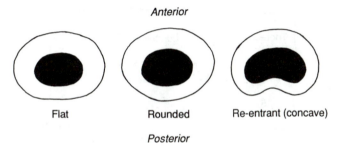

Fig. 2.5 Cross-sections of intervertebral discs showing variations in shape of posterior surface.

6–7 mm greater than the posterior height (Schmorl and Junghanns, 1971). In the thoracic region the discs are of nearly uniform thickness.

The discs are thickest in the lumbar region, where they are required to bear a greater proportion of the body weight, and thinnest in the upper thoracic region. The latter is normally a very stiff area of the spine where spondylosis commonly occurs.

Disc height also varies according to factors such as:

Age: There is a progressive loss of height in the spine with increasing age (Wood and Badley, 1983) and this is due to loss of height both in the discs and vertebral bodies.

Congenital anomalies: Joints with imperfect segmentation such as lumbarization or sacralization commonly have discs of reduced height, which appear to be developmental rather than degenerative in origin (Farfan, 1973).

Pathology: Marked degeneration in a disc, or prolapsed nuclear material, causes loss of disc height.

Diurnal variation: Overall body height decreases between 15–20 mm over a day (De Puky, 1935), principally due to loss of disc height. Prolonged loading of the spine has the same effect. In these instances, normal disc height will return following unloading of the spine (*see* pp. 76–8).

The height of the disc is an important factor controlling movement at the interbody joint: thicker discs allow more flexion-extension and lateral flexion. It is also thought that the *ratio* of disc height to vertebral body height (Fig. 2.6) may influence the movement possible in the sagittal plane (Kapandji, 1974). The cervical region is the most mobile with a ratio of disc/body height of 2:5. The lumbar region is slightly less mobile with a ratio of 1:3 and the thoracic region the least mobile with a ratio of 1:5. Studies done on cadavers by White (1969), however, failed to identify any correlation between disc/vertebral body height and sagittal mobility in the thoracic spine.

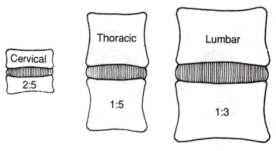

Fig. 2.6 Ratio of disc height to vertebral body height.

MICROSCOPIC STRUCTURE OF THE INTERVERTEBRAL DISC (Fig. 2.7)

The matrix of the disc principally consists of collagen fibres embedded in a proteoglycan/water gel with some elastic fibres. Also contained within it are chondrocytes and fibroblasts, whose functions are to maintain and repair it. The annulus and nucleus both have these constituents, but in different concentrations.

Proteoglycans

Proteoglycans are very large molecules which have the property of attracting and retaining water. Hence, the amount of proteoglycans in the nucleus (65%) is much greater (particularly in early life) than in the annulus (20%). They consist of glycosaminoglycan (GAG) chains linked to a central protein core and are densely packed between the collagen fibrils. The two major GAGs in the disc are chondroitin sulphate (CS) and keratan sulphate (KS), CS having twice the water-binding capacity of KS. The proteoglycans in the annulus are similar to those in the nucleus, although there are slight structural differences.

The fixed negative charges on CS and KS lead to an excess of cations in the matrix. This, and to a lesser extent the size of the proteoglycans, gives the disc a high osmotic pressure which maintains its fluid content and ensures that it remains inflated even under conditions of high vertical loading. With age or degeneration, the proteoglycan content in the disc decreases and the ratio of keratan sulphate to chondroitin sulphate increases; fluid is then lost more rapidly under a given load.

Collagen Fibres

The arrangement of collagen fibres in the annulus differs from that in the nucleus. In the annulus, the collagen is in parallel bundles arranged in concentric lamellae. In the nucleus, the collagen fibres are finer than in the annulus and are irregularly arranged in a loose meshwork.

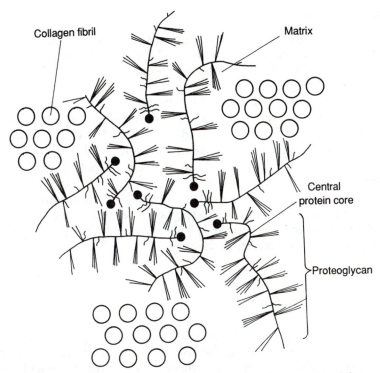

Fig. 2.7 Schematic view of microscopic structure of intervertebral disc.

Seven types of collagen have been identified in the disc, but only Types I and II are present in significant proportions. These are different both chemically and physically, reflecting the particular functions of the annulus (in sustaining tension) and the nucleus (in sustaining compression). Predominantly Type I collagen (skin and tendon collagen) is found in the outer annular fibres. This type of collagen gives the annulus considerable *tensile* strength. The fibres are relatively inextensible and will only stretch up to 3% of their length, but increased extensibility on loading is given to the annulus by virtue of the change in angle between fibres in adjacent lamellae, so that during flexion it may effectively 'extend' by 30% (Pearcy and Tibrewal, 1984).

Elastic Fibres

Elastic fibres are present in both the annulus and nucleus with a concentration at the annulus–nucleus junction. However, the elastic properties of the disc are due principally to the hydrostatic nature of the nucleus combined with the ability of the collagen fibres in the annulus to change their orientation. Elastic fibres may, nevertheless, play a role in helping the disc recover its shape after deformation. This may be particularly important as the disc, particularly the nucleus, becomes more fibrous with age and loses its normal elasticity (Ayad and Weiss, 1987).

Water

Water is the main constituent of the disc. In the nucleus the water content varies considerably with age and the state of health of the disc. It is over 85% in the juvenile disc, falling to approximately 70% in the mature disc. In the annulus, the content is 70–75% and this remains fairly constant throughout life. This variation in water content across the disc is thought to be related to the different concentrations of proteoglycans in the annulus and nucleus. The water is mostly extracellular, enabling transportation of dissolved solutes to the chondrocytes. The water content of the disc also varies in response to changes in loading (see pp. 76–8).

The water-binding capacity of the nucleus is of paramount importance in maintaining its elasticity. The rate at which water can pass in and out of the disc is influenced by the concentration of proteoglycans and by changes in intradiscal pressure.

INTRADISCAL PRESSURE

There is always an intrinsic pressure of about 0.7 kg/cm^2 (Nachemson and Evans, 1968) within the intervertebral discs even when they are unloaded. This 'prestressed' state of the disc provides it with some intrinsic stability. It is due to the compressive effect of the ligamentum flavum which consists principally of elastic fibres and which is at a distance from the motion centre of the disc. When the disc is subjected to external loading, such as from body weight, this resting pressure rises. The loading will vary depending on factors such as the position of the body (because of the effects of the force of gravity and muscular contraction) and whether or not a weight is being lifted or carried in the hands or on the back. When a vertical load is applied to a disc, the pressure in the nucleus is 50% higher than that applied externally, i.e. a load of 10 kg/cm^2 gives a pressure of 15 kg/cm^2 inside the disc (Nachemson, 1966). Forces acting in the annulus are related to those acting in the nucleus (Nachemson, 1965). The vertical stress in the annulus was calculated to be 50% of the applied external load per unit area, while the tangential, tensile strain was 4–5 times the applied external load, at least in its outer parts.

Intradiscal pressure also rises simply by flexion of the motion segment, whether or not it is loaded, which is surprising since its volume remains the same. In studies on autopsy specimens (Nachemson, 1965), when the discs were tilted forward by 8°, the intradiscal pressure was increased by 1.5 kg/cm^2, which corresponds to approximately 20 kg of external load. This increase is the same whatever load is borne by the disc and is, therefore, more significant proportionately for small loads than for larger ones. It may also be significant when considering the effect of 'passive flexion' exercises in supine-lying in the treatment of patients with disc disorders. On average, a disc flexed by 5.5° has a nuclear pressure 50% greater than a disc extended by 3° (calculated from Nachemson *et al.*, 1979 by Adams and Hutton, 1983).

Effect of the Position of the Body on Intradiscal Pressure

In a series of *in vivo* investigations, Nachemson and Morris (1964) and Nachemson (1966) measured the intradiscal pressures in the 2nd–4th lumbar discs with the subjects in various positions and performing different exercises (Fig. 2.8). The relationship between the different positions is of more significance than the absolute values.

Sitting

Of three of the positions tested – standing, sitting and reclining – intradiscal pressures were highest in the sitting position, varying between 100 and 180 kg. The particular position used was the upright unsupported sitting position.

The load on the disc was shown to be directly related to the body weight above the level of the disc measured, and was approximately three times that of the body weight above it. The lower the disc, therefore, the greater the load became. It is interesting to note that nearly 60% of the body weight is above the L4/5 disc (Ruff, 1950).

One reason for the relatively high intradiscal pressure in this position is the activity of the vertebral portion of psoas major, which has a stabilizing influence on the lumbar spine and, at the same time, a compressive effect. It thus contributes a considerable load in addition to gravitational forces. Another reason is that when a person sits on a horizontal surface, the lumbar spine is usually in some degree of flexion, which in itself increases the pressure, as well as transferring the load from the apophyseal joints more onto the discs.

In Nachemson's experiments, when the subjects leaned forward 20°, the load on the disc was increased by 40–60 kg. Although psoas activity was reduced, that of the erectores spinae increased considerably in order to prevent the trunk from falling further forward and, thereby, had a compressive effect on the discs. The method used did not permit measurements of intradiscal pressure at angles exceeding 20°.

There are, of course, many other postures that can be assumed when sitting, and the intradiscal pressure varies accordingly. These are considered, together with the effect on intradiscal pressure of lever arms and using a backrest, in the chapter on Posture on pp. 296–303.

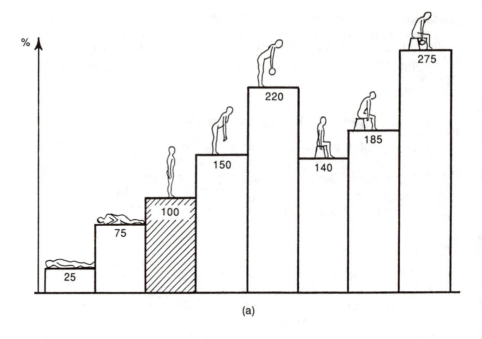

(a)

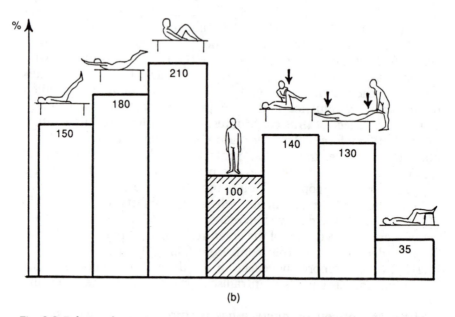

(b)

Fig. 2.8 Relative change in pressure (or load) in the 3rd lumbar disc. (a) in various positions; (b) in various muscle strengthening exercises. (From A. Nachemson, 1976. The lumbar spine: an orthopaedic challenge. *Spine*, **1**, 59–71 with permission of author and publisher, Harper and Row.)

Standing

In the upright standing position, a decrease from the pressure in the sitting position of about 30% was found, and values from 80–150 kg were noted. Again, leaning forward 20° further increased the intradiscal pressure.

Reclining

Problems with the method used for the *in vivo* measurements did not permit complete relaxation of the subjects in this position. Even so, the stress on the discs decreased by about 50% as compared with the sitting position, values being obtained between 35–85 kg.

Holding weights

Holding weights caused a further rise in intradiscal pressure. When the subjects held weights of 10 kg in each hand in the forward-leaning sitting position, the total amount of load varied between 230–270 kg. Similarly, in the forward-leaning standing position, when holding the same weights, loads of up to 250 kg were recorded. A combination of rotation and flexion also subjected the lumbar spine to considerable load, especially when a weight was held (Nachemson, 1987).

Exercises

During certain exercises, intradiscal pressures were greatly increased (*see* Fig. 2.8b), e.g. when the subjects performed sit-ups with their knees bent, *active* back hyperextension in prone-lying and bilateral straight-leg raising in lying. This is clearly of relevance when considering the treatment of patients in the acute stages of disc pathology.

Now that evidence points to certain discs being innervated (*see* p. 79), it is feasible that some tears in the outer annular fibres could give rise to pain because of increases in intradiscal pressure and subsequent tensile stresses on the annulus. Patients who say that their pain is absent when reclining, but comes on when standing and is much worse when sitting and during certain exercises, may well be describing the effects of stressing an annular tear.

Other findings with clinical application

Nachemson and Morris (1964) found that the *valsalva manoeuvre* (forced expiration against a closed glottis) produced intradiscal pressure increases in most cases. Those subjects who complained of discomfort while performing the manoeuvre also had the greatest increase in intradiscal pressure.

The effect on intradiscal pressure of wearing an inflatable *corset* was evaluated and there were decreases of about 25% in the total load on the disc. To achieve the same effect on a patient, the corset would need to be well fitted and tight.

NUTRITION OF THE INTERVERTEBRAL DISCS (Fig. 2.9)

Apart from its outermost annular fibres, the disc is avascular after the age of 10 years. For its nutrition, it then relies on the diffusion of nutrients such as glucose, sulphate and oxygen. These reach the disc by two routes: from the blood vessels surrounding the periphery of the annulus fibrosus (the annular route), and from the capillary plexuses beneath the end plates (the end plate route). The nucleus receives most of its nutrition through the end plate route.

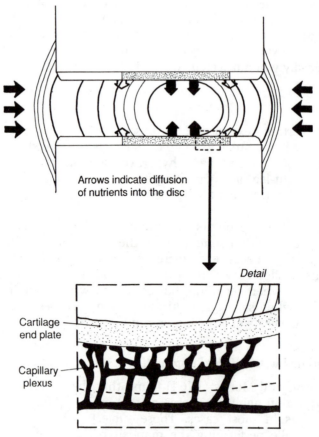

Arrows indicate diffusion of nutrients into the disc

Detail

Cartilage end plate

Capillary plexus

Fig. 2.9 Nutrition of the intervertebral disc.

Certain areas of the disc have a higher permeability: the periphery of the annulus and the inner one-third of the end plates in the region of the nucleus and inner annular fibres. There is a region 4.4–6 mm from the posterior border of the disc which has a deficient supply of nutrition from all sources (Maroudas et al., 1975). Overall, the anterior annulus receives a better nutrient supply than the posterior annulus (Adams and Hutton, 1986) which could help to explain why degenerative changes occur less frequently in the anterior part of the disc.

The chondrocytes are found in greater proportions close to the end plates and in the outer layers of the annulus, that is, near to a blood supply. However, those in the centre of the disc are further away from the blood vessels, and diffusion alone can barely supply them with nutrients (Maroudas et al., 1975).

Diffusion is more effective for transporting small molecules (Urban et al., 1982), while experiments performed on cadaveric lumbar discs have suggested that fluid flow may play some part in the transport of larger molecules such as proteins (Adams and Hutton, 1983). Fluid flows into and out of the disc in response to changes in posture and loading.

Effect of Posture on Fluid Flow

Certain postures were found to have different effects on fluid flow probably due to higher loads in some postures. The erect posture favoured diffusion into the anterior half of the disc compared to the posterior half. The fully flexed lumbar posture favoured diffusion into the posterior annulus, by thinning it and thus increasing its surface area, thereby decreasing the path from the nucleus to the periphery of the annulus. In life, however, this would be offset by a decrease in the supply to the end plate route because flexion increases the distance from the end plates to the midplane of the posterior nucleus. Adams and Hutton's experiments showed that flexion reduced the thickness of the posterior annulus by 37% on average, which would bring the whole of the 'deficient' region mentioned above to within 4.4 mm of the surface, and ensure a sufficient supply of glucose to all cells in the posterior annulus.

If the blood supply at the periphery of the disc is altered, this could affect the nutrition of the disc, and it is possible that this is one of the ways in which changes of posture affect the disc's nutrition. It has been shown, by experiments done on porcine intervertebral discs (Holm and Nachemson, 1988), that cigarette smoking adversely affects the circulation outside the disc by nicotine-induced vascular constriction, as well as cellular uptake rates and metabolic production within the disc. The inevitable consequence over a longer period of time will be deficient nutrition leading to degenerative metabolic processes. These effects, found in animals after a single exposure to smoking, do not, however, necessarily represent effects of chronic smoking in humans.

Experiments done on dogs showed that after several months' exercise training, the transport of nutrients into the disc was increased. Again, this could have been due to changes in the blood supply surrounding the discs (Holm and Nachemson, 1982).

It is important to consider the factors affecting the nutrition of the disc when giving prophylactic advice on back care to patients who have early disc pathology. Inadequate metabolite transport has been linked with disc degeneration (Holm and Nachemson, 1982; Nachemson et al., 1970) and it seems feasible that alternating periods of activity and rest, and frequent posture changes, would boost the fluid exchange in the discs, hence improving their nutrition. However, although the flexed posture has been shown to improve nutrition to the disc, it also increases the intradiscal pressure by about 50% compared with the lordotic posture (calculated from Nachemson et al., 1979) and this may be significant in some cases where disc pathology is more advanced. Exercises may well play an important part in improving nutrition to the disc, possibly by increasing the blood supply to its periphery, provided that they are carefully selected and do not exacerbate the patient's symptoms.

EFFECTS OF MOVEMENTS ON THE INTERBODY JOINTS

Movements in the interbody joints occur in conjunction with those in the other joints in the motion segments and can never be isolated from them. They include, therefore, the apophyseal joints in all regions of the spine; in addition, in the cervical spine, the joints of Luschka and, in the thoracic spine, the costovertebral and costotransverse joints. The movements at these accompanying joints are described in their relevant sections. It should be borne in mind, however, that in life, pure movement occurs less frequently than combined movements (see pp. 166–7).

Flexion

During flexion, the anterior annular fibres are compressed and tend to bulge, while the posterior fibres are under tensile stress.

The movement of the nucleus has been of particular interest because of the number of posterior herniations of the nucleus in the lumbar spine attributed to flexion injuries. Kapandji's theory (1974) was that the nucleus acted as a ball-bearing and was driven away from the side of movement, so that on flexion it was driven posteriorly (Fig. 2.10a). Bogduk and Twomey (1987) also described the posterior

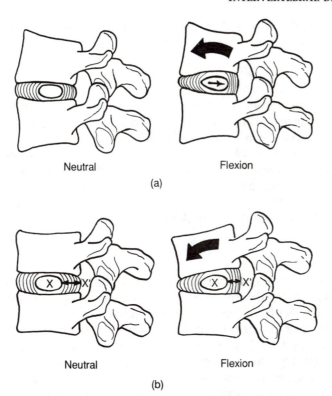

Neutral   Flexion

(a)

Neutral   Flexion

(b)

Fig. 2.10 Different theories of nuclear position during flexion. (a) Kapandji; (b) Dolan. X–X' = distance (nucleus to
outer fibres) decreases with flexion.

movement of the nucleus as it attempted to 'escape' from the anterior
compression which deformed it. More recently, Dolan (1989) stated
that in flexion the posterior annulus was stretched and thinned, so
that the distance between the nucleus and outer annular fibres was
decreased and the nucleus was relatively closer to the posterior margin
of the disc (Fig. 2.10b).

In life, when flexion of the spine occurs, it is often accompanied by
muscular activity, depending on the starting position of the movement. Through its compressive effect, this increases the intradiscal
pressure. However, intradiscal pressure rises even if the interbody joint
is flexed without being loaded (*see* p. 66).

What is of perhaps even more practical significance is what happens
on *repeated* flexion. Although a patient may describe an isolated flexion
movement causing injury to the lumbar spine, in many cases the
offending movement was probably the last in a succession of repeated
flexion movements. Studies carried out using cadaveric discs, which
were stressed repeatedly in compression and flexion (Adams and
Hutton, 1985), showed that there was distortion of the annular fibres

and nucleus (*see* Fig. 9.7, p. 280). The nucleus appeared to deform posterolaterally.

Extension

The reverse occurs, i.e. the posterior annulus is compressed and bulges, the anterior annulus is stretched and there is a tendency for the nucleus to deform forwards. Intradiscal pressure is lower than in flexion, but the effect of muscular activity must also be considered.

The anteroposterior deformation of the nucleus during movements in the sagittal plane has been the basis of an exercise regime described by McKenzie (1981) to relieve pain and restore function in patients with certain types of disc pathology.

Lateral Flexion

This has received, regrettably, relatively little attention, for combined with flexion, this movement occurs when stooping to one side to pick up an object from the floor – a common cause of back injuries (*see* p. 280). During the movement of lateral flexion, the annular fibres are compressed and tend to bulge on the side to which it occurs, while those on the opposite side have their attachments separated. There is presumably some deformation of the nucleus in a similar manner to that which occurs in flexion, i.e. deformation on the compressed side and a tendency to move towards the opposite side. Intradiscal pressure also rises (Nachemson, 1987).

Sliding

A small degree of sliding (1–2 mm) occurs at the interbody joints as an accessory movement in flexion, extension and lateral flexion. In flexion, *forward sliding* occurs and is resisted by the apophyseal joints and the annular fibres, in particular, half of the lateral annular fibres which are orientated in the direction of movement and are stretched principally longitudinally (Bogduk and Twomey, 1987). The anterior and posterior fibres offer relatively less resistance to forward sliding, because their orientation is not in the principal direction of the movement.

Rotation

Half of the annular fibres lie in the direction of rotation, while the other half lie in the opposite direction. Therefore, during rotation to one side, only half of the annular fibres have their points of attachment separated, while the other half have them brought closer together. Rotation puts more strain on the outer annular fibres than the inner

(Klein and Hukins, 1983) and the higher collagen concentration in the outer lamellae (Eyre, 1979) provide additional tensile strength. The inner fibres are the most oblique and, during rotation, they compress the nucleus, thereby raising the intradiscal pressure.

Distraction

Distraction of a motion segment can occur if a person hangs by the arms (for instance during gymnastic exercises) or during some therapeutic traction, if accurately applied. During distraction, every annular fibre has its points of attachment separated, disc height increases and intradiscal pressure decreases.

EFFECTS OF VERTICAL LOADING ON THE SPINE (Fig. 2.11)

Vertical loads are applied to the spine simply through the weight of the body, and additionally through the compressive effects of muscular activity and any weights if held.

On vertical loading of the spine, the nucleus pulposus and annulus

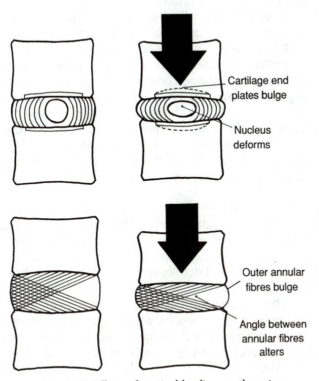

Cartilage end plates bulge

Nucleus deforms

Outer annular fibres bulge

Angle between annular fibres alters

Fig. 2.11 Effects of vertical loading on the spine.

fibrosus work in coordination to transmit weight from one vertebra to the next. The nucleus, being incompressible, tries to deform radially, but is resisted by the strong annular fibres, causing pressure in the nucleus to rise. Any resultant stresses are distributed radially to the annulus and end plates and, in a normal disc, these stresses are the same in all directions.

The direction of the annular fibres allows the resultant stresses to be absorbed. The angle that the fibres make with the horizontal becomes more acute (Pearcy and Tibrewal, 1984)—see Fig. 2.11. While the inner fibres are compressed, the outer fibres are put under tension, but the annulus bulges only slightly. Indeed, a load of 100 kg causes a lateral expansion of only 0.75 mm in a normal disc (Hirsch and Nachemson, 1954). However, increased bulging of the annulus occurs after prolonged loading (Köller et al., 1981). Evidently this occurs more readily in degenerated discs, since they lose more height than non-degenerated discs (see p. 275). Tensile stresses 4–5 times higher than the applied load are borne by the posterior annular fibres (Nachemson, 1965).

There is some deformation of the cancellous bone during vertical loading, and bulging of the end plates into the vertebral bodies may occur (Roaf, 1960)—see Fig. 2.11. Some of the compressive energy is dissipated by blood flowing out of the cancellous bone of the vertebral bodies into the perivertebral veins, providing some protection against fracture. These veins are unusual in that they have no valves, so that when the load is removed, some blood flows from the veins back into the vertebral bodies. If subjected to a sudden application of vertical loading, however, the cancellous bone may fracture. This could be due to there being insufficient time for blood flow to dissipate energy or for the posture to be altered to absorb the shock (Klein and Hukins, 1983). Similarly, during cyclic loading, the energy-dissipating mechanism eventually fails, if the period of loading is less than the time taken for the blood to flow back into the cancellous bone. It has been suggested that vibrations with a frequency of around 5 Hz could be damaging (Pope et al., 1980).

If a high vertical load is applied to the spine, damage usually results in collapse of the end plates (rather than herniation of the disc), suggesting that they are the weakest part of the disc in compression.

When a vertical load is maintained, the disc is said to 'creep': fluid passes from it at a slow and decelerating rate into the vertebral bodies and surrounding tissues until the disc is in equilibrium with the applied load. The heavier the load, the faster the rate of creep. The extent of the initial deformation for each load largely depends on the structure and integrity of the collagen network, but the rate and magnitude of the creep deformation is related more to the proteoglycan content of the disc.

Over the period of one day, body height decreases between 15–

20 mm (de Puky, 1935), principally due to loss of fluid from the discs. This is relatively more marked in children and least in elderly people. Conversely, increases in height of approximately 5 cm have been reported in astronauts, who were weightless for 3 months. Many factors influence disc height loss in each individual, such as the number of hours of sleep, the time of getting up, the time of day, the magnitude and duration of loads applied to it (which would include the particular postures assumed), previous loads and the condition of the disc. Disc height loss has been found to be related to the experience of discomfort, and also to the perception of exertion during physical exercises (Eklund and Corlett, 1987). In some patients, these symptoms may serve as a useful warning not to proceed with a particular activity.

As the disc loses height and bulges, the vertical and transverse dimensions of the intervertebral foramen are reduced, leaving less room for its contents, including the nerve root. The apophyseal joint surfaces are brought closer together and, in the lumbar spine at least, their tips begin to resist some of the intervertebral compressive forces (Dunlop *et al.*, 1984). These effects can give rise to symptoms if pathology is present.

The effect of disc height loss on mechanics in the lumbar spine has been postulated (Adams and Hutton, 1983). The approximation of the facets of the apophyseal joints is thought to reduce the range of axial rotation, since they normally limit this movement, and the range of extension may similarly be reduced. Conversely, the extra slack in the disc and ligaments is thought to decrease spinal stiffness in flexion and increase the range of flexion. This has clinical significance in that measurements of a patient's movements, if done at the start of a working day, are likely to differ from those done at the end of the afternoon if, for example, the spine has been subjected to reasonably heavy loading.

The rate at which fluid is lost from the disc tends to be slower than the rate at which it is imbibed, hence fluid lost in 16 h of daytime activity is replaced by 8 h of rest. At night, a rapid recovery of height occurs – approximately 70% of height being regained within 4 h (Fig. 2.12; Tyrrell *et al.*, 1985). On rising, the disc may be in a state of hyperhydration for the first few hours and, undoubtedly, this is related to the clinical observation that many patients say that their backs 'went' after a trivial incident during this particular period. It was found that when the fluid content of a cadaveric disc was artificially raised by saline injection, it became more resistant to bending stresses (Andersson and Schultz, 1979). Adams *et al.* (1987) hypothesized that perhaps the same thing happens in life, so that in the early morning a forward-bending movement may subject the lumbar ligaments and discs to damaging bending stresses, even though the movement would be perfectly safe later on in the day.

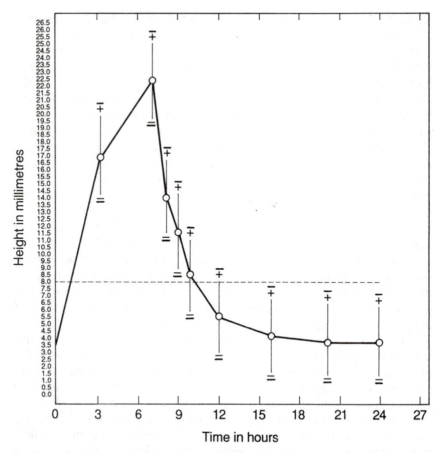

Fig. 2.12 Height gained and lost during a 24-h period from a midline baseline set at 3.5 mm. (From A.R. Tyrrell *et al.*, 1985. Circadian variation in stature and the effects of spinal loading. *Spine*, **10**, 2, 163, with permission.)

Unloading the spine during the day, even for short periods, results in a substantial recovery in disc height. This has practical implications when advising patients with disc or disc-related problems about their daily activities. Some rest positions result in more fluid imbibition than others: the lying position takes the load off the spine and encourages fluid intake, but flexing the lumbar spine has been shown to have a beneficial effect on the nutrition of the disc by aiding the transportation of metabolites (Adams and Hutton, 1986). So if the aim is simply to reinflate the disc, and there are no contraindications to flexing the disc, a flexed resting posture such as the Fowler position is apt. The rise in intradiscal pressure brought about by flexing an interbody joint needs to be taken into consideration.

NERVE SUPPLY OF THE INTERVERTEBRAL DISCS

Unmyelinated nerve endings are present in the immature intervertebral discs of the fetus and neonate (Tsukada, 1938, 1939; Ehrenhaft, 1943; Malinsky, 1959). In 1940, Roofe claimed to have found nerve endings in the outer annular fibres of mature lower lumbar discs. Much debate followed as to whether or not *normal* mature discs were innervated, most studies being done on lumbar discs. Wiberg (1949) failed to demonstrate any such nerve endings, a finding with which Wyke (1987) still agrees.

Other researchers, however, (Hirsch *et al.*, 1963; Jackson *et al.*, 1966) found evidence of innervation in the superficial layers of the annulus of mature discs, and Malinsky (1959) in its outer third. The nerve endings were reported to be unevenly distributed, more abundant in the lateral regions of the disc, less in the posterior region, and even less in the anterior region. Normal as well as degenerated discs were examined. No significant increase in nerve elements was observed in degenerated discs, nor were there any significant nerve endings in the areas where ingrowth of granulation tissue could be found (*see* p. 283).

The sources of these nerve endings are said to be the lumbar sinuvertebral nerves, branches of the lumbar ventral rami and the grey rami communicantes (Bogduk *et al.*, 1981). Each lumbar sinuvertebral nerve supplies the disc at the particular level at which it enters the vertebral canal and, in addition, the disc above. Outside the vertebral canal, the lumbar discs are innervated laterally by the grey rami communicantes, and posterolaterally by the grey rami communicantes and the ventral rami (Bogduk and Twomey, 1987).

The function of these nerve endings has not to date been confirmed, but there are three possibilities: (1) since there are similarities in the structure of the annulus fibrosus and that of a ligament, it is reasonable to assume that, like other ligaments in the body, the annulus could serve a proprioceptive function; (2) those that are associated with blood vessels could have either a vasomotor or vasosensory function (Malinsky, 1959); (3) it is possible that they have a nociceptive function, which would mean that, even in the absence of herniation, the disc could be a primary source of back pain. It is important for therapists to be aware of this possibility, so that relatively minor annular tears which are causing symptoms in a patient, hitherto considered to be of 'only muscular' origin, can be detected early so that correct treatment and prophylactic advice are given.

REFERENCES

Adams M.A., Hutton W.C. (1983). The effects of posture on the fluid content of lumbar intervertebral discs. *Spine*, **8**, 6, 665.

Adams M.A., Hutton W.C. (1985). The effect of fatigue on the lumbar intervertebral disc. *J. Bone Jt. Surg.*, **65-B**, 2, 199.

Adams M.A., Hutton W.C. (1986). The effect of posture on diffusion into lumbar intervertebral discs. *J. Anat.*, **147**, 121.

Adams M.A., Dolan P., Hutton W.C. (1987). Diurnal variations in the stresses on the lumbar spine. *Spine*, **12**, 2, 130.

Andersson G.B., Schultz A.B. (1979). Effects of fluid injection on mechanical properties of intervertebral discs. *J. Biomech.*, **12**, 453.

Ayad S., Weiss J.B. (1987). Biochemistry of the intervertebral disc. In *The Lumbar Spine and Back Pain*, 3rd edn. (Jayson M.I.V., ed.). Edinburgh: Churchill Livingstone, p. 122.

Bogduk N., Tynan W., Wilson A.S. (1981). The nerve supply to the human lumbar intervertebral discs. *J. Anat.*, **132**, 39.

Bogduk N., Twomey L. (1987). *Clinical Anatomy of the Lumbar Spine*, Edinburgh: Churchill Livingstone.

De Puky P. (1935). The physiological oscillation of the length of the body. *Acta Orthop. Scand.*, **6**, 338.

Dolan P. (1989). Written communication.

Dunlop R.B., Adams M.A., Hutton W.C. (1984). Disc space narrowing and the lumbar facet joints. *J. Bone Jt. Surg.*, (Br.), **66-B**, 706.

Ehrenhaft J.L. (1943). Development of the vertebral column as related to certain congenital and pathological changes. *Surg. Gynec. Obstet.*, **76**, 282.

Eklund J.A.E., Corlett E.N. (1987). Shrinkage as a measure of the effect of load on the spine. *Spine*, **9**, 2, 189.

Eyre D.R. (1979). Biochemistry of the intervertebral disc. *Int. Rev. Connect. Tissue Res.*, **8**, 227.

Farfan H.F. (1973). *Mechanical Disorders of the Low Back*. Philadelphia: Lea & Febiger.

Farfan H.F., Huberdeau R.M., Dubow H.I. (1972). Lumbar intervertebral disc degeneration. The influence of geometrical features on the pattern of disc degeneration – a postmortem study. *J. Bone Jt. Surg.*, **54-A**, 3, 492.

Hickey D.S., Hukins D.W.L. (1980). Relation between the structure of the annulus fibrosus and the function and failure of the intervertebral disc. *Spine*, **5**, 2, 106.

Hirsch C., Inglemark B.E., Miller M. (1963). The anatomical basis for low back pain. *Acta Orthop. Scand.*, **33**, 1.

Hirsch C., Nachemson A. (1954). New observations on mechanical behaviour of lumbar discs. *Acta Orthop. Scand.*, **23**, 254.

Holm S., Nachemson A. (1982). Nutritional changes in the canine intervertebral disc after spinal fusion. *Clin. Orthop.*, **169**, 243.

Holm S., Nachemson A. (1988). Nutrition of the intervertebral disc: acute effects of cigarette smoking. An experimental animal study. *Upsala J. Med. Sci.*, **93**, 91.

Jackson H.C., Winkelmann R.K., Bickel W.H. (1966). Nerve endings in the human lumbar spinal column and related structures. *J. Bone Jt. Surg.* (Am.), **48-A**, 1272.

Kapandji I.A. (1974). *The Physiology of the Joints, Vol. 3: The Trunk and the Vertebral Column*, Edinburgh: Churchill Livingstone.

Klein J.A., Hukins D.W.L. (1983). Functional differentiation in the spinal column. *Eng. Med.*, **12**, 2, 83.

Köller W., Funke F., Hartmann F. (1981). Das verformungsverhalten vom lumbalen menschlichen Zwischenwirbelscheiben unter langeinwirkender axialer dynamischer Druckkraft. *Z. Orthop.*, **119**, 206.

MacNab, I. (1977). *Backache*, Baltimore: Williams & Wilkins.

Malinsky J. (1959). The ontogenetic development of nerve terminations in the intervertebral discs of man. *Acta Anat.*, **38**, 96.

Marchand F., Ahmed A.M. (1990). Investigation of the laminate structure of lumbar disc anulus fibrosus. *Spine* **14**, 2, 166.

Maroudas A., Nachemson A., Stockwell R. *et al.* (1975). Some factors involved in the nutrition of the intervertebral disc. *J. Anat.*, **120**, 113.

McKenzie R.A. (1981). *The Lumbar Spine. Mechanical Diagnosis and Therapy.* New Zealand: Spinal Publications.

Mixter W.J., Barr J.S. (1934). Rupture of the intervertebral disc with involvement of the spinal canal. *New Engl. J. Med.*, **211**, 210.

Nachemson A. (1965). The effect of forward leaning on lumbar intradiscal pressure. *Acta Orthop. Scand.*, **35**, 314.

Nachemson A. (1966). The load on lumbar discs in different posiitions of the body. *Clin. Orthop.*, **45**, 107.

Nachemson A. (1987). Lumbar intradiscal pressure. In *The Lumbar Spine and Back Pain*, 3rd. edn. (Jayson M.I.V., ed.). Edinburgh: Churchill Livingstone, pp. 191–203.

Nachemson A., Morris J.M. (1964). *In vivo* measurements of intradiscal pressure, *J. Bone Jt. Surg.*, **46-A**, 5, 1077.

Nachemson A., Lewin T., Maroudas A. *et al.* (1970). *In vitro* diffusion of dye through the end-plates and the annulus fibrosus of human intervertebral discs. *Acta Orthop. Scand.*, **41**, 589.

Nachemson A., Schultz A., Berkson M. (1979). Mechanical properties of human lumbar spine motion segments: influences of age, sex, disc level and degeneration. *Spine*, **4**, 1.

Pearcy M.J., Tibrewal S.B. (1984). Lumbar intervertebral disc and ligament deformations measured *in vivo*. *Clin. Orthop.*, **191**, 281.

Pope M.H., Wilder D.G., Frymoyer J.W. (1980). Vibrations as an aetiologic factor in low back pain. In *Engineering Aspects of the Spine* (Institute of Mechanical Engineers Conference Publications, London), pp. 11–16.

Roaf R. (1960). A study of the mechanics of spinal injuries. *J. Bone Jt. Surg.*, **42-B**, 4, 810.

Roofe P.G. (1940). Innervation of annulus fibrosus and posterior longitudinal ligament. *Arch. Neurol. Psychiatr.*, **44**, 100.

Ruff S. (1950). Brief acceleration less than one second. In *German Aviation Medicine, World War II*, Washington, DC: US Government Printing Office, **1**, 584.

Schmorl G., Junghanns H. (1971). *The Human Spine in Health and Disease*, 2nd American edn. New York: Grune & Stratton.

Sylvén B. (1951). On the biology of nucleus pulposus. *Acta Orthop. Scand.*, **20**, 275.

Taylor J.R., Twomey L.T. (1985). Vertebral column development and its relation to adult pathology. *Aust. J. Physiother.*, **31**, 3, 83.

Tsukada K. (1938). Histologische Studien über die zwischenwirbelscheibe des Menschen: histologische Befunde des Foetus. *Mitt. Med. Akad. Kioto*, **24** (1057), 1172.

Tsukada K. (1939). Histologische Studien über die zwischenwirbelscheibe des Menschen: Alters-veränderungen. *Mitt. Med. Akad. Kioto*, **25** (1), 207.

Tyrrell A.R., Reilly T., Troup J.D.G. (1985). Circadian variation in stature and the effects of spinal loading. *Spine*, **10**, 2, 161.

Urban J.P.G. (1989). Written communication.

Urban J.P.G., Holm S., Maroudas A. *et al.* (1982). Nutrition of the intervertebral disc: effect of fluid flow on solute transport. *Clin. Orthop.*, **170**, 296.

White A.A. (1969). Analysis of the mechanics of the thoracic spine in man. *Acta Orthop. Scand.*, Suppl. 127.

Wiberg G. (1949). Back pain in relation to the nerve supply of the intervertebral disc. *Acta Orthop. Scand.*, **19**, 211.

Wood P.H.N., Badley E.M. (1983). An epidemiological appraisal of bone and joint disease in the elderly. In *Bone and Joint Disease in the Elderly* (Wright V., ed.), Edinburgh: Churchill Livingstone, pp. 1–22.

Wyke B. (1987). The neurology of low back pain. In *The Lumbar Spine and Back Pain* (Jayson M.I.V., ed.), 3rd edn., Edinburgh: Churchill Livingstone.

3

Muscles of the Vertebral Column

The trunk and pelvic musculature play a fundamental role in the functioning of the spine. Restoration of normal function is a primary defence against pain and the recurrence of musculoskeletal disorders. Although this may be acknowledged in theory, in practice the importance of good muscle function is often overlooked, especially if mobilization or manipulation of a joint has achieved a speedy and satisfactory relief of the patient's symptoms. It is, however, unlikely that mobilization or manipulation of joints alone can prevent the recurrence of spinal lesions.

From a mechanical point of view, the spinal column would be unstable in the sagittal plane without the support of its ligaments, tendons and muscles. These soft tissues act like guy ropes in tension to stabilize the spine in the upright posture, and, when under normal tension, increase the vertical compression on it. Adaptive shortening or lengthening of a muscle compromises its ability to function adequately in the stabilization of the trunk in a given posture, and in producing or controlling movements of the trunk and rib cage during activity of the upper limbs. The spinal muscles also play a part in the shock-absorbing mechanisms which help to relieve the spine of large loads, and have a protective function during trauma in which there is time for voluntary control.

Muscles are highly sensitive structures which react to all parts of the motor system. While the muscles themselves may be a source of local pain, the presence of pain or dysfunction in any element in the motion segment with the same segmental nerve supply causes a response – such as spasm and/or referred tenderness – in the muscles controlling it, e.g. experimental stimulation of the C5/6 interspinous ligament elicited spasm in the supraspinatus, infraspinatus and biceps muscles (Feinstein, 1977).

As well as considering the movements affected by individual muscles, it is particularly important to consider how the spinal muscles work over the whole vertebral column, because abnormalities in one spinal region may eventually give rise to a secondary set of symptoms in another. For instance, where there is leg length inequality, compensation occurs in the vertebral column, principally in the lumbar region, but it may also result in malalignment of head posture, resulting in the upper cervical region being held by tightened muscles in lateral flexion. The secondary problem may be more troublesome to the patient than the first, but treating the cervical spine alone would achieve limited and temporary results. Another example commonly seen in clinical practice is that of a patient with a limited range of extension in the lumbar spine, with compensation in the cervical spine of an exaggerated lordosis and with the head carried forward.

Some of the pressure techniques that are applied with the aim of passively mobilizing the joints also affect the overlying muscles. Sustained digital pressures are likely to bring about a temporary ischaemia of the muscle at the site of pressure, followed by hyperaemia due to the liberation of histamine as a sequel to minor damage to tissue. This hyperaemia sweeps away the metabolites of sustained contraction, enabling the muscles to relax.

MUSCLE TONE

Many of the skeletal muscles are, at any one time, in a state of reflex contraction known as muscle tone. This applies particularly to the muscles which are opposing the effects of gravity.

Motor Unit

The smallest group of muscle fibres employed voluntarily or in a reflex action is called a motor unit, and it constitutes a single motor neurone together with the muscle fibres which it innervates. These muscle fibres are often widely spread within a muscle, which means that even when only a few motor units are active, the force is generated diffusely. Each muscle is made up of several thousand motor units each with its own anterior horn cell in the spinal cord. In normal circumstances, only a proportion of the motor units are active at the same time. This proportion may, of course, increase when a muscle group is exercised, or it may decrease. An example of the latter, which may be seen clinically, is when a patient presents with paresis of muscles supplied by one spinal nerve following irritation and compression of the nerve by, for example, a prolapsed intervertebral disc. As most muscles are supplied by more than one spinal nerve, paresis rather than paralysis tends to occur.

The amount of tone present in striated muscle at any one time depends not only on the integral state of the motor units, some of which will be contracting, some relaxing, and some quiescent, but also on the impulse frequency in the neurone supplying each motor unit, and on the tension of the muscle's connective tissues.

Spasm

Hypertonus – or spasm – of a muscle can result either from injury to the muscle itself or as a reflex response to nociceptor irritation of joints and associated tissues. The severity of the spasm generally depends on the intensity of pain. It initially plays a protective role in splinting a painful lesion, and may be present over several segments or may span a whole vertebral region. In itself, spasm may be asymptomatic if short-lived. However, its presence may increase the compressive forces on the structures of the motion segment, the intervertebral disc in particular, thereby giving rise to greater pain and dysfunction.

Another mechanism whereby muscle spasm causes pain is through tension on its attachments to periosteum; a patient with a lumbar lesion giving rise to erector spinae spasm may complain of thoracic pain caused by the muscle's attachments into the rib angles. Muscle spasm may also be the primary mechanism involved in referred pain, e.g. piriformis spasm associated with a sacroiliac lesion causing buttock and trochanteric pain (Kirkaldy et al., 1979). If the spasm persists, implying a continuing source of deep pain, it results in a decrease in blood flow to the muscle leading to anoxia, and the accumulation of metabolic waste products which would normally be dispersed during relaxation. Fatigue and eventually pain in the muscle itself occur. Finally, internal changes take place in the muscle causing contracture.

An asymmetrical distribution of spasm may result in the classic deformity of a 'sciatic' scoliosis. Grieve (1981) postulated that this could be due to psoas spasm secondary to a vertebral joint disorder. Another example is unilateral spasm of sternocleidomastoid seen in some patients presenting with an acute 'wry neck'.

Neuromuscular Spindle

The *sensory* component important in the control of muscle contraction is the neuromuscular spindle. Each spindle consists of intrafusal and extrafusal muscle fibres. Intrafusal muscle fibres are innervated by both sensory and gamma motor neurones. Excitation by the gamma motor neurone causes contraction of the intrafusal fibres, which then applies tension to the sensory ending in the spindle, increasing activity in its nerve running to the spinal cord. This, in turn, increases contraction of the extrafusal fibres. This activity decreases muscle spindle activity. In some cases of voluntary movement, the activity in the alphamotor neurone may precede that in the gamma motor neurone, the spindle thereby detecting the degree of muscle contraction.

The gamma efferent system acts as a fine mechanism for adjusting the degree of contraction of the voluntary muscles. Changes in the gamma motor neurone activity reset the muscle spindles and the main muscle mass alters its degree of contraction to the new equilibrium position.

SPINAL REFLEXES

A spinal reflex is an involuntary response to a stimulus involving nerve pathways restricted to the spinal cord. Sensory nerves from the same and adjacent segments of the spinal cord give off branches which synapse with the anterior horn cells. Often there are one or more internuncial neurones along the route. Such synapses give rise to spinal reflexes which can cause muscular contraction even in the absence of higher control from the brain.

The stretch reflex is a simple spinal reflex involving only two neurones and one synapse. When a muscle is stretched, the stretch receptors in the muscle spindles are stimulated, and nerve impulses enter the spinal cord via the IA afferent nerves. These nerves synapse with the anterior horn cells supplying the same muscle, which responds with a short, involuntary contraction. The anterior horn cells are also under the influence of higher centres, and under normal circumstances the inhibitory component of the extrapyramidal system 'damps down' any spinal reflexes.

Maintenance of the upright standing posture depends on activation of the stretch reflex. The tendency is for the body to sway slightly the whole time. As it sways forwards, the muscles at the back of the legs are stretched, the muscle spindles are stimulated and, due to the stretch reflex, they contract, thereby bringing the body backwards. This then stretches the muscles of the front of the legs, the stretch reflex is stimulated, bringing the body forwards. Balance is, therefore, maintained by the alternate contraction and relaxation of these muscles.

In clinical practice, the stretch reflex is used to test conduction of certain spinal nerves, e.g. the knee jerk reflex is used to test the nerves supplying the quadriceps muscle. When the quadriceps tendon is tapped suddenly, the muscle spindles lying in the muscles are stimulated and the monosynaptic reflex causes the muscle to contract so that the knee is extended. The stretch reflex may be absent or depressed if the spinal nerve supplying the muscle is damaged due to a pathological process, e.g. osteophytic encroachment, disc prolapse. Inhibition from higher centres may be so great that it is difficult to elicit a knee jerk. This central inhibition can be reduced if the subject concentrates on some other voluntary movement, e.g. clasping his hands and then pulling outwards, whilst the test is being performed.

The mechanism of the stretch reflex may be used during treatment to stimulate voluntary contraction of a muscle. This principle is the basis of one of the proprioceptive neuromuscular techniques described by Voss *et al.* (1985).

SLOW AND FAST MUSCLE FIBRES

Most skeletal muscles show a mixture of two types of fibre known as Type I (slow) and Type II (fast) fibres (Gauthier and Schaeffer, 1974).

Type I These fibres are red, have a well-developed aerobic metabolism and are highly resistant to fatigue. They are adapted to produce a relatively slow, but repetitive, type of contraction which generates the sustained 'tonic' forces characteristic of postural muscles.

Type II These fibres are paler in colour and are called 'white'; they obtain energy primarily by glycolytic respiration, but are quite easily fatigued. These form the greater part of muscles which are primarily responsible for movement.

One type of fibre predominates in a muscle depending on its habitual activities.

TYPES OF MUSCLE CONTRACTION

There are two types of muscle contraction:

1. *Isometric* (from *iso-* = equal, and *-metric* = measurement) contraction occurs when a muscle contracts at a *fixed length*, creating tension at its attachments, but performing no external work (work being the product of force and the distance through which the force acts). The upper fibres of trapezius work isometrically to assist in stabilizing the scapula for the use of the upper limbs in activities such as typing. This type of muscle activity is usually termed *static* muscle work, as no external movement occurs.
2. *Isotonic* contraction occurs when there is an increase in intramuscular tension and a change in length of the muscle, either by shortening or lengthening, thereby performing work. This type of muscle activity is often called *dynamic* muscle work.

   If the muscle contracts isotonically in *shortening* to produce movement, drawing its attachments closer together, it performs *concentric* muscle work (*concentric* = *towards* the centre). The erectores spinae muscles work concentrically in the standing position during extension of the trunk from a flexed to a neutral position.

   If the muscle contracts isotonically in *lengthening*, the muscle attachments draw apart as it works to oppose the action of a force greater than that of its own contraction. It performs *excentric* or *eccentric* muscle work (*excentric from* the centre). For example, the erectores spinae work eccentrically from the erect standing posture when the trunk is slowly flexed. In this instance, these muscles are opposing the force of gravity.

The speed of action may influence which muscles work in a particular movement; for instance, in the last example, if the trunk is flexed at a more natural speed, the activity of erectores spinae is then absent except at the initiation and end of the movement.

If the aim is to re-educate fully a group of spinal muscles, consideration should be given to all of the different types of muscle work they have to perform during the everyday activities of the patient. Simply exercising the erectores spinae muscles concentrically fulfils only part of their normal function, and does not enhance their ability to work eccentrically.

STATIC AND DYNAMIC MUSCLE WORK

There are basic differences between static and dynamic muscle work.

Static

During static work, there is a rise of pressure within the muscles, which compresses the blood vessels, decreasing the amount of blood flowing into them in proportion to the force of contraction (Grandjean, 1971). When the applied force amounts to 60% of the maximum force, the blood supply is stopped completely; the muscle then receives neither sugar nor oxygen from the blood and it has to consume its reserves. In addition, waste products are not carried off but accumulate, causing acute pain from muscular fatigue. During a static effort of 15–20% of maximum, the blood supply to the muscle is thought to be normal. Static work with efforts of 50% and more of the maximum force can last for a minute at the most, while efforts of less than 20% will allow longer-lasting static muscular contractions. Static muscle work which demands a substantial effort in working life is, therefore, obviously unendurable and detrimental.

Static muscle work is less efficient (greater consumption of energy for smaller efforts) than dynamic muscle work.

Dynamic

In dynamic muscle work, contraction of a muscle is rhythmically followed by relaxation. Contraction causes an expulsion of blood from the muscle, and the subsequent relaxation allows a renewed flow of blood into the muscle. This increases the blood circulation to such an extent that it receives up to twenty times more blood during dynamic work than during static activity. During dynamic work, the muscle receives a good supply of sugar and oxygen which are rich in energy, and waste products are readily removed. So long as a suitable rhythm is chosen, dynamic work can be executed for a long time without fatigue.

RANGE OF MUSCLE WORK

Muscle fibres have the ability to shorten to almost half their resting length. Consequently, the arrangement of fibres within a muscle determines how much it can shorten when it contracts (Palastanga *et al.*, 1989). The muscular system is so arranged that habitual contractions involve only limited length changes in comparison with the overall length of the muscle.

The maximum excursion of a muscle that is possible, i.e. the amount of shortening and lengthening, is called the full range of muscle work. The terms inner, outer and middle range indicate in which part of the range the muscle contraction takes place.

Inner range is that nearest the point at which the muscle is shortest.

Outer range is that nearest the point at which the muscle is longest. If a muscle is very weak, a contraction is usually initiated more easily from stretch and, therefore, in its outer range.

Middle range lies between the two. This is the range in which muscles are most often used in everyday life and in which they are as a rule most efficient.

GROUP ACTIONS OF MUSCLES

Functionally, muscles work together in groups, although each muscle may have a specific role to play in relation to the action of the whole group. The integrated action of many groups is necessary for efficient movement to occur. The groups are named according to their function.

When muscles act to initiate and maintain a movement, they are classed as *prime movers* (or *agonists*). Muscles which would oppose such a movement are called *antagonists*. Except at the initiation and end of a movement, the antagonists usually remain quiescent, while the prime movers produce the movement.

When testing spinal movements, it is important to remember that virtually all of them are either opposed or assisted by the force of gravity. This has a profound effect upon the play of muscles during a particular movement. The activity of prime movers is always replaced by gravity whenever this is appropriate – in such cases the conventionally described role of muscles is often reversed.

Both prime movers and antagonists may contract together to hold a joint in one position, thereby acting as *fixators*. These muscles work to stabilize the position of a joint, often providing an immobile base from which other prime movers can act more efficiently. At the same time, the transarticular compression is increased.

When muscles pass over more than one joint, or with multiaxial joints, unrestrained contraction of the prime movers may produce additional unwanted movements. The contraction of *synergist* (*syn-* = with) muscles acting as partial antagonists to the prime movers eliminate these unwanted movements. For example, during trunk rotation, when the abdominals contract to produce the movement, they produce flexion simultaneously; multifidus, by producing extension (together with a small amount of rotation) balances the flexion moment generated by the abdominals, thereby acting synergically during rotation.

MUSCLE FATIGUE

Voluntary muscles become fatigued when contraction has been sustained for too long; anoxia and the accumulation of metabolites eventually cause the muscles to ache. These changes are, of course, normally offset by blood flow during the relaxation period, but sustained contraction causes a rise in intramuscular tension which tends to prevent the passage of blood. Even the postural muscles, which require less oxygen and can continue to contract for longer periods than the phasic muscles without fatigue, have their limit.

It is possible that prolonged contraction may lead to fibrous changes in the muscle.

MUSCLE DYSFUNCTION

In order for muscles to function efficiently, they must be supple and flexible, with an adequate blood and nerve supply. Any conditions depriving the muscles of these essentials will lead to an impairment of function, i.e. dysfunction.

Effects of Posture

During the mature lifespan of the individual, changes that occur in the soft tissues are largely adaptations to environmental factors

(Editorial, 1979). Mechanical stresses such as those imposed by prolonged asymmetrical postures have a marked effect on the muscles and soft tissues, causing fibroblasts along the lines of stress to multiply more rapidly and produce more collagen. These extra collagen fibres take up space in the connective tissue of the muscle, and begin to encroach on the space normally occupied by nerves, blood and lymphatic vessels. As a result of this trespass, the muscle loses its elasticity and may become painful when required to do work. In the long term, the collagen begins to replace the active fibres of the muscle. Since collagen is fairly resistant to enzyme breakdown, these changes tend to be irreversible.

Effects of Overuse/Misuse

Sustained muscle activity, as in strenuous exertion, leads to temporary swelling of the muscle, but this passes off unnoticed except in cases where the surrounding fascia is too tight, e.g. in the anterior tibial syndrome.

Excessive use of muscle will lead to hypertrophy; lack of use to atrophy. Certain occupations and activities, such as those which involve the persistent use of one arm as opposed to the other, as in operating machinery, can cause muscles to be overused. The effect may not necessarily be felt in the arm itself, but in the muscles which stabilize the scapula and vertebral column for the use of the arm, because of the fatiguing static contraction imposed on them. Excessive use of a particular muscle may also give rise to muscle imbalance (*see* p. 94–5).

Reductions in muscle flexibility may occur in sportsmen when defective training methods are used, and they are associated with a failure to take powerful joint movements to their extreme.

Trigger Points

The presence of spindle-shaped thickenings in muscle tissue is common, especially in the postural muscles. They used to be referred to as fibrositis – a misleading term because of the absence of inflammation in the muscle fibres – and they are now known as 'trigger points'. These are sustained contractions of isolated groups of muscle fibres; they lie in the line of the fibres and can be moved at right angles to them. They are tender on palpation.

There are several theories concerning their aetiology. The most likely causes are irritation of the nerve supply to the muscle, causing localized muscle spasm, or a reflex response to irritation of deeper structures which are supplied by the same segment. Although treatment directed at the cause is indicated in the early onset of these points, if they become chronic, then local treatment is also necessary.

Joint Disease or Trauma

The spinal muscles and joints are functionally interdependent. It therefore follows that dysfunction in either of them will sooner or later have an effect on the other. It has been shown that muscle dysfunction commonly accompanies degenerative joint disease (Jowett and Fidler, 1975). The presence of pain or a lesion in any element in the articular system influences the responses of the muscles controlling it, leading to altered patterns of movement which, in turn, perpetuate adverse strains.

The reverse mechanism can also occur, where muscle dysfunction precedes the joint problem. In people who are generally anxious and have excessive muscular tension, the compressive force across the joint surfaces is increased, and pain or strain eventually results from abnormal movement patterns.

When joints become stiff through trauma or disease, eventually the soft tissues surrounding them adapt by shortening. In some cases, this acts as a protective mechanism; for instance, if an intervertebral joint is mechanically unstable with excessive translatory movements, the soft tissues surrounding it will often eventually tighten (Kirkaldy Willis and Hill, 1979), and provide a certain amount of stability by limiting the available excursion of the joint.

In most cases, however, adaptive muscle shortening is undesirable and, when joint movement is restored by, for example, manipulation, it is essential that the flexibility and strength of the muscles controlling the motion segment are also regained as far as possible in order to restore motor coordination and function. The length to which a muscle is stretched before contraction has an effect on the strength of contraction (Thomas, 1975), which is why sportsmen stretch their muscles before performing.

Effects of Nervous Tension

Nervous tension has a profound effect on the physical body in chemical terms and also on the musculature. Whatever the cause of the tension – be it anxiety, depression, frustration or the general stresses of life – it expresses itself in muscular tension. The commonest site for this is in the cervical muscles at their attachment to the skull. Tension in the splenius capitis, semispinalis capitis, and trapezius gives rise to headache, neck ache, and shoulder ache. If the tension is maintained, pain is produced due to the accumulation of metabolites in the muscle. These metabolites can then be a source of irritation which perpetuates the contraction, thereby establishing a vicious cycle. Sustained tension can eventually lead to joint restrictions.

Neck pain which is due to tension can be relieved by manual treatment, but this may only be of temporary value unless the cause is also treated.

MUSCLE STRENGTH AND EXERCISES

It is of practical significance to the clinician whether or not having strong spinal and abdominal muscles is important in preventing back pain. Studies of spinal muscle strength in people with and without back pain vary in their findings but, in the main, show that in people with *chronic* back pain there is a reduction in strength when compared with normal subjects.

The lifestyle and occupation of each individual has a major effect on the strength of their musculature. Weak muscles render joints and their ligaments more vulnerable to strain, and it is clinically apparent that individuals who possess good neuromuscular function and are generally physically fit suffer less from certain types of spinal problems, such as the degenerative type of lesion, than individuals who sit for long periods during their working day and do minimal exercise. It must be stated, however, that partaking in some form of exercises, such as those in 'aerobic' classes, seem to precipitate back problems in some cases!

Appropriate exercise regimes to restore muscle strength can, in selected cases, be extremely beneficial to some patients. Good tone in the abdominal muscles is undoubtedly advantageous because of the important role they play in lifting (*see* pp. 117, 305–7). If real instability (*see* pp. 289–90) of a motion segment is present, exercises to improve its stability are vitally important in protecting it against strain during the activities of daily living. Unfortunately, there are various 'schools of thought' concerning spinal exercises: one school advocates giving flexion exercises to all patients with back pain, another advocates extension exercises. This indiscriminate use of exercises is unsafe and should be avoided. Incorrect use of exercises can aggravate a spinal disorder; in severe cases, it can even be the 'last straw' in prolapsing an intervertebral disc.

Careful assessment of the patient's condition by the therapist is necessary before prescribing even the most elementary spinal exercises, so that the aim of the exercise is clear: be it to strengthen muscles, stabilize joints, increase mobility, or relieve pain. An understanding of the patient's pathological condition is of paramount importance, and the *timing* of when exercises are given is equally so. For example, even if a patient does have weak abdominal muscles, there are times when specifically exercising them is contraindicated: all spinal muscular contractions lead to an increase in intradiscal pressure, which may be dangerous at a particular stage in the patient's pathology. Another example commonly seen in clinical practice is where hyperextension exercises have been given to a patient to ease a disc problem (*see* p. 68), but have caused pain in arthritic apophyseal joints.

The effects of collars and corsets on muscle strength are discussed on pp. 311–3.

MUSCLE IMBALANCE

There is normally an imbalance between the strength of the trunk extensors and flexors. The extensors are invariably dominant, the ratio being approximately 5:3 (Suzuki and Endo, 1983).

Habitually using certain muscle groups within a small and abnormally restricted amplitude of their available extensibility ranges can lead to them being in a state of overactivation, and hence they eventually shorten. Their antagonists respond by inhibition, weakness and lengthening. This process exaggerates the imbalance in the spinal muscles.

Muscles react in a consistent manner: those which tend to become tight are those which are stronger anyway, and they usually span more than one joint (Jull and Janda, 1987). A not uncommon finding in patients with chronic back pain is tightness of the hamstring muscles, which affects the biomechanics of the pelvis and, therefore, the lumbar spine. Typical patterns of exaggerated muscle imbalance can be found in the trunk. Muscles with a predominantly postural function shorten or tighten, while their antagonists, the phasic muscles, become weaker and tend to lengthen (Table 1). The reason for these differing reactions may be connected with the distribution of the two types of fibre in the muscles (see p. 87), although this has not been investigated thoroughly in man.

Exaggerated muscle imbalance may be caused by denervation, reflex inhibition due to pain or secondary to stress, or it may be imposed by ligamentous failure. Another cause appears to be the way in which the body is used. It is reasonable to assume, for instance, that a sedentary lifestyle could lead to tightening of the psoas muscles and weakening of the glutei. There is also the possibility of impaired control from the limbic system, which regulates muscle tone (Bannister, 1985) and which, in turn, can be influenced by emotional states.

One of the consequences of exaggerated muscle imbalance lies in its influence on the quality and control of movement. Tight muscles may be activated much more than is necessary during a particular movement (Jull and Janda, 1987), which lowers the degree of activation of muscles that would otherwise come into play, and establishes faulty movement patterns. Moreover, when an attempt is made to strengthen the inhibited and weakened muscles by resisting them, the results are disappointing. If, however, the length of the tightened muscles is regained by stretching them, a spontaneous disinhibition of the previously inhibited muscle occurs (Janda, 1978) and there is then a return to the normal responses when resistance is applied. This finding suggests that strengthening exercises for inhibited, weak muscles without first stretching their shortened antagonists may be ineffective.

Good control of movement also depends on adequate proprioceptive

Table 1
Muscle Imbalance

Postural muscles – tend to tighten
Sternocleidomastoid
Pectoralis major (clavicular and sternal parts)
Trapezius (superior part)
Levator scapulae
The flexor groups of the upper extremity
Quadratus lumborum
Erector spinae, perhaps mainly the longissimus dorsi and the rotatores
Iliopsoas
Tensor fasciae latae
Rectus femoris
Piriformis
Pectineus
Adductor longus, brevis and magnus
Biceps femoris
Semitendinosus
Semimembranosus
Gastrocnemius
Soleus
Tibialis posterior

Phasic muscles – tend to lengthen and weaken
Scaleni and the prevertebral cervical muscles
Extensor groups of the upper extremity
Pectoralis major, the abdominal part
Trapezius, the inferior and middle part
Rhomboids
Serratus anterior
Rectus abdominis
Internal and external abdominal obliques
Gluteal muscles (minimus, medius, maximus)
The vasti muscles (medialis, lateralis, intermedius)
Tibialis anterior
The peroneal muscles

(From Janda, 1976)

stimuli from muscles, joints, ligaments, skin, etc., as dysfunction in these structures reflexly affects motor control. The use of light corsets, backrests and adhesive strapping to the spinal extensors may well owe some of their effectiveness to proprioceptive stimulation of the skin.

CERVICAL MUSCLES

The cervical region is the most mobile in the spine. As well as producing and controlling the movements, the neck muscles have the important function of balancing the head on the neck. Many of the muscles are very small and deeply situated so that they are impossible to palpate in isolation.

During the coupled movements of lateral flexion and rotation in the lower cervical spine, the small, deep muscles also rotate the *cervical spine* to the *same* side. However, when the larger, superficial muscles attaching to the occiput (trapezius and sternocleidomastoid) contract unilaterally to produce lateral flexion, they also rotate the *head* to the *opposite* side.

The neck muscles contain a high proportion of afferent fibres – 80% – compared with most other striated muscles, which contain 50% (Abrahams, 1977). This makes them much more sensitive. Impaired function of the limbic system, such as that brought about by anxiety states, primarily affects these muscles (Bannister, 1985), and they react by going into spasm. This can cause a variety of symptoms not only in the neck, but also in the face and head. It is thought that it is one of the factors responsible for syndromes such as the tension headache. The area on the occiput which provides attachment for some of the neck muscles is a common site of pain and tenderness, which can be caused by spasm of the muscles pulling on the periosteum. Referred pain in the face, such as over the region of the temperomandibular joint, has also been noted clinically, due to spasm of cervical muscles. Movements of the jaw, as in chewing, are associated with static activity of the deep muscles in the upper cervical spine, and dysfunction in one will automatically affect the function of the other.

In modern times, the use of new technology such as word processors has resulted in a major problem regarding the neck – that of sustained static contraction, especially in the trapezius muscles (*see* p. 299). During examination and treatment, consideration of the static use of a patient's neck muscles may be of more significance in terms of pathogenesis than the dynamic use. Therapists in occupational health care are well aware of the importance of minimizing sustained static loads on the neck in employees who have to type for long periods.

In the following sections, the muscles are described in groups according to the prime movements they produce, without regard for their relative positions in the neck, after the style of Palastanga *et al.* (1989). During the examination of a patient's neck movements, it should be remembered, however, that the force of gravity may replace prime mover muscular activity, in which case the activity in the muscles will differ.

Muscles which flex the neck

- Longus colli
- Sternocleidomastoid
- Scalenus anterior (*see* p. 99)

Longus colli is the deepest of the anterior muscles and lies on the front and sides of the upper thoracic and cervical vertebral bodies. It has three sets of fibres:

1. *Inferior oblique* fibres – from anterior aspects of the 1st, 2nd and 3rd thoracic vertebral bodies – pass upwards and laterally to the anterior tubercles of the transverse processes of the 5th and 6th cervical vertebrae.
2. *Vertical fibres* – from the anterior part of the bodies of the upper three thoracic and lower three cervical vertebrae – to the anterior part of the bodies of the 2nd, 3rd and 4th cervical vertebrae.
3. *Superior oblique* fibres – from the anterior tubercles of the transverse processes of the 3rd, 4th and 5th cervical vertebrae – pass upwards and medially to the anterior tubercle on the anterior arch of the atlas.

NERVE SUPPLY
The ventral rami of C3, 4, 5 and 6.

ACTIONS
The main action of longus colli is flexion of the neck. The inferior and superior oblique fibres of one side also assist in laterally flexing the neck, and the inferior oblique fibres in rotating it to the opposite side.

Sternocleidomastoid (Fig. 3.1). Sternocleidomastoid has two

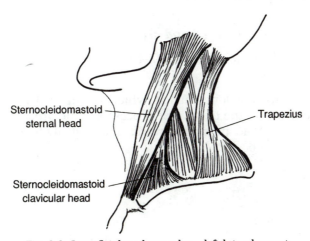

Sternocleidomastoid
sternal head

Trapezius

Sternocleidomastoid
clavicular head

Fig. 3.1 Superficial neck muscles – left lateral aspect. .

heads: the *sternal head* is attached to the upper part of the manubrium sterni; the *clavicular head* is attached to the upper surface of the medial third of the clavicle. The sternal head passes upwards, laterally and backwards; the clavicular head passes almost vertically upwards, behind the sternal head, blending with its deep surface. The sternocleidomastoid is attached by a short tendon into the lateral surface of the mastoid process of the temporal bone (especially the clavicular fibres) and lateral half of the superior nuchal line of the occipital bone (sternal fibres).

NERVE SUPPLY
The motor supply of sternocleidomastoid is by the spinal part of the accessory (eleventh cranial) nerve. It receives sensory fibres from the anterior rami of C2 and 3.

ACTIONS
Unilateral contraction of sternocleidomastoid laterally flexes the head on the neck, rotating it to the opposite side, and laterally flexes the cervical spine. The anterior fibres of the muscle are said to flex the head on the neck, while the posterior fibres may extend the head at the atlanto-occipital joint.

Bilateral contraction draws the head forwards and assists longus colli to flex the neck. If the head and neck are fixed, they assist in elevating the thorax in forced inspriation.

Spasm of sternocleidomastoid is a sigifinicant feature of several deformities seen in the neck. In *spasmodic torticollis* ('wry neck') shortening of this muscle is the deforming force, often accompanied by spasm of the clavicular portion of trapezius. In the deformity of *atlanto-axial rotatory fixation*, where there is fixation of the atlas on the axis in a rotatory position, the elongated sternocleidomastoid is in spasm (Fielding and Hawkins, 1978).

Muscles which flex the head and neck

- Sternocleidomastoid (*see* pp. 97–8)
- Longus capitis

Longus capitis is a long muscle which is attached below to the anterior tubercles of the transverse processes of the 3rd, 4th, 5th and 6th cervical vertebrae, passing upwards and medially to attach to the basilar part of the occipital bone.

NERVE SUPPLY
The ventral rami of C1, 2 and 3.

ACTIONS
Longus capitis flexes the head on the neck, and the upper cervical spine.

Muscles which flex the head on the neck

- Rectus capitis anterior

Rectus capitis anterior is a short muscle lying deep to longus capitis. It is attached to the anterior aspect of the lateral mass of the atlas up to the root of its transverse process, and passes upwards and medially to attach to the basilar part of the occipital bone.

NERVE SUPPLY
The ventral rami of C1 and 2.

ACTIONS
Rectus capitis anterior flexes the head on the neck. It may act as a postural muscle in stabilizing the atlanto-occipital joint.

Muscles which laterally flex the neck

- Scalenus anterior
- Scalenus medius
- Scalenus posterior
- Splenius cervicis
- Levator scapulae (*see* p. 106)
- Sternocleidomastoid (*see* pp. 97–8)

Scalenus anterior (Fig. 3.2) is attached to the anterior tubercles of the transverse processes of the 3rd–6th cervical vertebrae. Its fibres run almost vertically downwards to attach to the scalene tubercle on the 1st rib near the groove for the subclavian artery.

NERVE SUPPLY
The ventral rami of C4, 5 and 6.

ACTIONS
Unilateral contraction of scalenus anterior causes lateral flexion of the cervical spine to the same side, with a small amount of rotation to the opposite side. Bilateral contraction of the muscles produces flexion of the neck. If the upper attachment is fixed, scalenus anterior assists in elevating the 1st rib.

Scalenus medius (*see* Fig. 3.2) is the largest of the scalene muscles. Proximally, it is attached to the transverse process of the axis, often that of the atlas, and from the posterior tubercles of the transverse processes of the lower five cervical vertebrae. The fibres run downwards and laterally to be attached to the superior surface of the 1st rib just posterior to the groove for the subclavian artery.

NERVE SUPPLY
The ventral rami of C3–8.

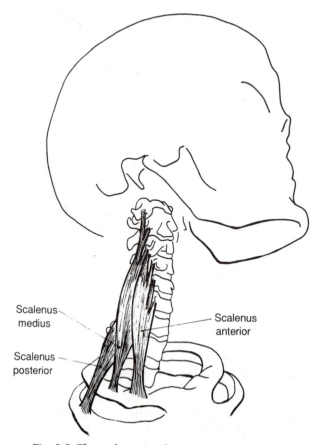

Fig. 3.2 The scalene muscles – anterolateral aspect.

ACTIONS

Unilateral contraction of scalenus medius produces lateral flexion of the cervical spine to the same side. If the upper attachment is fixed, it helps to elevate the 1st rib.

Scalenus posterior (*see* Fig. 3.2) is the smallest of the scalene muscles. Proximally it is attached to the posterior tubercles of the transverse processes of the 4th–6th cervical vertebrae. Its fibres run downwards and laterally to be attached to the outer surface of the 2nd rib.

NERVE SUPPLY

The ventral rami of C6, 7 and 8.

ACTIONS

Unilateral contraction of scalenus posterior produces lateral flexion of the lower part of the cervical spine to the same side. If its upper attachment is fixed, it helps to elevate the 2nd rib.

CLINICAL CONSIDERATION

Scalenus anterior and scalenus medius, together with the 1st rib, form the *scalene triangle*, through which the ventral roots of C5–T1 spinal nerves and the subclavian artery pass. These vessels are vulnerable to compression and may be affected by the presence of a cervical rib, a band of fascia, variations in the muscle attachments, or hypertrophy of the muscles, causing symptoms in the upper limb which simulate those from nerve root irritation and compression (*see* pp. 221–2).

The scalene muscles are active during inspiration, even during quiet breathing. In chronic respiratory conditions, the 1st rib may be elevated due to spasm in the muscles.

Splenius cervicis (Fig. 3.3) is attached distally to the spinous processes of the 3rd–6th thoracic vertebrae. Its fibres pass upwards and laterally to be attached to the posterior tubercles of the transverse processes of the upper three cervical vertebrae.

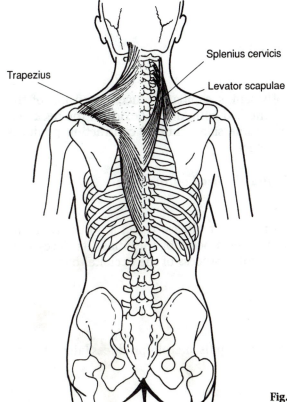

Trapezius

Splenius cervicis

Levator scapulae

Fig. 3.3 Trapezius, levator scapulae and splenius cervicis muscles.

NERVE SUPPLY
The dorsal rami of C5, 6 and 7.

ACTIONS
Unilateral contraction of splenius cervicis laterally flexes and slightly rotates the neck to the same side. Bilateral contraction extends the neck.

Muscles which laterally flex the head and neck

- Sternocleidomastoid (*see* pp. 97–8)
- Splenius capitis
- Trapezius (*see* pp. 105–6)
- Erector spinae (*see* pp. 123–130)

Splenius capitis lies deep to sternocleidomastoid and trapezius. Distally, it is attached to the lower half of the ligamentum nuchae, the spinous processes of the 7th cervical vertebra and upper four thoracic vertebrae. Its fibres run upwards and laterally to be attached just below the lateral third of the superior nuchal line, and mastoid process of the temporal bone.

NERVE SUPPLY
The dorsal rami of C3, 4 and 5.

ACTIONS
Unilateral contraction of splenius capitis produces extension of the head and neck, usually combined with lateral flexion of the neck and rotation of the face to the same side. Bilateral contraction produces extension of the head and neck.

Muscles which laterally flex the head on the neck

- Rectus capitis lateralis

Rectus capitis lateralis is a short muscle attaching distally to the upper surface of the transverse process of the atlas. Its fibres pass upwards to attach to the jugular process of the occipital bone.

NERVE SUPPLY
The ventral rami of C1 and 2.

ACTIONS
Unilateral contraction of rectus capitis lateralis produces lateral flexion of the head to the same side.

Muscles which extend the neck

- Levator scapulae (*see* p. 106)
- Splenius cervicis (*see* pp. 101–2)

Muscles which extend the head and neck

- Trapezius (*see* pp. 105–6)
- Splenius capitis (*see* pp. 102)
- Erector spinae (*see* pp. 123–130)

Muscles which extend the head on the neck

- Rectus capitis posterior major
- Rectus capitis posterior minor
- Obliquus capitis superior

With obliquus capitis inferior, these muscles are known as the *suboccipital* muscles.

Rectus capitis posterior major (Fig. 3.4) is attached distally to the spinous process of the axis and proximally to the lateral part of the inferior nuchal line of the occipital bone.

NERVE SUPPLY
The dorsal ramus of C1.

ACTIONS
Unilateral contraction of rectus capitis posterior major may rotate the head to the same side, but its main function is likely to be stabilization of the atlanto-occipital joint. Bilateral contraction produces extension of the head on the neck.

Rectus capitis posterior minor (*see* Fig. 3.4) is attached distally to the tubercle on the posterior arch of the atlas and proximally to the medial part of the inferior nuchal line of the occipital bone.

NERVE SUPPLY
The dorsal ramus of C1.

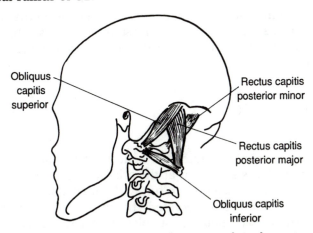

Fig. 3.4 The suboccipital muscles – posterolateral aspect.

ACTIONS

Rectus capitis posterior minor extends the head on the neck, and stabilizes the atlanto-occipital joint.

Obliquus capitis superior (*see* Fig. 3.4) is attached distally to the transverse process of the atlas, and proximally between the superior and inferior nuchal lines of the occipital bone lateral to semispinalis capitis.

NERVE SUPPLY

The dorsal ramus of C1.

ACTIONS

Obliquus capitis superior produces extension of the head on the neck and lateral flexion to the same side. It has an important role in stabilization of the atlanto-occipital joint.

Muscles which rotate the neck

- Semispinalis cervicis (*see* pp. 117–8)
- Multifidus (*see* pp. 122–3)
- Scalenus anterior (*see* p. 99)
- Splenius cervicis (*see* p. 101)

Muscles which rotate the head and neck

- Sternocleidomastoid (*see* pp. 97–8)
- Splenius capitis (*see* p. 102)

Muscles which rotate the head on the neck

- Obliquus capitis inferior
- Rectus capitis posterior major (*see* p. 103)

Obliquus capitis inferior (*see* Fig. 3.4) is the largest of the suboccipital muscles. It is attached distally to the spinous process of the axis and adjacent part of the lamina, and proximally to the transverse process of the atlas.

NERVE SUPPLY

The dorsal ramus of C1.

ACTIONS

Obliquus capitis inferior rotates the head to the same side. Bilateral contraction produces extension at the atlanto-axial joint.

The suboccipital muscles act to tune movements of the head finely. These muscles are highly innervated; the number of muscle fibres per neurone is small, each neurone supplying approximately 3–5 fibres.

These muscles are capable of rapid changes in tension, and they are able to control head posture with a fine degree of precision.

The suboccipital region is particularly prone to degenerative change, and the muscles have a strong tendency to tighten, resulting in the upper cervical spine being held in extension. In such instances, a compensatory flexion deformity often occurs in the lower cervical spine.

Muscles which Elevate the Shoulder Girdle

- Trapezius (upper fibres)
- Levator scapulae

Trapezius (*see* Figs. 3.1; 3.3) is the most superficial muscle in the cervico-thoracic spine. It is a large, triangular sheet of muscle extending from the occiput and spine medially to the pectoral girdle laterally. It is attached medially to the medial third of the superior nuchal line of the occipital bone, the external occipital protuberance, the ligamentum nuchae, and the spinous processes of the 7th cervical down to the 12th thoracic vertebra and connecting supraspinous ligaments. Its superior fibres pass downwards and laterally to be attached to the lateral third of the clavicle; its middle fibres pass almost horizontally to be attached to the medial margin of the acromion and spine of the scapula; its inferior fibres blend into an aponeurosis which is attached to the medial end of the spine of the scapula.

NERVE SUPPLY
Trapezius receives its motor supply from the accessory nerve (XI), and sensory branches from the ventral rami of C3 and 4.

ACTIONS
Trapezius has an important role both in stabilizing and moving the scapula during use of the arm, allowing a greater range of movement than would otherwise be possible. With serratus anterior, it rotates the scapula forwards so that the arm can be elevated. With the rhomboids, it acts to retract the scapula. With levator scapulae, its superior fibres elevate the scapula and maintain the posture of the shoulders when a heavy load is carried in the hand. In the unloaded arm, there is often little or no activity in the trapezius (Bearn, 1961).

When the scapula is fixed, the upper fibres of trapezius may laterally flex the neck to the same side and rotate it to the opposite side. Bilateral contraction produces extension of the head and neck.

CLINICAL CONSIDERATION
Spasm, tension or trigger points in the upper fibres of trapezius are common in patients with neck problems. Because of the rapid increase

in office automation, there is a growing tendency for operators of, for example, video display terminals to complain of pain, tenderness and stiffness in the neck (tension neck syndrome) due to sustained static loading of trapezius. The muscle's capacity for this type of work is very limited (*see* p. 299).

Levator scapulae (*see* Fig. 3.3) lies deep to sternocleidomastoid in its upper part and trapezius in its lower part. It is attached proximally to the transverse processes of the atlas and axis and the posterior tubercles of the transverse processes of the 3rd and 4th cervical vertebrae. Its fibres run downwards and laterally to be attached to the medial border of the scapula between its superior angle and the medial end of the spine of the scapula.

NERVE SUPPLY
The ventral rami of C3 and 4, and from C5 through the dorsal scapular nerve.

ACTIONS
Working with trapezius, levator scapulae helps to stabilize the scapula during movements of the arm. It helps to rotate the scapula so as to depress the point of the shoulder. When its proximal attachment is fixed, it assists in elevating the scapula. When its distal attachment is fixed, it laterally flexes the cervical spine and rotates it to the same side.

Bilateral contraction produces extension of the neck, working with trapezius.

MUSCLES OF RESPIRATION

- Diaphragm
- Intercostales
- Transversus thoracis
- Levatores costarum
- Serratus posterior superior
- Serratus posterior inferior
- Subcostales

These muscles all have some attachments to the ribs and, hence, are concerned in their movements and, consequently, respiration.

Diaphragm. The diaphragm is a musculotendinous sheet separating the thoracic from the abdominal cavity. Peripherally, its muscular fibres attach to the back of the xiphoid process, the internal surfaces of the cartilages and adjacent parts of the 7th–12th ribs, interdigitating with the transversus abdominis, from the medial and lateral arcuate ligaments and from the lumbar vertebrae by two crura.

The medial arcuate ligament is a thickening of the fascia covering psoas major; it is attached medially to the body of the 2nd lumbar vertebra and laterally to the transverse process of the 1st lumbar vertebra.

The lateral arcuate ligament is a thickening of the anterior layer of thoracolumbar fascia covering quadratus lumborum; it is attached medially to the transverse process of the 1st lumbar vertebra and laterally to the middle of the 12th rib.

The crura are attached to the anterolateral surfaces of the upper two (on the left) or three (on the right) lumbar vertebral bodies and their discs, and form an arch over the aorta.

These muscular fibres arch upwards and converge into a central strong aponeurosis or tendon, forming a dome-shaped sheet, which separates the thorax from the abdominal cavity. Openings in the diaphragm include those for the aorta, vena cava, oesophagus, splanchnic nerves and the sympathetic trunks.

NERVE SUPPLY
The diaphragm is supplied with motor and sensory fibres from the phrenic nerve (C3, 4 and 5). Additional sensory fibres to the periphery are supplied by the lower six intercostal nerves.

ACTIONS
The diaphragm is the main muscle of inspiration. On contraction of the muscle, the lower ribs are at first fixed, and the central tendon is drawn downwards and forwards, compressing the abdominal viscera which are prevented from bulging outwards by abdominal muscle tone. The central tendon then becomes the fixed point for the action of the diaphragm, which on further contraction elevates the lower ribs. The anterior ends of the vertebrosternal ribs are pushed forwards and upwards, elevating the sternum and upper ribs (see pp. 180–1).

The diaphragm also has an important part to play in increasing intra-abdominal pressure by resisting upward movement of the abdominal viscera on contraction of the abdominal muscles. It thereby assists in all expulsive actions such as coughing, sneezing, laughing, and prior to expulsion of faeces and urine, and of the fetus from the uterus. By this mechanism, it also supports the lumbar spine in lifting.

Intercostales (Fig. 3.5).   The intercostales are three thin layers of muscle lying between adjacent ribs.

Intercostales externi is the outer and thickest muscle layer. Its fibres pass from the lower border of the rib above to the upper border of the rib below, running obliquely downwards and medially anteriorly, and downwards and laterally posteriorly. Its attachments extend from the tubercles of the ribs posteriorly to the cartilages of the ribs anteriorly, where the muscle is replaced by the external intercostal membrane.

Intercostales interni is the middle muscle layer. Its fibres pass from the floor of the costal groove and costal cartilage of the rib above to the upper border of the rib below, running obliquely downwards and

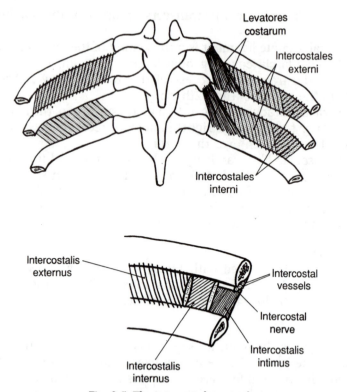

Fig. 3.5 The intercostales muscles.

laterally anteriorly, and downwards and medially posteriorly, at right angles to those of the intercostales externi. Its attachments may extend from the sternum to the costal angles posteriorly, where the muscle is replaced by the internal intercostal membrane.

Intercostales intimi is the deepest muscle layer. It runs from the internal aspects of two adjacent ribs in approximately the central two quarters. These muscles may be poorly developed or absent in the upper thoracic spine, but elsewhere in the thoracic spine they are better developed. The direction of muscle fibres is similar to that of the intercostales interni, from which they are separated by the intercostal nerves and vessels.

NERVE SUPPLY
The intercostales are supplied by the ventral rami of adjacent intercostal nerves.

ACTIONS
The actions of the intercostales are in dispute. Previously, it was considered that the intercostales externi elevated the ribs and were

thus inspiratory muscles, and that the intercostales interni depressed the ribs acting as expiratory muscles. As activity in the intercostales has been recorded during many trunk movements, it would seem that their role is to stabilize the thoracic cage.

Transversus thoracis (Sternocostalis). This muscle is located on the internal surface of the anterior part of the thorax. It is attached to the lower third of the deep surface of the sternum, xiphoid process and adjacent costal cartilages of the 4th–7th ribs. Its upper fibres pass upwards and laterally, while its lower fibres pass horizontally to attach to the inner surfaces of the costal cartilages of the 2nd–6th ribs.

NERVE SUPPLY
Transversus thoracis is supplied by the ventral rami of the adjacent intercostal nerves.

ACTIONS
Transversus thoracis depresses the costal cartilages, aiding expiration.

Levatores costarum (12 on each side) (*see* Fig. 3.5). The levatores costarum are small, strong bundles of muscle which lie between the 7th cervical and 11th thoracic vertebrae. Each muscle runs from the tip of the transverse process of the vertebra above to the rib of the next level below between the tubercle and angle. Each of the four lower muscles also has a second fasciculus attaching to the 2nd rib below its origin.

NERVE SUPPLY
Levatores costarum is supplied by the dorsal rami of the adjacent thoracic nerves.

ACTIONS
These small muscles elevate the ribs during inspiration. Acting from the ribs, they can also produce a slight degree of rotation and lateral flexion of the vertebral column.

Serratus posterior superior is a thin, quadrilateral muscle lying anterior to the rhomboids. Medially, it is attached to the lower part of the ligamentum nuchae, the spinous processes of the 7th cervical and upper three thoracic vertebrae and their supraspinous ligaments. The fibres pass downwards and laterally to be attached by four fleshy digitations lateral to the angles of the 2nd to 5th ribs.

NERVE SUPPLY
Serratus posterior superior is supplied by the ventral rami of the 2nd–5th intercostal nerves.

ACTIONS
These muscles could elevate the ribs to assist inspiration, but their role is unclear.

Serratus posterior inferior is a thin, quadrilateral muscle lying deep to latissimus dorsi. Medially, it is attached to the spinous processes of the 11th and 12th thoracic and 1st and 2nd lumbar vertebrae and their supraspinous ligaments via the thoracolumbar fascia. The fibres pass upwards and laterally to attach by four digitations into the lower four ribs, just lateral to their angles.

NERVE SUPPLY
The ventral rami of the 9th–12th thoracic spinal nerves.

ACTIONS
The serratus posterior inferior helps to pull the lower four ribs downwards and backwards, but its role is unclear.

Subcostales are usually best developed in the lower thoracic region. Each muscle passes from the internal surface of one rib near its angle to the internal surface of the 2nd and 3rd rib below. The direction of its fibres is the same as that of the internal intercostales.

NERVE SUPPLY
The ventral rami of the adjacent intercostal nerves.

ACTIONS
It is thought that the subcostales depress the ribs.

LUMBAR MUSCLES

The intersegmental nature of the deep back muscles (rotatores, multifidus, interspinales and intertransversarii), which connect adjacent vertebrae at appropriate angles, enables them to assist effectively in stabilizing the vertebral column. Because of their larger size, the superficial muscles of the back are better adapted to counterbalancing the external loads and to achieving the overall spinal posture and movement, but the quality of their performance is dependent on the integrated action of the deeper muscles.

Most of the back muscles are arranged more or less longitudinally, and, therefore, on contraction have a compressive effect on spinal structures in proportion to the strength of the contraction. Intradiscal pressure is particularly sensitive to differing strengths of muscle contraction, as is shown by increases recorded in certain postures and in lifting (*see* pp. 67–9 and 305).

Findings vary as to whether there is any difference in muscle strength in patients with low back pain compared to normal subjects. However, in patients with chronic low back pain, patterns of muscle imbalance can often be seen in this area, such as weakness of abdominal and gluteal muscles combined with tightness of erector spinae and psoas major. Not surprisingly, tests have shown that the abdominal muscles fatigue more easily than the back extensors, and this is even more marked in patients with back pain (Suzuki and Endo, 1983). However, Jull and Janda (1987) stress that attempts at strengthening weak muscles can prove futile, and their activity can decrease instead of increase, if the normal length of their tight antagonists is not regained first. Tightness of psoas major influences the mechanics of the lumbar spine, hip joint and sacroiliac joint, and may be one of the causative factors in this triad of joint problems which is not uncommonly seen in patients with chronic pain.

Where weakness of one muscle group exists, movement patterns alter in an attempt to accommodate for it, and so-called 'trick' movements occur. For instance, if gluteus maximus is weak, altering the pattern of hip extension which is, of course, a fundamental gait pattern, the hamstrings and erector spinae become overactivated. Similarly, in the trunk curl-up exercise, a tight psoas muscle can become the dominant prime mover over weakened abdominal muscles, making it essentially a hip flexion exercise, unless measures are taken to inhibit psoas activity by making the patient keep his feet on the couch while actively plantar flexing his ankles (Janda, 1983).

Muscle spasm, which initially usually has a protective function, can also be the primary mechanism involved in referred pain, e.g. spasm of piriformis associated with a sacroiliac lesion causing buttock and trochanteric pain (Kirkaldy Willis and Hill, 1979). Grieve (1981) has speculated that spasm of psoas major may sometimes be responsible for the deformity seen in a 'sciatic' scoliosis.

Muscles which produce flexion of the trunk

- Psoas major
- Psoas minor
- Obliquus externus abdominis ⎫
- Obliquus internus abdominis ⎬ the abdominal muscles
- Rectus abdominis ⎭

Psoas major (Fig. 3.6) is a long, deep muscle situated on the lateral aspect of the lumbar spine and the pelvic brim. It is attached proximally to the anterior surfaces of the transverse processes of all the lumbar vertebrae, the lumbar intervertebral discs and margins of their adjacent vertebral bodies (the highest being from the lower margin of the 12th thoracic vertebra; the lowest from the upper margin of the 5th lumbar vertebral body), and from fibrous arches between the above digitations, connecting the upper and lower margins of the vertebral bodies.

The muscle descends along the pelvic brim, passing posterior to the inguinal ligament and anterior to the capsule of the hip joint, having

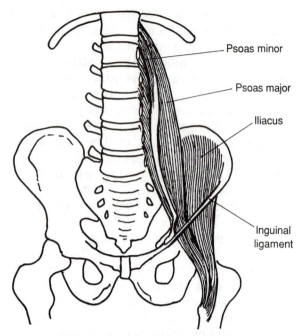

Fig. 3.6 Psoas and iliacus muscles.

received, on its lateral side, nearly all of the iliacus fibres. It converges into a tendon which is attached to the lesser trochanter of the femur.

NERVE SUPPLY
The ventral rami L1, 2 and 3. The lumbar plexus is situated posteriorly in the substance of the muscle.

ACTIONS
Acting from above with iliacus, psoas major flexes the hip joint. Its action in internal and external rotation, abduction and adduction of the hip joint is slight and somewhat variable, suggesting a stabilizing function.

Acting from below when the thighs are fixed, both psoas major muscles also have a powerful effect on flexion of the lumbar spine. In the 'sit-up' exercise, once the trunk has been raised slightly from the floor by contraction of the abdominal muscles, psoas major can then work to flex both the lumbar spine and hips. Unilateral contraction of the muscle when the thigh is fixed can also laterally flex the lumbar spine to the same side and produce contralateral rotation (Kapandji, 1974).

During quiet sitting, there is no activity in psoas major, but vigorous activity has been demonstrated in these muscles in controlling deviations of the trunk from the rest position, especially in lateral flexion of the trunk to the opposite side and leaning backwards (Keagy *et al.*, 1966). It is, therefore, probable that an important function of the muscle is as a trunk stabilizer. Marked activity has also been demonstrated when the foot is raised from the floor, as in lifting the foot to press the clutch pedal when driving.

During quiet standing there is no activity in psoas major, but it is active early in the swing phase in walking.

Spasm of psoas major may be one of the contributing factors in the classic deformity of a 'sciatic scoliosis' seen in some patients with intervertebral disc derangements or other pathology in the lumbar spine. The lumbar spine is held in a degree of lateral flexion and, usually, flexion, with a rotatory component.

Psoas minor (*see* Fig. 3.6) is inconstant. When present, it lies anterior to psoas major within the abdomen. It is attached proximally to the T12/L1 intervertebral disc and adjacent vertebral body margins and ends in a long tendon which is attached to the pecten pubis.

NERVE SUPPLY
The ventral ramus of L1.

ACTIONS
Psoas minor acts as a weak flexor of the lumbar spine.

Obliquus externus abdominis (Fig. 3.7) is the most superficial of the abdominal muscles and is situated on the anterolateral aspect of the abdominal wall. It is the strongest of the diagonal muscles. It is attached proximally to the external surface and inferior borders of the lower eight ribs and their costal cartilages, interdigitating with serratus anterior above and latissimus dorsi below.

The muscle fibres from the lower two ribs pass almost vertically downwards to attach to the anterior half of the iliac crest. Its upper and middle fibres pass downwards and medially to end in an aponeurosis which is broader below than above. The aponeuroses from both sides fuse in the midline at the linea alba, which runs from the tip of the xiphoid process of the sternum to the symphysis pubis. The lower border of the aponeurosis forms the inguinal ligament, extending from the anterior superior iliac spine to the pubic tubercle. An extension from the medial part of the inguinal ligament to the medial end of the pecten pubis is called the lacunar ligament.

NERVE SUPPLY
The ventral rami of the T7–12.

Obliquus internus abdominis (*see* Fig. 3.7). This muscle lies deep to the obliquus externus abdominis. Distally and laterally, it is attached to the lateral two-thirds of the inguinal ligament, the anterior two-thirds of the iliac crest and the thoracolumbar fascia.

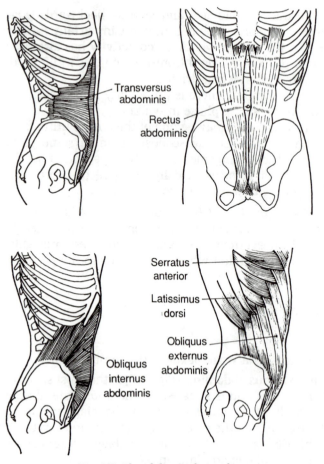

Fig. 3.7 The abdominal muscles.

Its posterior fibres pass upwards and laterally to attach to the inferior borders of the lower three or four ribs and are continuous with the intercostales interni; its middle fibres pass upwards and medially to attach to an *aponeurosis* (*see below*); the fibres from the inguinal ligament pass downwards and medially and, with the lower part of the aponeurosis of the transversus abdominis, form the conjoint tendon which attaches to the crest of the pubis and medial part of the pecten pubis.

The aponeurosis: In its upper two-thirds, the aponeurosis splits into two laminae at the lateral border of rectus abdominis. The laminae pass around rectus abdominis and reunite in the linea alba. The anterior lamina blends with the aponeurosis of the obliquus externus abdominis, while the posterior lamina blends with the aponeurosis of transversus abdominis. The upper part of the aponeurosis attaches to the cartilages of the 7th–9th ribs. In the lower third, the aponeuroses of the obliquus externus abdominis and transversus abdominis pass in front of rectus abdominis to the linea alba.

NERVE SUPPLY
The ventral rami of T7–12 and L1.

Rectus abdominis (*see* Fig. 3.7) is a long muscle running vertically on the front of the abdomen, separated from its fellow by the linea alba. It is attached distally by two tendons: to the pubic crest laterally, and to ligamentous fibres covering the front of the symphysis pubis. Proximally it attaches to the 5th, 6th and 7th costal cartilages. Laterally, it may extend to the 3rd and 4th costal cartilages and, medially, it occasionally attaches to the costoxiphoid ligaments and the side of the xiphoid process.

At three levels, transverse fibrous bands, known as tendinous intersections, cross the muscle fibres. They are normally situated opposite the umbilicus, the xiphoid process, and midway between the xiphoid process and the umbilicus. There may be incomplete intersections below the umbilicus.

The muscle is enclosed between the aponeuroses of the obliqui and transversus abdominis.

NERVE SUPPLY
The ventral rami of T6/7–12.

Muscles which raise intra-abdominal pressure

- Obliquus externous abdominis (*see* p. 113)
- Obliquus internus abdominis (*see* pp. 113–5)
- Rectus abdominis (*see* above)
- Transversus abdominis

Transversus abdominis (*see* Fig. 3.7) is the innermost flat muscle of the abdominal wall and has horizontally arranged fibres. It is attached laterally to the lateral third of the inguinal ligament, the anterior two-thirds of the iliac crest, the thoracolumbar fascia between the iliac crest and the 12th rib, and the internal aspects of the lower six costal cartilages, where it interdigitates with the diaphragm.

The muscle fibres pass horizontally around the abdominal wall to attach to an aponeurosis which blends with the linea alba. In the upper three-quarters it blends with the posterior lamina of the aponeurosis of the obliquus internus abdominis and passes behind rectus, whereas, in the lower quarter, it passes in front of rectus. The upper muscular fibres of transversus abdominis passing behind rectus are sometimes continuous in the midline with the transversus of the opposite side.

The lower fibres which attach to the inguinal ligament arch downwards and join with those of the obliquus internus abdominis to attach to the pubic crest and pecten pubis forming the conjoint tendon.

NERVE SUPPLY
The ventral rami of T7–12 and L1.

ACTIONS OF THE ABDOMINAL MUSCLES
Although the eight abdominal muscles (four on each side) work as a group during some activities, each also plays a more specific role, and this should be borne in mind when giving exercises aimed at strengthening them. The muscles form a firm elastic wall which helps to keep the abdominal viscera in place, the obliquus internus abdominis being particularly important for this purpose.

The combined action of the abdominal muscles has the effect of raising intra-abdominal pressure. This occurs as contraction of the muscles pulls via their aponeuroses on the rectus sheath and compresses the abdominal viscera. The oblique muscles play a much more significant role in this respect than the recti. The increase in intra-abdominal pressure plays an important part in expulsive efforts: the increased pressure on the bladder assists micturition; on the rectum, defaecation; on the stomach, vomiting; and during childbirth, the compressive force of the abdominal muscles helps to expel the fetus from the uterus. The significance of raised intra-abdominal pressure in lifting is discussed on pp. 305–7.

The abdominal muscles also assist in expiration, coughing and sneezing: when the diaphragm relaxes, it is pushed upwards by pressure on the viscera from contraction of the abdominal muscles; this increases the intrathoracic pressure so that, when the glottis is opened, air is expelled from the lungs. If the pelvis and spine are fixed, the act of coughing is further reinforced by the external obliques depressing the lower ribs and compressing the lower part of the thorax.

Electromyographic studies have shown that during most trunk movements in the standing and sitting positions, there is very little activity in the abdominal muscles. Depending on the location of the centre of gravity, in normal standing, there is either slight constant or intermittent activity in the abdominal muscles in about 25% of individuals; the remaining 75% show similar activity in the erectores spinae (Floyd and Silver, 1951). Activity is increased if considerable resistance is applied to the trunk and during extension from the upright position.

In the curl-up exercise from the supine to the sitting position, the recti are most important, and they contract as soon as the head is raised. Further flexion activates the obliques, but to a lesser extent. However, if the abdominals are weak in the presence of an overactive iliopsoas, the movement pattern of this exercise can be altered, and to reduce iliopsoas activity the hip joints should be flexed by at least 60°. If the thorax is fixed, the recti and obliques tilt the pelvis backwards and flex the lumbar spine (*see* pelvic tilting, pp. 132–3).

The oblique muscles show greatest activity in twisting and compressive actions. The external oblique rotates the trunk to the opposite side, the internal oblique to the same side, so that in rotation of the trunk to the right, for example, the right internal oblique works with the left external oblique to produce the movement. Unilateral contraction of the abdominal muscles laterally flexes the trunk to the same side.

Accurate electromyographic investigations on the transversus abdominis have proved difficult to carry out. Probably, it does not participate to any appreciable extent in the movements of the trunk, but through its attachments to the thoracolumbar fascia it has a stabilizing effect on the flexed lumbar spine and, therefore, assists in lifting (*see* p. 307). Together with the oblique abdominal muscles in particular, it also compresses the abdominal viscera and raises intra-abdominal pressure.

Muscles which produce rotation of the trunk

- Obliquus internus abdominis (*see* pp. 113–5)
- Obliquus externus abdominis (*see* p. 113)
- Multifidus (*see* pp. 122–3)
- Rotatores (*see* p. 131)
- Semispinalis

Semispinalis is present in the thoracic and cervical regions only and consists of three parts:

Semispinalis thoracis arises from the transverse processes of the 6th–10th thoracic vertebrae and attaches to the spinous processes of the upper two thoracic and lower two cervical vertebrae.
Semispinalis cervicis arises from the transverse processes of the upper 5–6 thoracic vertebrae and attaches to the spinous processes of the 2nd–5th cervical vertebrae.
Semispinalis capitis arises from the tips of the transverse processes of the upper 6–7 thoracic and 7th cervical vertebrae and from the articular processes of the 4th–6th cervical vertebrae. It attaches between the superior and inferior nuchal lines of the occipital bone. The medial part of this muscle is named spinalis capitis.

NERVE SUPPLY
The dorsal rami of the adjacent cervical and thoracic spinal nerves.

ACTIONS
Semispinalis thoracis and cervicis contract bilaterally to produce

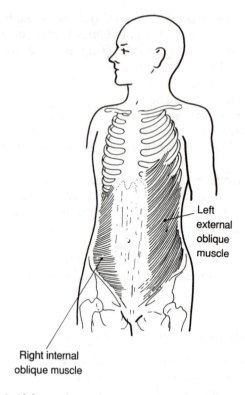

Left external oblique muscle

Right internal oblique muscle

Fig. 3.8 Abdominal muscles which rotate the trunk to the right.

extension of the thoracic and cervical vertebral column. Unilateral contraction causes rotation of the trunk and neck towards the opposite side.

Spinalis capitis extends the head and turns the face slightly towards the opposite side.

Thoracolumbar Fascia (Fig. 3.9)

The thoracolumbar fascia covers the deep muscles of the back of the trunk and is continuous above with the deep cervical fascia. In the lumbar spine, it consists of three layers which separate the muscles into three compartments.

1. The *anterior layer* is attached medially to the anterior surfaces of the lumbar transverse processes and intertransverse ligaments, inferiorly to the iliolumbar ligament and adjacent iliac crest, and superiorly it forms the lateral arcuate ligament. It covers the anterior surface of quadratus lumborum, lateral to which it blends with the other layers of the thoracolumbar fascia.

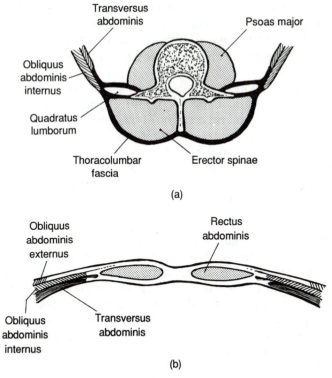

Fig. **3.9** The thoracolumbar fascia. (a) transverse section; (b) transverse section of anterior abdominal wall.

2. The *middle layer* is attached medially to the tips of the lumbar transverse processes and the intertransverse ligaments, superiorly to the 12th rib and inferiorly to the iliac crest. It lies behind quadratus lumborum and laterally gives rise to the aponeurosis of the transversus abdominis.

3. The *posterior layer* is attached in the midline to the lumbar and sacral spinous processes and to the supraspinous ligaments. It consists of two laminae: the fibres of the superficial lamina are directed caudomedially and provide attachment for latissimus dorsi, while those of the deep lamina are directed caudolaterally, giving the posterior layer a cross-hatched appearance (Bogduk and Macintosh, 1984). This deep lamina consists of bands of collagen fibres, which form a series of distinct ligaments which anchor the 4th and 5th lumbar and 1st sacral spinous processes to the posterior superior iliac spines, and the 3rd lumbar spinous process to the ilia via the lateral raphe. The laminae form a retinaculum over the back muscles, preventing their displacement dorsally (Bogduk and Twomey, 1987).

At the lateral margin of erector spinae, the middle and posterior layers form a dense union called the *lateral raphe*. They are joined by the anterior layer at the lateral border of the quadratus lumborum and give origin to transversus abdominis and part of the obliquus internus abdominis.

In the thoracic region, the thoracolumbar fascia is thin. It covers the extensor muscles of the trunk, separating them from the muscles which connect the vertebral column to the upper limbs. It is attached medially to the spinous processes of the thoracic vertebrae and laterally to the angles of the ribs.

The thoracolumbar fascia – in particular its posterior layer – plays an important role in the stability of the lumbar spine, especially in the flexed posture and in lifting, when it functions in three ways (Bogduk and Twomey, 1987):

1. The deep lamina fibres which connect the 4th and 5th lumbar vertebrae to the ilia play a *passive ligamentous role*. During lumbar spine flexion, these fibres are taut, and as the hips are extended and the pelvis rotated backwards during the return to the upright posture, the fibres help to transmit the force to the lumbar spine, and subsequently to the thorax, which can then be extended, assisting the lift. In this way, the deep lamina fibres complement the role of the interspinous and iliolumbar ligaments (*see* p. 307).

2. The connections of the posterior layer with the transversus abdominis through the lateral raphe allow this muscle to exert an *'antiflexion' effect* on the lumbar spine. This mechanism works in the following manner:

   > From any point in the lateral raphe, fibres from the superficial lamina pass downwards and medially, and from the deep lamina pass upwards and medially. Consequently, the posterior layer can be seen as consisting of a series of overlapping triangles of fibres with the apex of each triangle in the lateral raphe and the base, which is about two segments long in the midline. When lateral tension is applied to the apex of the triangle, it is transmitted upwards through the deep fibres and downwards through the superficial fibres to the corners of the triangle in the midline, tending to approximate them. This tension on the fascia can be exerted by contraction of transversus abdominis and to a lesser extent obliquus internus abdominis. It has the effect of resisting separation of the 2nd and 4th, and 3rd and 5th spinous processes and, therefore, flexion of these vertebrae. In this way, contraction of transversus abdominis when lifting braces the lumbar spine by resisting flexion of its lower vertebrae. The effect of abdominal muscle contraction

on raising intra-abdominal pressure is independent of this mechanism and is discussed on pp. 116, 306.

3. The third way in which the posterior layer stabilizes the flexed lumbar spine is through its retinacular structure and is called the *hydraulic amplifier mechanism* (Gracovetsky *et al.*, 1977). When the lumbar back muscles contract they shorten and expand. The posterior layer enveloping them resists the expansion, and tension develops within the fascia. This allows the back muscles to act synergistically with their fascia in resisting flexion.

In addition to contraction of transversus abdominis, this mechanism enables tension in the thoracolumbar fascia to be sustained throughout a lift.

Muscles which produce lateral flexion of the trunk

- Obliquus externus abdominis (*see* p. 113)
- Obliquus internus abdominis (*see* pp. 113–5)
- Rectus abdominis (*see* p. 115)
- Erector spinae (*see* pp. 123–30)
- Multifidus (*see* pp. 122–3)
- Quadratus lumborum
- Intertransversarii (*see* pp. 131–2)

Quadratus lumborum is a wide, quadrilateral muscle running between the ilium and 12th rib, deep to erector spinae. It is attached distally to the 5th lumbar transverse process, the iliolumbar ligament and adjacent iliac crest. The majority of its fibres are attached proximally to the medial half of the lower anterior surface of the 12th rib. The remaining fibres are attached to the anterior surface of the transverse processes of the upper four lumbar vertebrae.

NERVE SUPPLY
The ventral rami of the 12th thoracic and upper 3–4 lumbar spinal nerves.

ACTIONS
Quadratus lumborum acts as a muscle of inspiration by fixing the 12th rib, thereby stabilizing the origin of the diaphragm. Unilateral contraction produces lateral flexion of the lumbar spine to the same side. Bilateral contraction assists extension of the lumbar spine.

Muscles which produce extension of the trunk

- Quadratus lumborum (*see* above)
- Multifidus
- Semispinalis (*see* pp. 117–8)
- Erector spinae
- Interspinales (*see* p. 131)

Multifidus (Fig. 3.10) consists of a number of tendinous fascicles which lie deep to semispinalis and erector spinae, filling in the groove at the sides of the spinous processes of the vertebrae from the sacrum to the axis.

At each spinal level from the axis to L5 a fascicle arises from the caudal end of the spinous process. The fascicles diverge caudally and laterally and have different areas of attachment in the different spinal regions:

Sacral attachments: to the back of the sacrum as low as the 4th sacral foramen, to the erector spinae aponeurosis, the medial surface of the posterior superior iliac spine and the dorsal sacroiliac ligaments.

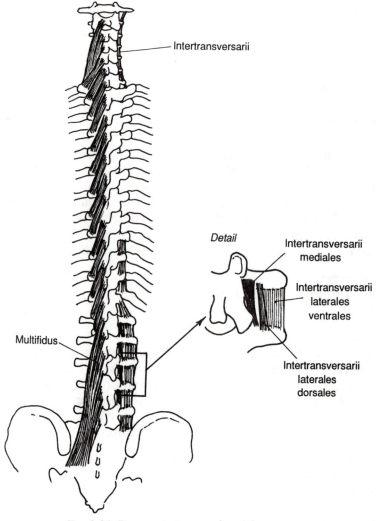

Fig. 3.10 Deep posterior muscles of the spine.

Lumbar attachments: **Short** fascicles arise from each lamina and insert into the mamillary process two levels below. The short fascicles from L5 attach just above the 1st dorsal sacral foramen. **Larger** fascicles attach onto the mamillary processes. It is noteworthy that some of the deeper fibres attach to the capsules of the apophyseal joints next to the mamillary process. These attachments prevent the joint capsules from being trapped inside the joints during movements executed by the multifidus.

Thoracic attachments: to all the transverse processes.

Cervical attachments: to the articular processes of the lower 4 or 5 vertebrae.

The fascicles at all levels vary in length, the longest extending over 3–4 vertebrae, while the shortest attach onto adjacent vertebrae.

NERVE SUPPLY
The dorsal rami of adjacent spinal nerves.

ACTIONS
The direction of the fibres is oblique, and therefore three actions may be possible:

1. When working bilaterally, multifidus may produce posterior sagittal rotation of its vertebra of origin, i.e. the 'rocking' component of extension, or control this component during flexion. Macintosh and Bogduk (1986) demonstrated that each fascicle of the lumbar multifidus is at right angles to its spinous process of origin and is ideally placed to do this, but is unable to produce the posterior translation which normally accompanies extension. While multifidus acts principally on individual spinous processes, some of its fascicles extend over several segments and have an indirect effect on the vertebrae interposed between its attachments. In the lumbar spine it has a bowstring effect which accentuates the lumbar lordosis.

2. Multifidus is active in contralateral and ipsilateral axial rotation of the trunk (Donisch and Basmajian, 1972). However, its role is not to produce rotation; the oblique abdominal muscles are better suited to do this, but when they contract they also simultaneously produce flexion. With the erector spinae, multifidus opposes this flexion effect, thereby maintaining pure axial rotation. It, therefore, acts during rotation as a stabilizer.

3. Multifidus is also active in lateral flexion of the trunk to the same side.

Erector spinae (Fig. 3.11) is a large, powerful musculotendinous mass consisting of three columns: iliocostalis, longissimus and spinalis. It extends from the dorsal aspect of the skull to the sacrum, lying

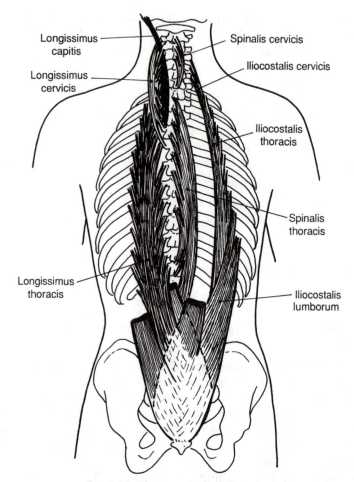

Fig. 3.11 The erector spinae muscles.

lateral to multifidus and forming the prominent contours on either side of the spine.

The erector spinae arises principally from a wide, flat *aponeurosis* which is attached to the 11th and 12th thoracic spinous processes, and the lumbar and sacral spinous processes, their supraspinous ligaments, the medial aspects of the iliac crests and the sacrum. The aponeurosis is mainly formed by the tendons of muscles acting on *thoracic* levels: longissimus thoracis and iliocostalis thoracis, but it also receives a few of multifidus's fibres from the upper lumbar spine. The lumbar fibres of erector spinae do not themselves attach to the aponeurosis, and it can consequently move freely over them, which suggests that they are able to act independently from the rest of the erector spinae.

From this extensive origin, the erector spinae passes upwards deep

to latissimus dorsi and in the upper lumbar spine splits into three
columns:

Lateral – iliocostalis
Intermediate – longissimus
Medial – spinalis

Each column also receives fibres from the different spinal regions, and
is itself divided into three parts.

1. **Iliocostalis**
   a. *Iliocostalis lumborum* has been described as having both lum-
      bar and thoracic components. The thoracic component, which
      is traditionally described, inserts, by flattened tendons, into the
      angles of the lower 8–9 ribs. In other words, this part of the
      muscle spans the lumbar spine, but has no direct attachment
      to it. More recent research (Macintosh and Bogduk, 1987)
      shows that there is a lumbar component to the muscle, called
      iliocostalis lumborum pars lumborum. These intrinsic lumbar
      fibres arise from the tips of the L1–4 transverse processes and
      the thoracolumbar fascia and insert independently of the
      erector spinae aponeurosis into the iliac crest and the posterior
      aspect of the posterior superior iliac spine. They constitute a
      substantial portion of the total muscle mass acting directly on
      the lumbar vertebrae.
   b. *Iliocostalis thoracis* arises medial to iliocostalis lumborum from
      the upper borders of the angles of the 7th–12th ribs and inserts
      into the upper borders of the angles of the 1st–6th ribs and the
      posterior aspect of the transverse process of the 7th cervical
      vertebra.
   c. *Iliocostalis cervicis* arises medial to iliocostalis thoracis from the
      angles of the 3rd–6th ribs and inserts into the posterior
      tubercles of the transverse processes of the 4th–6th cervical
      vertebrae.

NERVE SUPPLY
The dorsal rami of adjacent spinal nerves.

ACTIONS
Iliocostalis contracts bilaterally to extend the spine. In the case of
iliocostalis lumborum, bilateral contraction exerts an indirect
'bowstring' effect on the lumbar spine, causing an increase in its
lordosis.

Unilateral contraction of iliocostalis laterally flexes the respective regions of the spine to the same side. Iliocostalis lumborum,
in addition to laterally flexing the thoracic spine, also indirectly
laterally flexes the lumbar spine.

Iliocostalis lumborum has little effect on ipsilateral rotation because the distance between the ribs does not shorten very much. However, in contralateral rotation, this distance is greatly increased and the muscle can serve to derotate the thoracic cage and, therefore, the lumbar spine (Bogduk and Twomey, 1987).

Iliocostalis lumborum pars lumborum acts with multifidus in opposing the flexion effect, which occurs when the lumbar spine is rotated by the oblique abdominal muscles. As iliocostalis lumborum pars lumborum contracts to produce axial rotation, it simultaneously acts as an extensor.

2. **Longissimus**

a. *Longissimus thoracis*. This muscle is the largest of the erector spinae group. It is attached distally to the lumbar and sacral spinous processes and the sacrum between the spinous processes of the 3rd sacral vertebra and the posterior superior iliac spine. Its tendons form the main part of the erector spinae aponeurosis. Proximally, it is attached to the transverse processes of the 1st–12th thoracic vertebrae and between the tubercle and angle of the 2nd–12th ribs.

Intrinsic fibres of longissimus, called *longissimus thoracis pars lumborum* have been identified by Bogduk (1980), who refuted the standard description of the muscle and vindicated that by Charpy (1912). These fibres arise from the accessory and transverse processes of all the lumbar vertebrae and insert into the ilium, posterior superior iliac spine and sacroiliac ligament. They are covered by the lumbar intermuscular aponeurosis, an anteroposterior continuation of the erector spinae aponeurosis.

b. *Longissimus cervicis*. This muscle runs from the transverse processes of the upper 4–5 thoracic vertebrae to the posterior tubercles of the transverse processes of the 2nd–6th cervical vertebrae, medial to longissimus thoracis.

c. *Longissimus capitis* lies between longissimus cervicis and semi-spinalis capitis. It arises from the transverse processes of the upper 4–5 thoracic vertebrae and the articular processes of the lower 3–4 cervical vertebrae and inserts into the posterior margin of the mastoid process.

NERVE SUPPLY

The dorsal rami of the spinal nerves according to their position.

ACTIONS

Bilateral contraction of longissimus thoracis acts principally on the ribs and thoracic vertebrae, producing extension. It also acts indirectly on the lumbar spine, causing an increase in the lumbar lordosis. Unilateral contraction laterally flexes the thoracic spine and, thereby, indirectly the lumbar spine to the same side.

Bilateral contraction of longissimus thoracis pars lumborum produces lumbar extension, but because its attachments are closer to the axes of sagittal rotation, it is less efficient in this action than multifidus. The fibres of longissimus thoracis pars lumborum are so orientated that it also produces posterior translation of the vertebrae, more so at the lower lumbar levels, restoring the anterior translation that occurs during flexion.

Unilateral contraction of the muscle produces lateral flexion of the lumbar spine.

Bilateral contraction of longissimus cervicis produces extension of the cervical spine, while unilaterally it laterally flexes it to the same side.

Bilaterally, longissimus capitus contracts to extend the head on the neck. Unilaterally, it acts to turn the face towards the same side.

3. **Spinalis**
   a. *Spinalis thoracis* is the most clearly demarcated of the spinales and is attached distally to the spinous processes of a varying number of upper thoracic vertebrae (4–8), and proximally to those of the 11th and 12th thoracic vertebrae and the 1st and 2nd lumbar vertebrae.
   b. *Spinalis cervicis* is an inconstant muscle. When present, it is attached distally to the lower part of the ligamentum nuchae and the spinous processes of the 7th cervical vertebra and occasionally those of the 1st and 2nd thoracic vertebrae. It is attached proximally to the spinous process of the axis and sometimes those of the 3rd and 4th cervical vertebrae.
   c. *Spinalis capitis* is poorly developed and blends with semispinalis capitis.

NERVE SUPPLY
The dorsal rami of adjacent spinal nerves.

ACTIONS
The spinales extend the respective regions of the vertebral column.

ACTIVITY OF ERECTORES SPINAE
1. *During maintenance of posture.* Dysfunction in the erectores spinae muscles, such as through spasm or tightness, is often present in patients with back problems and, therefore, a more detailed account of its static postural role and its dynamic functions will have practical significance when considering the patient's activities of daily living and ergonomics.

In the normal *standing* position, there is very little erectores spinae activity, the mobile vertebral column being well balanced on the sacrum by joints and soft tissues. In about 75% of individuals, the line of gravity passes anterior to the 4th lumbar vertebra (Asmussen and Klausen, 1962) and consequently the erectores spinae show slight constant or intermittent activity as they counterbalance the tendency of the vertebral column to fall forwards (Floyd and Silver, 1951; 1955). Longissimus thoracis is more active than iliocostalis lumborum, suggesting that it has a greater postural role. The line of gravity may pass behind the lumbar spine in a significant number of individuals, and in these people abdominal muscle activity is recruited to prevent the vertebral column extending.

This low level of erectores spinae activity is increased when either the head or the upper limbs are moved forwards. If a load is held, erector spinae activity is also increased in proportion to its weight and the further in front of the body the load is held (Kippers and Parker, 1985). Holding a low density, light object can still necessitate increased erectores spinae activity if it is so large that, even when held close to the body, its centre of mass is a significant distance in front of it (Fig. 3.12).

When carrying a load, the distribution of the stresses in the spine is dependent on the position of the load. If it is carried high on the back, e.g. a rucksack, the trunk compensates by leaning forwards, so there is more erectores spinae activity than in normal standing. If the load is carried low on the back, erectores spinae activity decreases to less than in normal standing, but there is increased activity in psoas major, indicating that the load is causing the vertebral column to extend (Klausen, 1965). With knowledge of the muscular responses to the different positions in which a load can be carried, strategies can then be devised to rest muscle groups when they begin to fatigue.

When the centre of gravity is displaced sideways, as when holding a weight in one hand, the contralateral erector spinae contracts to prevent undesired lateral flexion.

Erectores spinae activity in *sitting* varies with the position. In an unsupported sitting position (without a backrest), activity in the lumbar erectores spinae is at a constant low level, but there is an increase in the thoracic erectores spinae activity. Muscle activity is greater in anterior sitting (leaning forward) than in posterior sitting. In supported sitting – when a backrest is used or the arms rest on a desk – erector spinae activity is reduced. The angle of the backrest has a significant influence; increasing its backward inclination reduces erectores spinae activity (*see* p. 301).

2. *During trunk movements from the upright position.* As the spine moves forward into flexion, there is an increase in erectores spinae activity in proportion to the angle of flexion. If a load is carried, activity in erector spinae increases proportionately with the size of the load (Andersson *et al.*, 1977).

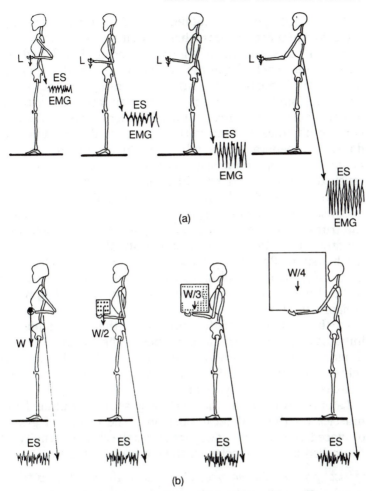

Fig. 3.12 Activity of erectores spinae. (a) a load (L) requires increased erectores spinae tension (ES) when it is held further in front of the body; (b) objects of different size and weight which require the same response from the erectores spinae when held in front of the body. The length of arrow (ES) indicates the erectores spinae tension relative to the weight of the object represented by the length of each arrow (W, W/2, W/3, W/4). (Modified from Tichauer, 1971, 1978.)

Gravity produces the movement, but its rate is controlled by erectores spinae and multifidus eccentrically contracting. Longissimus thoracis and iliocostalis lumborum control the movement of the thorax on the lumbar spine, anchoring them to the pelvis. In the lumbar region, multifidus, longissimus thoracis par lumborum and iliocostalis lumborum par lumborum also control anterior sagittal rotation and anterior translation of the lumbar vertebrae.

At about 90% of maximal flexion of the lumbar spine, a point is reached in most subjects where activity ceases in the erectores spinae. This is known as the *critical point* (Floyd and Silver, 1955). The vertebral column is then braced by the approximation of the apophyseal joints and tension in the posterior ligaments, but there is no active muscular protection of the spine or neuromuscular control of the movement. This implies, and is borne out clinically, that working in stooped postures is hazardous. As a general guide, when the finger tips are below knee height there is a high probability that the critical point has been reached (Watanabe, 1980). If a weight is carried, the critical point occurs later in the range of vertebral flexion.

Considerable erectores spinae activity occurs in extension of the trunk from the flexed position. Iliocostalis and longissimus act around the thoracic kyphosis to bring the thorax back on the lumbar spine. Posterior sagittal rotation of the lumbar vertebrae is brought about by multifidus which causes the superior surface of the lumbar vertebrae to be progressively tilted upwards to support the thorax.

Further extension of the trunk from the upright position is initiated by erectores spinae but, once the line of gravity has been displaced, the trunk moves under the effect of gravity and erector spinae activity ceases. If the movement is forced or resisted, the muscles come into play again.

Lateral flexion from the upright position is initiated by the muscles on the ipsilateral side; once the centre of gravity is displaced, the movement occurs under the effect of gravity and is controlled by the muscles on the contralateral side.

Intradiscal pressure during erectores spinae activity.   When the erectores spinae contract, they exert longitudinal compression on the lumbar vertebral column which raises the intradiscal pressure. Increased muscular activity through certain activities is associated with an increase in intradiscal pressure (*see* pp. 66–70).

In stressed, tense individuals, the normal resting muscle activity is higher than average (Lundervold, 1951). It therefore follows that intradiscal pressure would also be greater in these individuals.

Muscles which Stabilize the Spine

- Multifidus (*see* pp. 122–3)
- Rotatores
- Interspinales
- Intertransversarii

These deep, short muscles probably act principally as postural muscles, stabilizing adjacent vertebrae, and control their movements, allowing the longer, more superficial muscles to act efficiently.

Rotatores are best developed in the thoracic region where there are 11 on each side. Here they are attached distally to the upper and posterior part of the transverse process of the vertebra. The fibres pass upwards and medially to attach to the lower border and lateral surface of the lamina of the next vertebra above as far as the root of its spinous process.

In the cervical and lumbar regions, the rotatores are represented by variable muscle bundles with attachments similar to those in the thoracic region.

NERVE SUPPLY
The dorsal rami of adjacent spinal nerves.

ACTIONS
Theoretically, the rotatores can produce rotation at each spinal segment in the thoracic region, but their main function is probably stabilization of that part of the vertebral column.

Interspinales are short muscles lying on either side of the interspinous ligament. They connect the spinous processes of adjacent vertebrae between the axis and the 1st or 2nd thoracic vertebrae, and between the 11th or 12th thoracic vertebra and the 5th lumbar vertebra.

NERVE SUPPLY
The dorsal rami of adjacent spinal nerves.

ACTIONS
The interspinales produce posterior sagittal rotation of the vertebra above, and play a significant role in stabilizing the vertebrae during movement.

Intertransversarii (see Fig. 3.10, p. 122). The intertransversarii are small slips of muscle between the transverse processes of adjacent vertebrae in the cervical, lower thoracic and lumbar regions.

In the *cervical* region, they consist of anterior and posterior slips which are separated by the ventral rami of the spinal nerves. The posterior muscles are divisible into medial and lateral parts. The anterior muscles and the lateral parts of the posterior muscles connect the costal processes of adjacent vertebrae, while the medial parts of the posterior muscles connect the transverse processes. There are seven pairs of muscles between the atlas and the 1st thoracic vertebra.

In the *thoracic* region, they consist of single muscles connecting the transverse processes of the 10th thoracic and 1st lumbar vertebrae.

In the *lumbar* region, the intertransversarii consist of two muscles – *intertransversarii mediales* and *intertransversarii laterales*.

The intertransversarii mediales connect the accessory process and mamillary process of one vertebra proximally to the mamillary process of the vertebra below.

The intertransversarii laterales are divisible into anterior and posterior parts. The anterior part connects the margins of adjacent transverse processes, and the posterior part connects the accessory process of one vertebra to the transverse process below.

NERVE SUPPLY

The medial parts of the posterior transversarii in the cervical region, the thoracic intertransversarii and the intertransversarii mediales in the lumbar region are supplied by the dorsal rami of adjacent spinal nerves. The remainder are supplied by the ventral rami and are, therefore, not traditionally included among the back muscles which are all innervated by the dorsal rami.

ACTIONS

The intertransversarii on one side could theoretically produce lateral flexion to the same side of their respective regions. However, it is more likely that they function as stabilizing muscles during movement.

The cervical intertransversarii contain a particularly high density of muscle spindles (Abrahams, 1977), and it has been suggested that they act as large, proprioceptive transducers by monitoring spinal movements and providing feedback to the surrounding muscles, thereby influencing their action.

Muscles which Control Anteroposterior Pelvic Tilting (Fig. 3.13)

Forward tilting

- Erector spinae (*see* pp. 123–30)
- Psoas major (*see* pp. 111–3)

Backward tilting

- Rectus abdominis (*see* p. 115)
- Obliquus internus abdominis (*see* pp.113–5)
- Obliquus externus abdominis (*see* p. 113)
- Gluteus maximus
- The hamstrings:
    Semitendinosus
    Semimembranosus
    Biceps femoris

The exercise of tilting the pelvis on the femoral heads in an anteroposterior direction is frequently given in the treatment of low back pain. Imbalance between shortened and tight lumbar erectores spinae and psoas major muscles, and weakened gluteal and abdominal muscles is often evident in patients with low back pain.

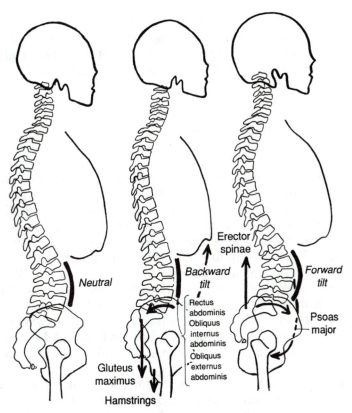

Fig. 3.13 Pelvic tilting.

Movement of the anterior part of the pelvis proximally is referred to as *backward* tilting, and distally as *forward* tilting. In the standing position, backward pelvic tilting is produced anterosuperiorly by concentric contraction of the recti and oblique abdominals, working posteroinferiorly with gluteus maximus and the hamstrings, which pull the posterior part of the pelvis downwards. At the same time, the lumbar spine is flexed and intradiscal pressure increased. Forward tilting is produced principally by erector spinae raising the posterior part of the pelvis. The lumbar lordosis is then increased and intradiscal pressure decreased.

The muscle work involved will, of course, vary depending on the starting position used.

Gluteus maximus is a powerful, quadrilateral muscle forming the prominence of the buttock. Proximally, it is attached to the gluteal surface of the ilium behind the posterior gluteal line, the posterior border of the ilium and adjacent part of the iliac crest, the aponeurosis of erector spinae, the posterior aspect of the sacrum, including the upper part of the sacrotuberous ligament, and the side of the coccyx.

Its muscle fibres pass downwards and laterally, the majority of the fibres (three-quarters) forming a separate tendinous lamina which narrows down and attaches to the iliotibial tract of the fascia lata. The remaining one-quarter of the muscle fibres attach to the gluteal tuberosity of the femur.

NERVE SUPPLY
The inferior gluteal nerve, L5, S1 and 2.

ACTIONS
When acting from the pelvis, gluteus maximus is a powerful extensor of the flexed thigh, laterally rotating it at the same time, and plays a major role in activities such as climbing the stairs and running, when it is intermittently active. In ordinary walking, the muscle shows some intermittent activity. Its upper fibres are active in powerful abduction of the thigh. When acting from its distal attachments, gluteus maximus working with the hamstrings helps to raise the trunk from a flexed position by rotating the pelvis backwards on the head of the femur. These muscles play an important role in balancing the pelvis on the femoral heads. Weakness of gluteus maximus combined with tightness of erector spinae promotes a forward tilting of the pelvis and can adversely affect both the static posture and dynamic function of this region.

Through its attachments to the iliotibial tract, gluteus maximus provides a powerful support on the lateral side of the knee. Its ability to rotate the femur laterally when standing assists in raising the medial longitudinal arch of the foot.

The hamstrings are the posterior femoral muscles – semitendinosus and semimembranosus (the medial hamstring) and biceps femoris (the lateral hamstring).

Semitendinosus.   The proximal attachment of this muscle is to the ischial tuberosity from a tendon shared with the long head of biceps femoris, and from an aponeurosis connecting the two muscles. The muscle fibres soon end in a long tendon which attaches to the upper part of the medial condyle of the tibia.

NERVE SUPPLY
The sciatic nerve through its tibial division, L5, S1 and 2.

Semimembranosus.   This muscle lies deep to semitendinosus. It is attached proximally to the ischial tuberosity by a tendon which spreads into an aponeurosis from which muscular fibres arise. It is attached distally mainly to the posterior aspect of the medial tibial condyle, but also sends slips in different directions, particularly upwards and laterally forming the oblique popliteal ligament.

NERVE SUPPLY
The sciatic nerve through its tibial division, L5, S1 and 2.

Biceps femoris. This muscle is situated on the posterolateral aspect of the thigh. Proximally it arises by two heads: a *long head* from the ischial tuberosity from a tendon shared with semitendinosus, and the lower part of the sacrotuberous ligament; a *short head* from the linea aspera on the femur and from the lateral supracondylar line. The fibres of the long head cross the sciatic nerve and receive those of the short head on its deep surface. The muscle gradually narrows down into a tendon which is attached to the head of the fibula, the fibular collateral ligament and the lateral condyle of the tibia.

NERVE SUPPLY
The sciatic nerve – the long head through the tibial part and the short head through the common peroneal part L5, S1 and 2.

ACTIONS OF THE HAMSTRINGS
The hamstrings act upon both the hip and knee joints. Acting from above, they flex the knee joint. Acting from below, the muscles, in particular biceps femoris, help to raise the trunk from a flexed position by extending the hip joint. They also play an important role in balancing the pelvis on the femoral heads. Working with the abdominal muscles anterosuperiorly and gluteus maximus posteroinferiorly, they can tilt the pelvis backwards, which consequently flexes the lumbar spine.

When the knee is flexed or the hip extended, biceps femoris can produce lateral rotation of the hip, and semitendinosus and semimembranosus can produce medial rotation.

The length of the hamstrings varies markedly in different individuals. In symptom-free subjects, straight-leg raising in the lying position can vary from 45–120°. Functionally, tight hamstrings indirectly have a marked effect on posture of the lumbar spine (*see* pp. 40, 300) by causing backward tilting of the pelvis. Spasm in the hamstrings often accompanies low back and/or leg pain.

Other Muscles which are Relevant in Spinal Disorders

- Latissimus dorsi
- Piriformis
- Rectus femoris

Latissimus dorsi (Fig. 3.14) is a large, flat, triangular sheet of muscle extending from the trunk to the upper arm. Although it is principally a muscle acting on the shoulder joint, a description of it is included here, because of the effect on the lumbar spine when the muscle is stretched.

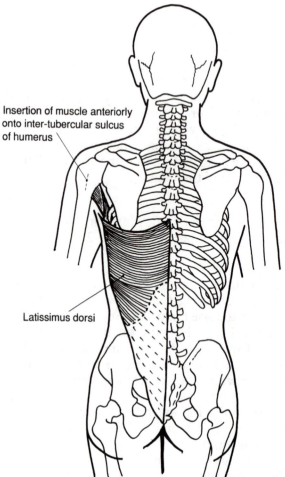

Insertion of muscle anteriorly
onto inter-tubercular sulcus
of humerus

Latissimus dorsi

Fig. 3.14 Latissimus dorsi.

It is attached distally by tendinous fibres to the spinous processes of the 7th–12th thoracic vertebrae anterior to trapezius, and from the posterior layer of thoracolumbar fascia which is attached to the spinous processes of all the lumbar and sacral vertebrae, supraspinous ligaments and iliac crest. It also has muscular fibres arising from the iliac crest, and is attached to the lowest 3–4 ribs, interdigitating with obliquus abdominis externus.

The muscular fibres of latissimus dorsi pass laterally and the lower ones almost vertically upwards to converge into a thick fasciculus. This crosses and attaches to the inferior angle of the scapula and then wraps round the teres major, forming with it the posterior fold of the axilla. It ends in a long tendon which is attached to the lower end of the intertubercular sulcus of the humerus.

NERVE SUPPLY

The thoracodorsal nerve, C6, 7 and 8.

ACTIONS

Latissimus dorsi is a strong adductor, extensor and medial rotator of the arm. With pectoralis major and teres major, it depresses the elevated arm against resistance as, for instance, in climbing, when these muscles pull the trunk upwards and forwards. It has an important function during the downstroke in swimming. Through its attachment to the ribs, it also takes part in all sudden expiratory movements such as coughing or sneezing.

If the arms are elevated in the prone-lying position, the latissimus dorsi muscles are stretched and tension is applied to the lower thoracic and lumbar spines through the thoracolumbar fascia. This is often undesirable when treating a patient, and to gain relaxation of the lower thoracic and lumbar spines, the arms should be lowered.

Piriformis is a triangular muscle lying deep inside the buttock, with its base within the pelvis and its apex posterior to the hip joint. Medially, its base is attached to the front of the sacrum between and lateral to the 1st and 4th sacral foramina, the gluteal surface of the ilium near the posterior superior iliac spine, the capsule of the sacroiliac joint and the pelvic surface of the sacrotuberous ligament. Its fibres pass downwards, laterally and forwards, through the greater sciatic foramen, narrowing into a tendon which is attached to the upper border of the greater trochanter of the femur. As the muscle passes out of the greater sciatic foramen, it lies just above the sciatic nerve, and is often pierced by its common peroneal portion.

NERVE SUPPLY

The ventral rami of L5, S1 and 2.

ACTIONS

Piriformis laterally rotates the extended thigh, and helps to stabilize the pelvis in the standing position. If the hip joint is flexed as in the sitting position, the muscle can abduct the thigh, for instance when getting out of a car.

Spasm or tightness of piriformis is sometimes one of the features of sacroiliac joint pathology.

Rectus femoris. This muscle is the part of the quadriceps femoris group which has an attachment to the pelvis. Its proximal attachment is by two tendons from the anterior inferior iliac spine and above the acetabulum and capsule of the hip joint. The two heads spread into an aponeurosis from which muscular fibres arise. About two-thirds of the way down the thigh, the muscle starts to narrow down into a thick tendon which is attached to the base of the patella.

NERVE SUPPLY

The femoral nerve, L2, 3 and 4.

ACTIONS

The quadriceps femoris is the main extensor of the knee joint. Rectus femoris can also assist in flexing the hip joint or, if the thigh is fixed, it helps to flex the pelvis. Tightness in the muscle can affect the mechanics of the pelvis and is sometimes associated with disorders of the sacroiliac joint.

REFERENCES

Abrahams V.C. (1977). The physiology of neck muscles; their role in head movement and maintenance of posture. *Can. J. Physiol. Pharmacol.*, **55**, 332.

Andersson G.B.J., Ortengren R., Nachemson A. (1977). Intradiscal pressure, intra-abdominal pressure and myoelectric back muscle activity related to posture and loading. *Clin. Orthop.*, **129**, 156.

Asmussen E., Klausen K. (1962). Form and function of the erect human spine. *Clin. Orthop.*, **25**, 55.

Bannister R. (1985). *Brain's Clinical Neurology*, 64th edn. London: Oxford University Press.

Bearn J.G. (1961). An electromyographic study of the trapezius, deltoid, pectoralis major, biceps and triceps muscles, during static loading of the upper limb. *Anat. Rec.*, **140**, 103.

Bogduk N. (1980). A reappraisal of the anatomy of the human lumbar erector spinae. *J. Anat.*, **131**, 525.

Bogduk N., Macintosh J.E. (1984). The applied anatomy of the thoracolumbar fascia. *Spine*, **9**, 164.

Bogduk N., Twomey L.T. (1987). *Clinical Anatomy of the Lumbar Spine*. Edinburgh: Churchill Livingstone.

Charpy A. (1912). Muscles de la region postérieure du tronc et du cou. In *Traité d'Anatomie Humaine*, 3rd edn. (Charpy A., Nicolas A., eds.) Paris: Masson, Vol. 2, Fasc 1, pp. 124–127.

Donisch E.W., Basmajian J.V. (1972). Electromyography of deep back muscles in man. *Am. J. Anat.*, **133**, 25.

Editorial (1979). Stay young by good posture. *New Scientist*, **82**, 544.

Feinstein B. (1977). Referred pain from paravertebral structures. In *Approaches to the Validation of Manipulation Therapy* (Buerger A.A., Tobis J.F., eds.). Springfield, Illinois: Thomas, p. 139.

Fielding J.W., Hawkins R.J. (1978). Atlanto-axial rotatory deformities. *Ortho. Clin. N. Am.*, **9**, 995.

Floyd W.F., Silver P.H.S. (1951). Function of erectores spinae in flexion of the trunk. *Lancet*, **i**, 133.

Floyd W.F., Silver P.H.S. (1955). The function of the erectores spinae muscles in certain movements and postures in man. *J. Physiol.* **129**, 184.

Gauthier G.F., Schaeffer S.F. (1974). Ultrastructural and cytochemical manifestations of protein synthesis in the peripheral sarcoplasm of denervated and newborn skeletal muscle fibres. *J. Cell Sci.*, **143**, 113.

Gracovetsky S., Farfan H.F., Lany C. (1977). A mathematical model of the lumbar spine using an optimal system to control muscles and ligaments. *Orthop. Clin, N. Am.*, **8**, 135.

Grandjean E. (1971). *Fitting the Task to the Man. An Ergonomic Approach.* London: Taylor & Francis.

Grieve G.P. (1981). *Common Vertebral Joint Problems.* Edinburgh: Churchill Livingstone.

Janda V. (1976). The muscular factor in the pathogenesis of back pain syndrome. Physiotherapy Symposium, Oslo.

Janda V. (1978). Muscles, motor regulation and back problems, 27. In *The Neurologic Mechanisms in Manipulative Therapy* (Korr I.M., ed.). New York: Plenum.

Janda V. (1983). *Muscle Function Testing.* London: Butterworths.

Jowett R.L., Fidler M.W. (1975). Histochemical changes in multifidus in mechanical derangements of the spine. *Orthop. Clin. N. Am.*, **6**, 45.

Jull G.A., Janda V. (1987). Muscles and motor control in low back pain: assessment and management. In *Physical Therapy of the Low Back* (Twomey L.T., Taylor J.R., eds.) Ch. 10. Edinburgh: Churchill Livingstone.

Kapandji I.A. (1974). *The Physiology of the Joints, 3, The Trunk and the Vertebral Column.* Edinburgh: Churchill Livingstone.

Keagy R.D., Brumlik J., Bergan J.L. (1966). Direct electromyography of the psoas major muscle in man. *J. Bone Jt. Surg.*, **48-A**, 1377.

Kippers V., Parker A.W. (1985). Electromyographic studies of erectores spinae: symmetrical postures and sagittal trunk motion. *Aust. J. Physiother.*, **3**, 95.

Kirkaldy Willis W.H., Hill R.J. (1979). A more precise diagnosis for low back pain. *Spine*, **4**, 102.

Klausen K. (1965). The form and function of the loaded human spine. *Acta Physiol. Scand.*, **65**, 1–2, 176–190.

Lundervold A.J.S. (1951). *Electromyographic Investigations of Position and Manner of Working in Typewriting.* Oslo: W. Brøggers Boktrykkeri A/S.

Macintosh J.E., Bogduk N. (1986). The biomechanics of the lumbar multifidus. *Clin. Biomechan.*, **1**, 205.

Macintosh J.E., Bogduk N. (1987). The morphology of the lumbar erector spinae. *Spine*, **12**, 7, 658.

Palastanga N., Field D., Soames R. (1989). *Anatomy and Human Movement*, Oxford: Heinemann Medical Books.

Suzuki N., Endo S. (1983). A quantitative study of trunk muscle strength and fatigability in the low back pain syndrome. *Spine*, **8**, 69.

Thomas V. (1975). *Exercise Physiology.* London: Crosby Lockwood Staples.

Voss D., Ionta M., Myers B. (1985). *Proprioceptive Neuromuscular Fascilitation*, 3rd edn. Philadelphia: Harper and Row.

Watanabe K. (1980). Biomechanical implications of EMG activity of erector spinae and gluteus maximus muscles in postural changes of the trunk. In *Biomechanics VII-B* (Morecki A., Fidelus K., Kedzior K. *et al.*, eds.). Baltimore: University Park Press, pp. 23–30.

4

Blood Supply of the Spinal Cord and Vertebral Column

BLOOD SUPPLY OF THE SPINAL CORD

The spinal cord has been described as a solitary integrated organ which extends nearly the whole length of the spine (Schmorl and Junghanns, 1959). The metabolic demands of the brain and spinal cord are high, and together they consume about 20% of the available oxygen in the circulating blood. The spinal cord grey matter has a higher metabolic demand than the white matter; consequently, blood flow within the grey matter is 15.4 times greater than in the white matter. If the blood flow to the spinal cord is occluded for three minutes, an infarct develops in its grey matter.

The blood supply of the cord is provided via the aorta, medullary feeder arteries, longitudinal arterial trunks of the cord, small arteries, arterioles, precapillaries and capillaries (Dommisse, 1986).

Longitudinal Arterial Trunks (Fig. 4.1)

The arterial supply of the cord is derived from one anterior and two posterolateral longitudinal arterial trunks (anterior spinal artery and posterior spinal arteries). The anterior longitudinal trunk lies over the anterior median sulcus. In its upper part, it communicates with the small anterior spinal arteries and branches of both vertebral arteries. The posterior longitudinal trunks are paired vessels extending the length of the cord. They pass around and between the posterior nerve rootlets. In their upper part, they communicate with the posterior inferior cerebellar branches of both vertebral arteries by means of two posterior spinal arteries.

Medullary Feeder Arteries

The longitudinal trunks are supplied and maintained by medullary feeder arteries. The site, number and source of origin of the medullary feeders varies in each individual. The medullary feeders are particularly numerous in the region of the brachial and lumbosacral plexuses.

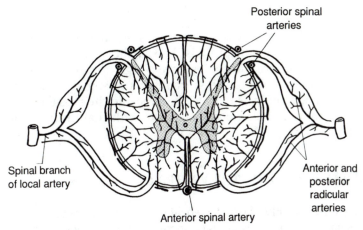

Fig. 4.1 Intrinsic arteries of the spinal cord – transverse section. (Adapted from P.L. Williams and R. Warwick, 1980. In *Gray's Anatomy*, 36th edn. Edinburgh: Churchill Livingstone, p. 896.)

There are relatively fewer medullary feeders in the thoracic region and, as it has the narrowest spinal canal lumen, it is a critical vascular zone. Medullary feeders arise from the segmental arteries and enter the intervertebral foramen to join the longitudinal arterial trunks on the cord surface.

Perforating Arteries

Three sets of perforating arteries penetrate the spinal cord:

1. Anterior perforating arteries arise from the anterior longitudinal arterial trunk and penetrate the median sulcus to supply the major portion of the cord substance. The anterior perforators are largest and most numerous in the region of the brachial and lumbosacral plexuses. The anterior perforators and anterior longitudinal arterial trunk are vital for normal function. Occlusion of these vessels will result in 'anterior spinal artery syndrome' with motor paralysis and impairment of thermal and pain sensations, although tactile and pressure senses are preserved.
2. Small posterior perforating arteries enter the cord substance with the posterior rootlets, and are distributed in the posterior one-third of the cord. They anastomose with the capillary plexus.
3. Small perforating arteries provide surface communications between the anterior and posterior perforating arteries. They also anastomose with the capillary plexus.

Capillaries of the Spinal Cord

An uninterrupted plexus of capillaries extends from the medulla oblongata to the conus medullaris. The capillary density is greatest in the grey matter where the nerves have a high metabolic demand. The dorsal root ganglia, spinal nerve rootlets and spinal nerves have an abundant blood supply. However, the supply to the dorsal root ganglia is particularly rich, being commensurate with that of the spinal cord grey matter.

ARTERIAL SUPPLY OF THE VERTEBRAL COLUMN

The arterial supply of the vertebral column is derived from branches of the segmental arteries. The cervical region receives branches from the vertebral and ascending cervical arteries; the thoracic column branches arise from the costocervical and posterior intercostal arteries; the branches to the lumbar region arise from the lumbar and iliolumbar arteries while the pelvis takes its supply from the lateral sacral arteries.

Lumbar Spine

Each lumbar artery passes laterally and back around the vertebral body until it reaches the intervertebral foramen. Branches of the lumbar arteries supply the vertebral bodies (*see* pp. 143–5).

Branches of the lumbar arteries

Just outside the intervertebral foramina each lumbar artery divides into several branches.

1. Anterior branches supply the abdominal wall.
2. Posterior branches supply the paravertebral muscles, the apophyseal joints and bony arch of the vertebral bodies.
3. Three spinal canal branches arise from the lumbar arteries opposite the intervertebral foramen.

   a. The *anterior spinal canal branch* enters the canal and bifurcates into ascending and descending branches. The ascending branch crosses the outer third of the intervertebral disc and joins the descending branch from the artery above. These branches form an arcade system on the anterior wall of the spinal canal.

   b. The *posterior spinal canal branches* are also disposed in an arcuate pattern, forming a closely woven network over the anterior surface of the lamina and ligamenta flava. Branches also pass to the laminae, spinous processes, extradural fat and the anterior plexus on the dura mater.

c. The third type of spinal canal branches are the *radicular branches* which supply the lumbar nerve roots.

Blood supply of the spinal nerve roots

The lumbar nerve roots are supplied, proximally, by vessels from the conus medullaris of the spinal cord and, distally, in the intervertebral foramina from radicular branches of the lumbar arteries.

At their attachment to the conus medullaris, the ventral and dorsal rootlets are supplied by five branches from the conus medullaris for a few centimetres. The remainder of the root is supplied by the proximal and distal radicular arteries.

The proximal radicular arteries arise from the anterior and posterior spinal arteries. Each proximal radicular artery passes with its root embedded in its own pial sheath. The artery enters the root, several millimetres from the spinal cord and follows one of the main nerve bundles along its length.

The radicular artery is a branch of the lumbar artery. It enters the spinal nerve, dividing into branches that enter the ventral and dorsal roots, becoming the distal radicular artery. The dorsal distal radicular artery forms a plexus around the dorsal root ganglion. The distal radicular artery passes proximally along the root until it meets and anastomoses with the proximal radicular artery.

Branches of the distal and proximal artery communicate with one another. These communicating branches are coiled (Parke and Watanabe, 1985). The arteries themselves are also coiled proximal and distal to the origin of these branches. These coils accommodate the stretching of the nerve root that occurs during lumbar spinal movements.

The nerve roots have proximal and distal radicular veins. The proximal veins tend to drain towards the spinal cord, while the distal veins drain towards the intervertebral foramina, where they anastomose with the lumbar veins. The radicular veins lie deep in the nerve and take a wavy course.

Blood supply of the vertebral bodies (Fig. 4.2)

The segmental arteries (lumbar arteries, intercostal arteries, deep cervical arteries) pass around the vertebral bodies, giving rise to ascending and descending branches called the *primary periosteal arteries*. These branches supply the periosteum of the vertebral bodies. Periosteal branches also arise from the anterior spinal canal arteries to supply the posterior wall of the vertebral bodies.

Interosseous arteries

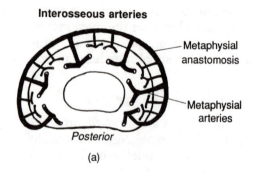

(a)

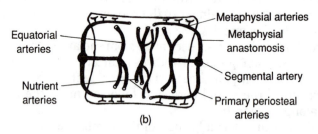

(b)

Interosseous veins of the lumbar vertebral bodies

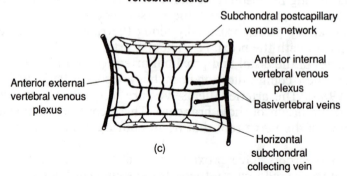

(c)

Fig. 4.2 Blood supply of the vertebral bodies. (a) transverse section of superior or inferior end of vertebral body; (b) frontal section through the middle of vertebral body. (After Ratcliffe, 1980); (c) sagittal section through a lumbar vertebra. (Adapted from H.K. Crock and H. Vashizaw, 1976.)

At the superior and inferior borders of each vertebra, the primary periosteal arteries form an anastomotic ring called the *metaphysial anastomosis*. Branches of this anastomosis, the *metaphysial arteries*, supply the superior and inferior borders of the vertebral body.

The centre of the vertebral body derives its blood supply from branches of the segmental arteries and the anterior spinal canal arteries.

Branches of the anterior spinal canal arteries are named *nutrient arteries*; they pierce the middle of the posterior surface of the vertebral body. Branches of the segmental arteries are named *equatorial arteries*; they pierce the anterior and lateral aspect of the vertebral body.

Branches of the nutrient and equatorial arteries form an arterial grid in the centre of the vertebral body. These branches form pathways towards the respective vertebral end plates.

During ageing, atherosclerosis of the arteries occurs, so that the lumen of the blood vessels is reduced or obliterated, resulting in a reduction or cessation of blood flow. Arteries which follow a tortuous course are particularly affected and the nutrient and metaphysial arteries of the vertebral bodies are among the first to undergo these changes. As ageing occurs, the periphery of the vertebral body, therefore, receives a better blood supply than the central region (Palastanga *et al.*, 1989). Reduced blood supply to the centre of the vertebral body will affect the nutrition of the centre of the intervertebral disc.

At the vertebral end plate, terminal branches of the metaphysial arteries and nutrient arteries form a dense capillary network in the subchondral bone. It has been noted in dogs that the capillary ends over the nucleus are large and globular, while the capillary terminals over the annulus fibrosus are smaller, less numerous and simpler in appearance (Crock and Goldwasser, 1984). Consequently, the blood supply to the nucleus is probably greater ensuring that nutrition of the centre of the disc is adequate.

The principal veins of the vertebral body are the *basivertebral veins* which are situated in the centre of the vertebral body. The basivertebral veins run horizontally in the middle of the vertebral body forming a large-scale venous grid into which the vertebral veins of the vertebral body flow from above and below.

The basivertebral veins drain primarily posteriorly into the anterior internal vertebral venous plexus. They also drain anteriorly into the anterior external vertebral venous plexus. The basivertebral veins receive vertical tributaries from the upper and lower halves of the vertebral body, and these tributaries receive oblique tributaries from peripheral parts of the vertebral body.

At the vertebral end plate, small vertical capillaries drain into a horizontal network of small veins that lie parallel to the end plate. This is the *subchondral postcapillary venous network*. Short veins drain from this plexus into a larger venous channel, the *horizontal subarticular collecting vein system*. This system of veins also lies parallel to the end plate. Veins from this network pass vertically towards the centre of the vertebral body.

Blood Supply of the Thoracic Spine and Ribs

Nine pairs of *posterior intercostal arteries* arise from the thoracic aorta and are distributed in the nine lower intercostal spaces. The 1st and 2nd intercostal spaces are supplied by the *superior intercostal artery.*

Branches of the posterior intercostal arteries

Muscular branches pass to the intercostal and pectoral muscles and to serratus anterior.

Lateral cutaneous branches pass with the lateral cutaneous branches of the thoracic nerves.

The *collateral intercostal branch* arises from the posterior intercostal artery near the angle of the rib. It crosses to the upper border of the rib below to anastomose with an intercostal branch of the thoracic artery.

Mammary branches arise from the arteries at the 2nd, 3rd and 4th spaces.

The *dorsal branch* passes back between the necks of the ribs superiorly and inferiorly, lateral to the vertebral body and medial to the superior costotransverse ligaments. Opposite the intervertebral canal, it gives rise to spinal canal branches. These branches (anterior spinal canal branch, posterior spinal canal branch, radicular branch) follow a similar course to those of the lumbar spine (*see* pp. 142–3) to supply the vertebra, spinal cord and nerve roots. The dorsal branch also supplies the paravertebral back muscles.

Blood Supply of the Cervical Column

Vertebral artery (Figs. 4.3; 4.4)

The vertebral artery has four parts:

Part 1. It arises from the upper and posterior area of the first part of the subclavian artery and runs backwards between longus colli and scalenus anterior. The vertebral vein and common carotid artery lie in front of it, and behind it lies the inferior cervical ganglion and the ventral rami of the 7th and 8th cervical nerves.

Part 2. It enters through the foramen transversarium of the 6th cervical vertebra and passes through each cervical vertebra to the foramen transversarium of the axis, where it passes upwards and laterally to the foramen transversarium of the atlas.

As it ascends, it is accompanied by a branch of the inferior cervical ganglion and a plexus of veins, which eventually form the vertebral vein. It lies in front of the ventral rami of the 2nd–6th cervical nerve roots and lateral to the joints of Luschka.

Part 3. The artery emerges from the foramen of the atlas, medial to rectus capitis lateralis, and curves backwards behind the lateral

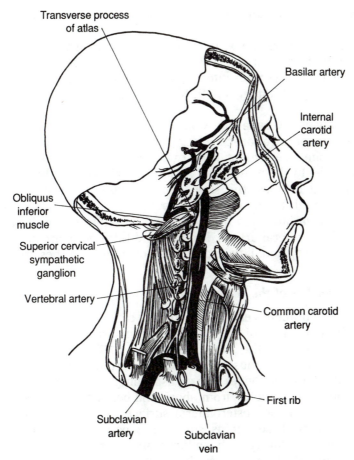

Transverse process
of atlas

Basilar artery

Internal
carotid
artery

Obliquus
inferior
muscle

Superior cervical
sympathetic
ganglion

Vertebral artery

Common carotid
artery

First rib

Subclavian
artery

Subclavian
vein

Fig. 4.3 Course of the right vertebral and carotid arteries. (Adapted from P.L. Williams and R. Warwick, 1980. In *Gray's Anatomy*, 36th edn. Edinburgh: Churchill Livingstone, p. 689.)

mass of the atlas with the ventral rami of C1 medial to it. The artery then lies on a groove in the posterior arch of the atlas and passes below the arched border of the posterior atlanto-occipital membrane to enter the spinal canal. The dorsal ramus of C1 lies between the artery and the posterior arch of the atlas.

Part 4.   After entering the spinal canal, the artery pierces the dura and arachnoid mater and inclines medially to the front of the medulla oblongata where, at the lower border of the pons, it unites with the opposite artery to form the basilar artery.

Variations of the vertebral artery

The origin of the artery may vary depending on side. On the left, it can originate from the arch of the aorta, between the left common carotid and subclavian arteries. Occasionally, it may arise from the descending aorta.

The artery enters the 6th cervical foramen transversarium – not infrequently it may enter via the 7th or 5th cervical vertebra, and it has even been reported entering the foramen as high as the 3rd cervical vertebra (Taitz *et al.*, 1978). This variation may or may not be symmetrical.

In a study of 150 cadavers, Stopford (1916) found that the vertebral arteries were of unequal size in 92% of instances. In 22 cadavers, the vessel on one side was at least twice the size of the vessel on the opposite side. In the presence of a marked difference in the calibres of the vertebral arteries, the supply to the basilar artery is virtually entirely through the dominant artery.

There are variations in the elastic and muscular tissues in different parts of the vertebral artery. The first and third parts are adapted for greater elasticity, mobility and the lack of support in these regions.

Spinal branches of the vertebral artery

The spinal branches enter the vertebral canal through the intervertebral foramina and divide into two branches. One branch passes along the roots of the nerve to supply the spinal cord and its membranes. It anastomoses with the other arteries of the spinal cord.

The other branch divides into an ascending and descending branch which join with branches from above and below to form two anastomotic chains on the posterolateral surfaces of the vertebral bodies. Branches from these chains supply the periosteum and vertebral bodies, communicating with similar branches from the opposite side. These communications give rise to small branches, which join similar branches above and below to form a central anastomotic chain on the posterior surfaces of the vertebral bodies.

Muscular branches of the vertebral artery

As the vertebral artery passes around the lateral mass of the atlas, muscular branches are given off and supply the deep muscles of the region.

Cranial branches of the vertebral artery

In the cranium, the main branches form the anterior and posterior spinal arteries.

The posterior inferior cerebellar artery is the largest branch of the vertebral artery in the cranium and supplies the lateral aspect of the medulla, choroid plexus of the 4th ventricle and the lower surface of the cerebellar hemisphere. Meningeal branches and the medullary artery also arise from the vertebral artery.

The two vertebral arteries unite at the lower border of the pons to form the basilar artery, and branches supply the medulla, pons, brainstem and cerebellum.

Circle of Willis (Fig. 4.4)

The vertebral arteries and the circulus arteriosus (circle of Willis) supply a large area of the brain.

The circle is situated at the base of the brain. It is formed in front by two anterior cerebral arteries which are joined together by the

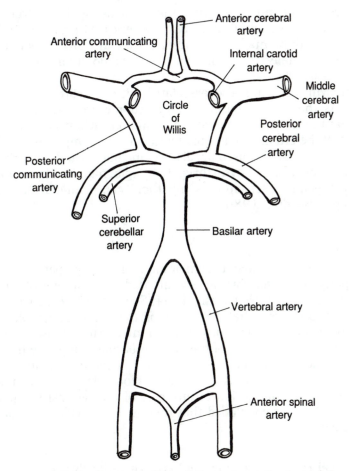

Fig. 4.4 Schematic view of principal arteries at the base of the brain. (Adapted from P.L. Williams and R. Warwick, 1980. In *Gray's Anatomy*, 36th edn. Edinburgh: Churchill Livingstone, p. 691.)

anterior communicating artery. Behind, the basilar artery divides into two posterior cerebral arteries, each of which is joined to the internal carotid artery of the same side by the posterior communicating artery.

The arteries forming the circle vary enormously and some are often absent: 60% of individuals have anomalies of the circle of Willis.

The direction of blood flow within the circle varies. Physical and chemical factors are thought to determine the direction of flow.

VERTEBROBASILAR INSUFFICIENCY

Symptomology

The vestibular nuclei receive their blood supply entirely from branches of the vertebral and basilar arteries (Fisher, 1967). If the blood flow to these nuclei is reduced, vestibular function is impaired. Dizziness is usually the commonest and predominant symptom of vertebrobasilar disease.

Other symptoms are also associated with vertebrobasilar insufficiency. As the vertebrobasilar arteries supply areas other than the vestibular nuclei, any accompanying symptoms will vary according to the area of the brainstem affected by ischaemia. Symptoms associated with vertebrobasilar vascular disease include visual disturbances, diplopia, 'drop attacks', dysarthria, dysphagia, nausea, ataxia, impairment of trigeminal sensation, sympathoplegia, hemianaesthesia and hemiplegia (Bogduk, 1986).

Pathology

It has been suggested that irritation of the sympathetic plexus accompanying the vertebral artery can produce symptoms of vertebrobasilar insufficiency (Neuworth, 1954; Stewart, 1962; Lewit, 1969). It was hypothesized that irritation of the sympathetic plexus by osteophytic encroachment or prolapsed intervertebral disc could lead to spasm of the distal part of the vertebrobasilar complex which may result in brainstem ischaemia. However, in experiments on monkeys (Bogduk et al., 1981), the vertebral blood flow was completely unresponsive to stimulation of any part of the cervical sympathetic system, and it was concluded that there was no evidence to support this theory.

Mechanical Factors Affecting the Vertebrobasilar System

Pathological changes in the cervical spine or within the vertebral artery may influence blood flow within the artery and hence the blood supply to the brain. These mechanical disorders may be classified as either intrinsic or extrinsic.

Extrinsic disorders are those which compress the external wall of the vertebral artery, thereby narrowing the lumen of the vessel and compromising the blood flow within it. Soft tissue thickening, lipping of the vertebral body, and osteophytic impingement are examples of mechanical factors which may impinge the vertebral artery or displace it. Displacement of the artery can be slight or so marked that the course of the artery is altered considerably and, consequently, the blood flow within it may be affected.

The vertebral artery is particularly susceptible to trauma at three locations:

1. During its ascent through the foramina transversaria, the vertebral artery may be subject to compression or angulation by osteophytes projecting laterally from the uncinate processes. In a review of the literature on vertebrobasilar insufficiency caused by uncinate osteophytes, Bogduk (1986) highlights several interesting points. Compression of the vertebral artery is seen most commonly at the C5/6 level with a lesser incidence at the C4/5 and C6/7 levels. When the neck is in the neutral position, osteophytic encroachment may or may not distort the vertebral artery but, as the neck is rotated, distortion of the artery is either produced or increased. In most instances the vertebral artery on the side to which the head is rotated is most likely to be affected by uncinate osteophytes. Dizziness is the commonest symptom of osteophytic impingement within the foramina transversaria. At operation, in addition to bony outgrowths, adhesions circumventing the vertebral artery have frequently been observed. Resection of the osteophytes is not always sufficient to restore adequate blood flow, and patency of the vessel may only be achieved by removal of the adventitial adhesions as well.

2. The atlanto-axial joint is the site where damage to the vertebral artery most frequently occurs. Stretching of the vertebral artery can occur if the atlas subluxes on the axis (e.g. in rheumatoid arthritis, aplasia of the odontoid process). In these cases, postmortem studies have shown thrombosis of the atlanto-axial section of the vertebral artery – thrombus formation is probably initiated by the distortion of the vessel (Webb *et al.*, 1968).

    The vertebral artery may be subjected to considerable stretching at the atlanto-axial joint during physiological neck movements. In an angiographic study of the vertebral arteries in a cadaver (Tatlow and Bammer, 1957), it was found that rotation of the head was accompanied by narrowing of the contralateral artery in its atlanto-axial segment. As the vertebral artery becomes stretched during physiological movement, the lumen of the vessel decreases and blood flow may be reduced or occluded.

    In its path through the foramina transversaria of the atlas and axis, the vertebral artery is relatively fixed. This fixity in combination with the large range of movement at the C1/2 joint makes the artery vulnerable to stretching at this point.

3. Damage to the vertebral artery may also occur at the occipito-atlanto joint. The artery lies on the posterior arch of the atlas and may be enclosed by an anomalous bony ring; this bony ring is present in one-third of the population and does not necessarily give rise to symptoms.

In the first part of the vertebral artery, three types of anomalies may compromise the vessel (Bogduk, 1986):

1. An anomalous origin of the vertebral artery from the subclavian artery so that during rotation of the neck the artery becomes distorted and occluded (Power *et al.*, 1961);
2. Bands of cervical fascia crossing the vertebral artery which constrict the vessel during rotation of the neck (Hardin and Poser, 1963);
3. An anomalous course of the artery between the fascicles of longus colli or scalenus anterior at their attachment to the C6 transverse process. During neck rotation the artery may be squeezed by the muscle bundles (Husni and Storer, 1967).

Atherosclerosis is the major *intrinsic* disorder to affect the vertebro-basilar system. Atheromatous changes have been noted in all the arteries of the body, and are commonly found in the vertebral and basilar arteries. In the vertebral artery, narrowing may occur at focal points due to the formation of isolated plaques or it may be more widespread so that considerable parts of its length are affected. These changes within the artery increase the likelihood of obstruction or stenosis occurring. If the vertebral artery is narrowed intrinsically due to arteriosclerosis, and it also becomes compromised by an extrinsic factor, such as osteophytic encroachment, blood flow will be particularly at risk.

Thrombosis of the vertebral and basilar arteries is a complication of atherosclerosis and emboli tend to lodge in the distal branches of the vertebrobasilar system, particularly the posterior cerebral artery (Fisher and Karnes, 1965).

Brown and Tatlow (1963) carried out angiographic studies on 41 cadavers to observe the effect of head positions on the vertebral arteries. They found extension alone did not affect the vertebral arteries, but rotation and extension together occluded the vessels in five specimens. When traction was applied with the head rotated and extended, occlusion was noted in 17 out of 21 specimens.

It is also noteworthy that in 24 out of 41 specimens, occlusion did not occur on rotation and extension of the neck. When occlusion did occur, in each case the artery on the contralateral side was occluded, and it was always at or above C2.

The use of traction in conjunction with manipulative procedures has been advocated (Cyriax, 1978) as it is thought to increase the safety of the procedure – the findings of Brown and Tatlow (1963) would seem to contradict this view.

The effect of head positions on the flow of perfused water within the carotid and vertebral arteries of cadavers was studied in an attempt to quantify the reduction of blood flow on neck rotation (Toole and Tucker, 1980). In most specimens, flexion, extension and rotation all affected the arterial flow, but rotation to less than 45° was the principal compromising manoeuvre. Whenever decreased flow was noted, a further 5–10° of movement occluded the vessel completely. Decreased flow was noted at points well within the normal physiological range of the neck. It was found that flow in the vertebral artery could be reduced to 10% of the initial rate by neck rotation.

In contrast, an *in-vivo* study (Hardesty *et al.*, 1963) measured vertebral blood flow during rotation of the neck in two patients and recorded a reduction in blood flow of 23% and 9% respectively.

Partial or complete occlusion of the vertebral artery, while compromising blood flow, will not be symptomatic unless there is a critical reduction in the blood supply to the brainstem. Angiographic studies on two patients who complained of dizziness and brainstem symptoms revealed that the contralateral vertebral artery was narrowed when the head was rotated, but that this position failed to reproduce the patient's symptoms of brainstem ischaemia (Barton and Margolis, 1975). Reduction of blood flow itself may not be critical in an individual with a normal healthy vertebrobasilar system, where adequate collateral flow is available. For example, occlusion of one vertebral artery in the neck may be compensated for by collateral blood flow from the opposite vertebral artery, the occipital artery, the ascending and deep cervical arteries and blood flow via the circle of Willis.

Symptoms of vertebrobasilar insufficiency are more likely to occur when the compensating mechanisms are not available due to congenital anomalies or concurrent disease (Bogduk, 1986).

It has already been noted that the vertebral arteries are of unequal size in 92% of individuals. Damage to or compression of the dominant artery may lead to brainstem ischaemia if the contralateral artery is unable to maintain an adequate blood supply. Studies have shown that when blood flow within one vertebral artery is occluded, symptoms of brainstem ischaemia have been produced when the contralateral artery is rudimentary or poorly filling (Husni *et al.*, 1966; Pasztor, 1978). These mechanical lesions may not have been symptomatic if the opposite artery had provided an adequate blood flow.

Clinical Implications

A number of cases of trauma to the vertebral artery following manipulative treatment have been reported (Kanshepolsky *et al.*,

1972; Parkin *et al.*, 1978; Fast *et al.*, 1987). Grant (1988) summarizes the details of 58 cases reported in the English language literature of vertebrobasilar complications following cervical manipulation.

Complications were experienced by young adults (mean age 37.3 years, range 7–63 years) and symptoms varied from transient light-headedness to infarction of the brain with neurological damage or death. In 45 cases, the neurological symptoms developed within minutes of the manipulative procedures being applied. The most frequent technique used was a rotation manipulation.

Angiographic data available for 32 subjects indicated that the atlanto-axial segment had been damaged in 19 instances. In 23 out of 26 subjects, cervical X-rays taken after the incident showed no abnormality or minor degenerative changes.

Another literature review of complications following cervical manipulation also highlighted that many of the subjects were at a young age (Krueger and Okazaki, 1980). They stated that there is a poor correlation between stroke after manipulation and the incidence of cervical spondylosis. Many of the patients were at an age when uncinate osteophytes are unlikely to be present. Any bony impingement is most likely to compromise the vertebral artery in its path through the foramina transversaria between C2–6, but the most frequent site of trauma in the subjects under review was the atlanto-axial segment of the vertebral artery. As there are no uncovertebral joints at the atlanto-axial segment, bony exostosis at this level is unlikely to be the cause of vertebrobasilar symptoms. Atheroma is also unlikely to be a significant factor in the young adult, and it has not been found to be a feature at autopsy in the subjects reviewed.

Experimental studies of atlanto-axial occlusion and premanipulative tests adopted by clinicians for patients with brainstem ischaemia use passive head rotation as the principal testing procedure. This manoeuvre differs from manipulative thrusts in two respects: force and speed. It seems probable that these two factors increase the likelihood of the intima tearing. It should be considered that a passive neck rotation test prior to manipulation will not give any indication as to the susceptibility of vascular injury to the vertebral artery on a forceful rotation.

Treatment techniques for the cervical spine should only be used in the full knowledge of contraindications to their use and after comprehensive examination and testing procedures have been employed. Grant (1988) gives a detailed account of dizziness testing and its application in treatment, concluding with the following statements:

1. There is always an element of unpredictability. Complications have arisen in patients even when premanipulative testing was negative or previous manipulative treatment was uneventful.
2. The test procedures themselves hold certain risks.

3. All dizziness testing should be fully recorded.
4. Patients should be made aware of risks involved in manipulative procedures (informed consent). The manipulative therapist may still be legally viable if commonly known screening measures are not employed.

VEINS OF THE VERTEBRAL COLUMN

The venous drainage of the vertebral column is derived from intricate plexuses that lie both inside and outside the vertebral canal. The veins of the plexuses do not have valves, hence the direction of blood flow is reversible. The plexuses anastomose with each other. Variations in the gross anatomy are common.

External Vertebral Venous Plexuses

These are most developed in the cervical region. The *anterior* external vertebral venous plexus lies in front of the vertebral bodies anastomosing with the basivertebral veins, intervertebral veins and tributaries from the vertebral bodies. The *posterior* external vertebral venous plexus lies over the posterior surfaces of the laminae, the spinous processes, the transverse processes and the articular processes. They anastomose with the internal vertebral venous plexus and end in the vertebral, posterior intercostal and lumbar veins.

Internal Vertebral Venous Plexuses

These are also known as Batson's plexus (Batson, 1940). These plexuses lie within the spinal canal and extend from the basiocciput to the coccyx. They subserve the venous drainage of the brain and spinal cord. The plexuses are orientated around the anterior and posterior walls of the spinal canal and are arranged as four longitudinal veins: two anterior and two posterior.

The *anterior* internal vertebral venous plexus lies on the posterior surface of the vertebral bodies and intervertebral disc on each side of the posterior longitudinal ligament. The veins are disposed in an arcuate system on either side, joining in the midline. The veins are thin-walled, but have a large calibre when distended. They anastomose with the basivertebral veins.

The *posterior* internal vertebral venous plexuses lie posterolaterally within the spinal canal and join in the midline.

The internal and external vertebral venous plexuses anastomose around the emerging nerve root at the intervertebral foramen.

These plexuses provide a place for storage of blood, but also allow outflow of blood under all conditions. A large proportion of the cardiac output is directed at the brain and spinal cord: inflow must be matched by outflow to maintain an effective circulation.

The plexuses act as pressure absorbers. Any unequal pressure in adjacent veins is quickly equalized. The plexus itself has no pressure, thereby ensuring that cerebral flow is not interrupted during normal conditions, e.g. breathing, coughing, sneezing.

These thin-walled sinuses can be a serious source of bleeding and are potential contributors to postoperative arachnoiditis and radiculo-pathy (Dommisse and Grobler, 1976).

The *basivertebral veins* emerge from the intervertebral foramina on the posterior surfaces of the vertebral bodies (*see* blood supply of vertebral bodies, p. 145). The veins enlarge in old age.

The *intervertebral veins* accompany the spinal nerves through the intervertebral foramina, draining the veins from the spinal cord and the internal and external vertebral venous plexuses. These veins end in the vertebral, posterior intercostal, lumbar and lateral sacral veins.

It is not known whether the intervertebral veins have effective valves, but experimental studies suggest that blood flow in them may be reversed (Batson, 1957). This may explain how neoplasms may lead to metastases in the vertebral bodies and spread from pelvis and lungs to the brain.

VEINS OF THE SPINAL CORD

The veins are situated in the pia mater. There are two *median longitudinal* veins, one in front of the anterior median fissure and the other behind the posterior median septum of the spinal cord.

Two anterolateral and two posterolateral longitudinal channels run behind the ventral and dorsal roots respectively. This plexus drains into the internal vertebral venous plexus.

Factors Influencing Blood Flow to Nervous Tissue

The spinal cord, dorsal root ganglia and spinal nerve roots are critical zones of vascular supply. Blood flow to these structures may be affected by congenital, traumatic, inflammatory, neoplastic, meta-bolic, degenerative or iatrogenic factors.

Spinal stenosis has been defined as narrowing of the spinal canal, nerve root canals or intervertebral foramina. It may be local, segmen-tal or generalized, and can be caused by bony or soft tissue narrowing (Arnoldi *et al.*, 1976). The spinal cord, dorsal root ganglia and spinal nerve roots may be compromised by spinal stenosis.

Lumen of the Spinal Canal (Fig. 4.5)

The cross-sectional area of the spinal canal varies in shape and dimensions in the different spinal areas. The canal is largest in the cervical spine and at the thoraco-lumbar junction. It becomes narrow between the 4th and 9th thoracic vertebrae, the narrowest point being at the 6th thoracic vertebra. The spinal column in this region is a critical vascular zone. A minimal reduction in the space will result in compression and ischaemia.

In the lumbar spine the vertebral canal is flattened in the anteroposterior direction, and wider laterally to accommodate the cauda equina.

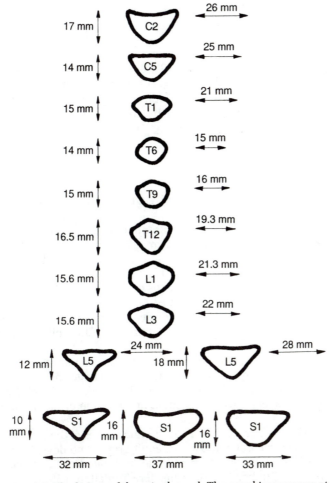

Fig. 4.5 The lumen of the spinal canal. The canal is narrower at the 6th thoracic vertebra. The narrow zone extends from T4 to T9 vertebral levels. (Adapted from G.F. Dommisse, 1986. The blood supply of the spinal cord. In *Modern Manual Therapy*, Grieve G.P., ed. Edinburgh: Churchill Livingstone, pp. 37–52.)

The Neural Canals

The spinal nerves and dorsal root ganglia are vulnerable within the neural canal. The length of the canal varies in the different spinal regions. In the cervical spine the neural canals are 10–15 mm in length, in the thoracic region the canals are just small openings, and in the lumbar region the canals are 20–35 mm in length.

In the lumbar spine, the neural canals contain many veins and arteries, the dorsal root ganglia and the spinal nerves. The contents of the canal may be compressed by soft tissue or bone, e.g. herniating disc, osteophytes. Compression of the neural structures will give rise to ischaemic pain and permanent fibrotic changes will occur if the pressure is not relieved.

Arachnoiditis

The dura mater is a highly vascular structure. If it is damaged following invasive procedures, e.g. surgery, myelograms, an inflammatory reaction takes place which results in permanent fibrotic changes. The spinal nerve sheaths are no longer patent – these changes are irreversible (Dommisse, 1986).

REFERENCES

Arnoldi C.C., Brodsky A.E., Cauchoix J. *et al.* (1976). Lumbar spinal stenosis. *Clin. Orthop.*, **115**, 4.

Barton J.W., Margolis M.T. (1975). Rotational obstruction of the vertebral artery at the atlanto-axial joint. *Neuroradiology*, **9**, 117.

Batson O.V. (1940). The function of the vertebral veins and their role in the spread of metastases. *Ann. Surg.*, **112**, 138.

Batson O.V. (1957). The vertebral vein system. Caldwell Lecture, 1956. *Am. J. Roentgenol. Radium Ther. Nucl. Med.*, **78**, 195.

Bogduk N. (1986). Cervical causes of headaches and dizziness. In *Modern Manual Therapy* (G.P. Grieve, ed.), Edinburgh: Churchill Livingstone **27**, 289–302.

Bogduk N., Lambert G., Duckworth J.W. (1981). The anatomy and physiology of the vertebral nerve in relation to cervical migraine. *Cephalalgia*, **1**, 1.

Brown B. St. J., Tatlow W.F.T. (1963). Radiographic studies of the vertebral arteries in cadavers: effects of position and traction of the head. *Radiology*, **81**, 80.

Crock H.V., Goldwasser M. (1984). Anatomic studies of the circulation in the region of the vertebral end-plate in adult greyhound dogs. *Spine* **9**, 702.

Cyriax J. (1978). *Textbook of Orthopaedic Medicine.* Vol. 1. *Diagnosis of Soft Tissue Injuries*, 7th edn. London: Baillière Tindall, p. 159.

Dommisse G.F. (1986). The blood supply of the spinal cord. In *Modern Manual Therapy* (Grieve G.P., ed.) Edinburgh: Churchill Livingstone, Ch. 4, pp. 37–52.

Dommisse G.F., Grobler L. (1976). Arteries and veins of the lumbar nerve roots and cauda equina. *Clin. Orthop., Relat. Res.*, **115**, 22.

Fast A., Zinicola D.F., Marin E.L. (1987). Vertebral artery damage complicating cervical manipulation. *Spine*, **12**, 9, 840.

Fisher C.M. (1967). Vertigo in cerebrovascular disease. *Arch. Otolaryngol.*, **85**, 529.

Fisher C.M., Karnes W.E. (1965). Local embolism. *J. Neuropath. Exp. Neurol.*, **24**, 174.

Grant R. (1988). Dizziness testing and manipulation of the cervical spine. In *Physiotherapy of the Cervical and Thoracic Spine*. Edinburgh: Churchill Livingstone, Ch. 7.

Hardesty W.H., Whiteacre W.B., Toole J.F. *et al.* (1963). Studies on vertebral artery blood flow in man. *Surg. Gynaecol. Obstet.*, **116**, 662.

Hardin, C.A., Poser C.M. (1963). Rotational obstruction of the vertebral artery due to redundancy and extraluminal cervical fascial bands. *Ann. Surg.*, **158**, 133.

Husni E.A., Bell H.S., Storer J. (1966). Mechanical occlusion of the vertebral artery: a new clinical concept. *J. Am. Med. Ass.*, **196**, 475.

Husni E.A., Storer J. (1967). The syndrome of mechanical occlusion of the vertebral artery. *J. Am. Med. Ass.*, **196**, 101.

Husni E.A., Storer J. (1967). The syndrome of mechanical occlusion of the vertebral artery: further observations. *Angiol.*, **18**, 106.

Kanshepolsky J., Danielson H., Flynn R.E. (1972). Vertebral artery insufficiency and cerebellar infarct due to manipulation of the neck. *Bull. Los. Ang. Neurol. Soc.*, **37**, 62.

Krueger B.R., Okazaki H. (1980). Vertebral-basilar distribution infarction following chiropractic cervical manipulation. *Proc. Mayo Clin.*, **55**, 322.

Lewit K. (1969). Vertebral artery insufficiency and the cervical spine. *Br. J. Geriatr. Pract.*, **6**, 37.

Neuworth E. (1954). Neurologic complications of osteoarthritis of the cervical spine. *N.Y. State J. Med.*, **54**, 2583.

Palastanga N., Field D., Soames R. (1989). *Anatomy and Human Movement: Structure and Function*. Oxford: Heinemann Medical.

Parke W.W., Watanabe R. (1985). The intrinsic vasculature of the lumbosacral spinal nerve roots. *Spine*, **10**, 508.

Parkin P.J., Wallis W.E., Wilson J.L. (1978). Vertebral artery occlusion following manipulation of the neck. *N.Z. Med. J.*, **88**, 441.

Pasztor E. (1978). Decompression of the vertebral artery in cases of cervical spondylosis. *Surg. Neurol.*, **9**, 371.

Power S.R., Drislane T.M., Nevin S. (1961). Intermittent vertebral artery compression: a new syndrome. *Surgery*, **49**, 257.

Schmorl G., Junghanns H. (1959). *The Human Spine in Health and Disease*. New York: Grune and Stratton.

Stewart D.Y. (1962). Current concepts of 'Barre syndrome' or the 'posterior cervical sympathetic syndrome'. *Clin. Orthop. Relat. Res.*, **24**, 40.

Stopford J.S.B. (1916). The arteries of the pons and medulla oblongata: part 1. *J. Anat.*, **50**, 131.

Taitz C., Nathan H., Arensburg B. (1978). Anatomical observations of the foramina transversaria. *J. Neurol. Neurosurg., Psychiatr.*, **41**, 170.

Tatlow W.F.T., Bammer H.G. (1957). Syndrome of vertebral artery compression. *Neurology*, 7, 331.

Toole J.F., Tucker S.H. (1960). Influence of head position on cerebral circulation. *Arch. Neurol.*, 2, 616.

Webb F.W.S., Hickman J.A., Brew D. St. J. (1968). Death from vertebral artery thrombosis in rheumatoid arthritis. *Br. Med. J.*, 2, 537.

5

Normal Movement

Normal movements between two adjacent vertebrae are relatively small, but the cumulative effect of these movements gives a considerable range to the vertebral column as a whole.

Numerous studies have attempted to measure intersegmental and regional spinal movement, but huge variations in 'normal' movement have been recorded. Figures 5.1 and 5.2 table the estimated range and representative degrees of rotation around three axes based on a review

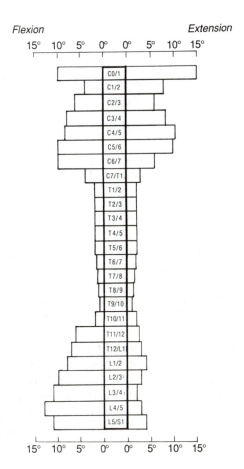

Fig. 5.1 Average ranges of segmental movement. These are *average* values. Wide variations occur according to age, body structure, pathology, etc. (*see* text).

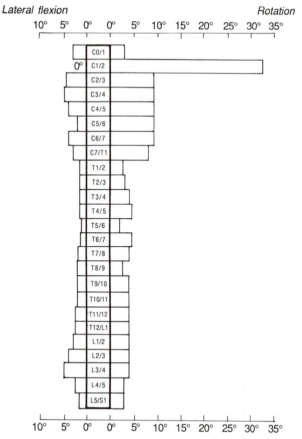

Fig. 5.2 Average ranges of segmental movement (values given are to *one* side). These are *average* values. Wide variations occur according to age, body structure, pathology, etc. (*see* text).

of literature and the authors' analysis (White and Panjabi, 1978a). Many factors influence movement, and variations in range recorded reflect differences in the age, race, sex, numbers of subjects and also differences in experimental design such as various methods of measurement, lack of reliability and validity, and errors in measurement.

Studies of cadavers have provided valuable insight into intersegmental motion, but it is not known how closely these movements reflect *in vivo* movement at the motion segment. Functional interdependence of the bony and muscular elements of the spine was highlighted by Campbell and Parsons (1944). Inevitably, normal muscle tone and muscles acting in their functional capacity as prime movers, antagonists and fixators will affect spinal movement. A precise, non-invasive *in vivo* measurement technique that carries no risk and allows three-dimensional analysis has yet to be developed. Clinically, it is useful to have a working knowledge of relative spinal ranges, but as there is considerable disparity in mean ranges recorded, too much emphasis should not be placed on these values. The essence of a good spinal examination is being able to observe movement abnormalities and relate these firstly to the patient's signs and symptoms, and secondly to what would be expected from that subject when age, sex, race and body type are taken into account.

Movement is often thought of as motion between two rigid vertebral bodies. Subchondral bone and articular cartilage deform equally under pressure (Radin *et al.*, 1970) and bone deformation contributes a small proportion to vertebral movement. If the bony posterior elements are fused, there is still enough plasticity in the bone anterior to the pedicles to allow movement between the vertebral body and disc on vertical loading. A posterior spinal fusion will, therefore, stabilize an unstable segment, but it will not completely immobilize the segment.

PLANES OF THE BODY AND AXES OF MOVEMENT (Fig. 5.3)

A three-dimensional coordinate system allows analysis and definition of any position or movement in space. There are three principal planes of the body. Each plane is perpendicular to the other two planes.

Planes
1. The *sagittal* or *median* plane is a vertical plane passing through the body, dividing it into right and left halves.
2. The *frontal* or *coronal* plane is a vertical plane, which divides the body into anterior and posterior halves.
3. The *horizontal* or *transverse* plane divides the body into an upper and lower half.

An external force acting on the spine can be resolved into component forces and movements acting along or about three axes. Each axis is perpendicular to the plane in which movement occurs.

Axes
1. The *vertical* axis is perpendicular to the ground (X axis).
2. The *frontal* axis passes horizontally from side to side (Y axis).
3. The *sagittal* axis passes horizontally from front to back (Z axis).

The movement of a mass around an axis is described as *rotation*. The

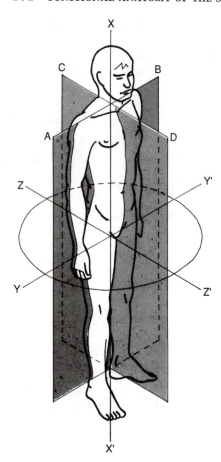

Fig. 5.3 Planes of the body and axes of movement. AB = frontal plane; CD = sagittal plane; ○ = horizontal plane; XX′ = vertical axis; YY′ = frontal axis; ZZ′ = sagittal axis.

axis may be inside or outside the rotating body. A body is in rotation when all particles along some straight line within the body (or hypothetical extension of it) have a zero velocity to a fixed reference point. A body is in *translation* when all particles in the body at a given time have the same velocity relevant to some reference.

A *degree of freedom* is motion in which a rigid body has the possibility of translating forwards and backwards along a straight line or rotating back and forward in a clockwise and counterclockwise direction about a perpendicular axis (White and Panjabi, 1978a).

At a segmental level, the vertebral body can move in the sagittal, vertical and frontal planes, and it also rotates around the three same axes. Each vertebral body, therefore, has six degrees of movement and can move in six different ways:

1. Glide forwards and backwards in the sagittal plane (i.e. anterior and posterior translation);

2. Tilt forwards and backwards around a frontal axis (i.e. anterior and posterior sagittal rotation);
3. Glide laterally in the frontal plane (lateral translation);
4. Tilt laterally in the frontal plane around a sagittal axis, e.g. during lateral flexion;
5. Distract and compress in the horizontal axis of the spine;
6. Rotate in a horizontal plane around a vertical axis (axial rotation).

When a vertebral body moves, the axis or 'centre of rotation' of the body is different from one instant to the next. This point around which movement occurs is termed the *instantaneous axis of rotation*. It represents a mean axis around which coupled accessory movements occur during motion in a cardinal plane.

At one instant, motion of a rigid body in three-dimensional space can be analysed as a simple screw motion. This motion is a combination of rotation and translation about and along the same axis. The axis has the same direction as the resultant of the three rotations given sequentially about the X, Y and Z axes. It describes movements among the three planes and is known as the *helical axis of motion*.

MOTION SEGMENTS (Fig. 5.4)

Between the skull and sacrum there are 25 levels at which movement may occur. The term 'motion segment' is used to describe an intervertebral disc and its articulations with the adjacent vertebral bodies above and below. The motion segment is the traditional unit of study in spinal kinematics.

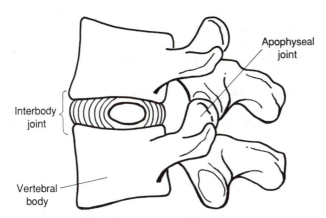

Fig. 5.4 The motion segment – lumbar region.

A typical motion segment consists of:

- Symphyses between the intervertebral disc and the adjacent vertebral bodies, i.e. the interbody joints
- Articular processes of the apophyseal joints
- Joints of Luschka (cervical spine only)
- Articulations of the ribs (thoracic spine only)

It should be noted that movement of any individual joint of a specific motion segment cannot occur in isolation. This is of particular significance in mobilization or manipulation of a spinal joint. Manual therapy directed at a specific apophyseal joint will inevitably result in movement of the other joints of that particular motion segment.

It has been suggested that movement at each motion segment is directly related to the proportion of disc height to vertebral body height (*see* p. 63). However, investigations of the relationship (in the thoracic spine) of the disc/body height ratio to the amount of movement did not show any significant correlation (White, 1969).

The direction of movement at each vertebral level is primarily determined by the orientation of the apophyseal joints. This varies in the different spinal regions. (For direction of apophyseal joints, *see* Ch. 1.) Other factors that also influence movement include the annulus fibrosus, longitudinal ligaments and the posterior bony elements.

The orientation of these joints does not exactly coincide with the plane of movement, and commonly two or more types of movement occur at the same time. Rotation or translation of a vertebral body about one axis is consistently associated with rotation or translation of the same vertebral body about another axis – this is known as *coupling*. For example, rotation of the spine is always accompanied by some degree of lateral flexion. Likewise, lateral flexion of the spine is accompanied by some degree of vertebral rotation (Stoddard, 1962).

When examining movement of the vertebral column, the combination of movements that normally occur must be considered. It is often inadequate and inaccurate to observe in isolation the physiological movements of flexion, extension, lateral flexion and rotation. All spinal physiological movements exhibit either coupled or 'tripled' movement, so in order to understand normal and abnormal movement patterns in relation to pathology, it is important that combinations of movement patterns are examined. It therefore follows that it may also be desirable to use a combination of movement patterns for treatment purposes.

REGIONAL CHARACTERISTICS OF NORMAL MOVEMENT

Movement in one direction may either restrict or allow movement in another direction.

Cervical Spine

Between C2–7, in neutral, in flexion or in extension, lateral flexion to one side makes rotation to the same side easier, e.g. lateral flexion of the neck to the right is accompanied by rotation to the right.

Thoracic Spine

Stoddard (1962) states that below the 3rd thoracic vertebra, if the spine is in neutral or extension, lateral flexion to one side is accompanied by rotation to the opposite side. When the thoracic spine is flexed, lateral flexion to one side is accompanied by rotation to the same side. In a series of cadaveric experiments, White (1969) demonstrated that in the upper thoracic spine, during lateral flexion, the vertebral body rotated axially into the concavity of the lateral curve. In the middle and lower thoracic spine the same pattern predominated, but was not as marked as in the upper thoracic spine. It was also noted in some cases that the reverse coupling occurred as axial rotation of the vertebra was towards the convexity of the lateral curve.

Lumbar Spine

In the upper four segments, axial rotation of the vertebrae is normally accompanied by lateral flexion to the opposite side, and lateral flexion is accompanied by rotation to the opposite side.

Conversely, at the joints between the 5th lumbar vertebra and the sacrum, axial rotation of the vertebra is accompanied by lateral flexion to the same side, and lateral flexion of the joint is accompanied by rotation to the same side (Bogduk and Twomey, 1987).

If there is any degree of tropism (*see* pp. 52–3) at the lumbo-sacral junction, the coupling of movements will be affected accordingly.

GENERAL CHARACTERISTICS OF NORMAL MOVEMENT

When one physiological movement has occurred, it has the effect of reducing other additional movements, for instance:

1. In flexion, the amount of lateral flexion and rotation possible is reduced;
2. Extension reduces the amount of lateral flexion and rotation possible;
3. Lateral flexion restricts flexion and extension;
4. Rotation restricts flexion and extension.

These characteristics of normal movement are of particular relevance in patients presenting with a spinal deformity. For example, lateral flexion and rotation to the opposite side will be reduced in a subject with a kypho-scoliosis. Similarly, flexion and extension will be reduced in a patient with a lateral deviation of the lumbar spine.

If treatment is aimed at gaining physiological range, it is essential that the patient is placed in a position that allows optimum gain in range. For example, if posteroanterior vertebral pressures are applied to lumbar spinous processes with the aim of increasing lumbar extension, the treatment is less likely to be effective if the patient has been carelessly positioned so that the pelvis is shifted to one side and the spine is not straight.

Normal mobility of the spinal column varies considerably. It may be influenced by one or more of the following factors: age, sex, ligamentous laxity, genetics, pathology.

Age

There is a decline in spinal mobility of all ranges with increasing age. As hormonal differences reduce with increasing age, the sexual differentiations in vertebral shape, posture and spinal range of movement disappear, so that in old age lumbar movement in men and women is almost identical (Twomey and Taylor, 1987). Histological and biochemical changes within the disc increase disc stiffness by as much as 40%, and this is associated with a decrease in physiological range. Changes that affect disc stiffness include an increase in the number of collagen fibres and in the ratio of Type I to Type II collagen, a change in the proteoglycan ratios and a subsequent decrease in water content. 'Fatigue failure' of the collagen in older cartilage may also occur, but it is unclear as to whether the individual collagen fibres fatigue or if the bonds between adjacent fibres break down (Stockwell, 1979). The ageing disc is less able to act as a shock absorber and transmit loads along the vertebral column.

Moll and Wright (1971) state that thoracic and lumbar mobility increases between the ages of 15 and 24. After 25, there is a general decrease in movement which may eventually decline by as much as 50%. In a study done on cadavers and living subjects, Twomey and Taylor (1987) also noted decreasing mobility in both the lumbar sagittal and horizontal planes after the age of 25.

Sex

There are conflicting views as to whether males or females have greater spinal mobility. Studies of a normal population of males and females showed that up to the age of 65 men had a greater total sagittal mobility, but after 65 women had greater total sagittal mobility (Sturrock et al., 1973).

Range of movement is greater when a combination of relatively greater disc height and relatively shorter vertebral end plates occurs. Disc heights in males and young adult females are the same but, as vertebral end plates in young female adults are shorter, the latter are more likely to have greater range of movement.

In a cadaveric study, Twomey and Taylor (1987) found that adolescent and young adult females had between 13–26% more sagittal mobility than males of the same age. Both sexes had substantially the same range of sagittal movement in middle-aged and elderly groups. However, young adults measured in a live study did not show the sex differential in the total sagittal range, which was demonstrated with the cadavers, suggesting that muscles play an important role in limiting the amount of possible movement.

Ligamentous Laxity

Ligamentous laxity causing hypermobility of a joint may be present as a single joint entity, or it may affect just peripheral joints or just spinal joints, or it may be generalized. There are various causes of ligamentous laxity, including an inherited disorder of collagen synthesis secondary to a hypomobile area, or due to degenerative processes.

In a survey of the diagnoses of 9275 consecutive patients attending a rheumatology clinic, 2% (185) were diagnosed as suffering from the hypermobility syndrome. Eighty-five per cent (157) of the patients were female, compared with 57% of the clinic sample as a whole. Thus of all the clinic attenders, 3.25% of the females and 0.63% of the males were considered to have this disorder (Beighton et al., 1983). The incidence of generalized hypermobility in the population as a whole is likely to be much higher, as not all cases are symptomatic, and some that are do not necessarily attend a rheumatology clinic. Ethnic variation is evident and a study of joint mobility among university students in Iraq demonstrated its presence in 25.4% of males and 38.5% of females (Beighton et al., 1973).

Hypermobility may or may not produce symptoms but, where joints are lax, they may suffer adverse effects of trauma and overuse. Until recently, it was thought that hypermobility was advantageous for activities such as ballet and gymnastics, but it is now evident that hypermobile joints are more prone to injury and trauma.

Genetics

Spinal mobility will be affected by factors such as height, obesity or race.

Congenital anomalies, e.g. sacralization of the 5th lumbar vertebra, or congenital fusion of adjacent vertebrae, will prevent movement at the segment involved.

Pathology

Degenerative changes of the spine do not necessarily affect range of movement. However, pathology that alters the normal alignment of the apophyseal joints or the intervertebral discs will inevitably affect the range and type of movement possible at the affected segment.

SEGMENTAL MOVEMENT

Experiments in which intervertebral movements are examined are often carried out on a motion segment *in vitro*. It should be remembered that such work can only truly represent *in vitro* movement, and other factors such as active muscle work, position of the limbs and body weight have a significant effect on movement *in vivo*.

Cervical Spine

Unlike the thoracic and lumbar regions, the upper and lower parts of the cervical spine can move independently of each other, so that in the sagittal plane independent sagittal rotation of the upper or lower cervical spine is possible.

The two sections of the cervical spine may also move in opposite directions, e.g. the upper cervical spine may be extended and the lower cervical spine flexed simultaneously. This particular combination of segmental postures is often seen clinically in degenerate necks.

A greater degree of upper cervical flexion can be achieved if the lower cervical spine is held in a relatively extended position rather than when the whole of the cervical spine is flexed. There are several possible explanations for why this difference in upper cervical range occurs. In some individuals, when the neck is fully flexed, the chin approximates the sternum so that the occiput may be deflected into extension at the end of range (Dirheimer, 1977). It has been suggested that passive insufficiency of sternocleidomastoid is more likely to cause the upper cervical deflexion during full neck flexion (Kapandji, 1974). Passive insufficiency of a muscle occurs when full range of movement at a joint is limited by the length of the muscle which crosses it. During upper and lower cervical flexion, the length of sternocleidomastoid may be insufficient to allow full cervical flexion, so that the upper cervical spine moves into slight extension. Insufficient length of the cervical ligaments may have a similar effect by passive coordination of the joints. Passive coordination occurs when at least one of the participating bones is not acted upon directly by muscles or there is a physical link across two or more joints (Barnett *et al.*, 1961). If there is insufficient length of the ligamentum nuchae to allow maximum separation of all the spinous processes, as well as separation of the occiput from the posterior tubercle of the atlas, then, in full flexion, the gap between the basiocciput and the posterior atlantal arch will appear less than in the neutral position (Worth, 1988).

Structures within the spinal canal may also affect cervical flexion. The spinal cord and meninges extend throughout the length of the cervical spine and are attached above to the bodies of the 2nd and 3rd cervical vertebrae. Insufficient length or restricted movement of the spinal cord and meninges may prevent full flexion of both the upper and lower cervical spine. The upper cervical spine may extend at the end of the movement to relieve this stretch and it does so by the mechanism of passive coordination (Worth, 1988).

For clarity, the cervical spine will be divided into two distinct segments: the upper segment from C0 to C2 and the lower segment from the inferior facets of C2 to the superior facets of C7. Anatomically, C1 and 2 are different from the rest of the cervical spine: movements at C0/1 and C1/2 are described first, followed by the resulting combined movements at the upper cervical segment.

Movements of the Craniovertebral Joints

There is marked variability in the reported ranges of movement at the craniovertebral joints. This may be in part due to differences in experimental method and measurement techniques, lack of reliability and validity studies and errors of measurement (Worth and Selvik, 1986). It has been shown that asymmetry of the bony and ligamentous structures of this region is very common, e.g. joint surfaces on the superior surface of the atlas may not lie in the same plane, or one of the occipital condyles may be smaller than the other (Dalseth, 1974). Any such asymmetry or anomalies of these joints would inevitably affect the range and direction of movement possible. Attempts by the physiotherapist to measure *in vivo* movements of the craniovertebral joints with any degree of accuracy are fraught with difficulty. Placing a goniometer on a subject's head will only measure head movement and not demonstrate three-dimensional vertebral movement. Orthodox radiographic views of the cervical spine are only two-dimensional, and the complexity of movement in this region can only be truly revealed by methods which allow three-dimensional analysis of movement. A study of the three-dimensional kinematics at the occipito-atlantal and atlanto–axial joints (Worth and Selvik, 1986) showed that rotation occurs around any of three axes at these joints with concomitant rotations about and translations along the other axes at these joints.

C0/1: **The two atlanto-occipital joints.** Maximum movement in these joints occurs in the sagittal plane, i.e. flexion and extension, or nodding of the head. Penning (1978) gave the average range for this movement as 30°, while Fielding (1954) reported 10° of flexion and

25° of extension. Worth and Selvik (1986) recorded an average of 18° when the head was moved from extension to flexion.

During normal physiological flexion of the head and neck, the occipital condyles roll and translate *forwards* on the lateral masses of the atlas, while the atlas translates *backwards* relative to the occiput. The atlas also tilts upwards and posteriorly so that the posterior arch of the atlas and the occiput are approximated. The movement is limited by tension in the articular capsules, the posterior atlanto-occipital membrane and ligamentum nuchae.

This sequence of events may not occur if the rest of the cervical spine is fixed and movement takes place at the C0/1 segment only. Clinically, this can happen in severe cases of ankylosing spondylitis or gross degenerative changes, when the rest of the spine becomes fused, or if the therapist examines the movement of flexion at the C0/1 joint in isolation by fixing the remainder of the cervical spine. In these circumstances, the posterior arch of the atlas and the occiput may be felt to gap; as the occipital condyles roll and translate *backwards* on the atlas, the atlas moves *forwards* and the posterior arch of the atlas and occiput move apart (Gutmann von G., 1970).

During extension, the reverse of the above movements occurs. Quantative values for the amount of forward and backward transla-tion which accompanies flexion and extension vary from 10 mm (Steindler, 1955) to a mean of 5.46 mm ± 0.20 mm (Worth and Selvik, 1986).

Controversy still exists as to whether axial rotation around a vertical axis occurs at the atlanto-occipital joints. Many authors believe that rotation cannot occur because of the direction and configuration of the bony surfaces (Last, 1972; White and Panjabi, 1978b; Jeffreys, 1980). Kapandji (1974) describes rotation at C0/1 which is secondary to rotation occurring at C1/2. He states that rotation of the occiput to the left is accompanied by an anterior movement of the right occipital condyle on the right lateral mass of the atlas and a 2–3 mm displacement of the condyle to the left, resulting in lateral flexion to the right. Worth and Selvik (1986) measured 3.43° ± 0.39° of rotation occurring around a vertical axis at the occipito-atlantal joint. Findings supported flexion with lateral flexion to the opposite side.

A small amount of lateral gliding occurs at the atlanto-occipital joint. The occipital condyles glide laterally towards the convexity on the superior facets of the atlas and approximately 3° of lateral gliding can occur to each side.

C1/2: The two lateral atlanto-axial joints and the median atlanto-axial joint. This is the most mobile segment in the spine: rotation to one side being 30–35°. The movement occurs at all three joints, the axis of movement being the odontoid peg.

Median atlanto-axial joint. The transverse ligament and atlas form an osseoligamentous ring which pivots around the odontoid during rotation.

Lateral atlanto-axial joints.   During rotation to the left, the right lateral mass of the atlas moves forwards on the superior facet of the axis and the left lateral mass moves backwards. Rotation to the left is limited by tension of those fibres of the left alar ligament which are attached to the dens in front of the axis of movement and those of the right alar ligament which attach to the dens behind the axis of movement.

Rotation to the left is accompanied by slight lateral flexion to the left due to a degree of offset of the atlas on the axis.

It has been noted that rotatory movement and returning to the neutral position alternately decrease and increase the vertical height of the atlas on the axis by 2–3 mm (Hohl and Baker, 1964). However, experiments by Worth and Selvik (1986) showed that there was no significant vertical approximation during axial rotation at C1/2.

Flexion/extension.   The total range is 15°. The transverse ligament maintains the odontoid peg in apposition to the anterior arch of the atlas and, in an adult, there should be no more than a 3 mm distance between these bony points (4–5 mm in children). If this distance is greater, there may be some instability in the craniovertebral region. In severe cases of rheumatoid arthritis with resulting laxity of the transverse ligament, this distance can be considerably more, leading to subluxation of the joint. The posterior arch of the atlas and spinous process of the axis separate during flexion and approximate on extension.

Lateral flexion.   The downward oblique orientation of the lateral atlanto-axial joints restricts movement in the frontal plane. Kapandji (1974) states that no lateral flexion occurs at the atlanto-axial joint, but Worth and Selvik (1986) measured a mean of 4.07° ± 2.01° of lateral flexion at C1/2.

C0/1/2 combined movements.   During *rotation* of the head, e.g. to the left, the occiput and atlas move as one unit on the axis, pivoting on the odontoid. Towards the end of C1/2 rotation at approximately 30°, rotation then occurs at C0/1; in addition the axis starts to rotate to the left on C3 and the spinous process of C2 can be felt to move to the right. Lateral flexion to the left accompanies the left rotation.

On *lateral flexion* of the head, e.g. to the left, there is minimal movement at C0/1 when the occipital condyles glide to the right and a small degree of lateral flexion may also occur at C1/2 (Worth and Selvik, 1986). It is accompanied by rotation of the body of C2 to the left: its spinous process can be felt to move towards the right.

The relationship between the atlas and axis alters during lateral flexion. Lateral flexion of the head and neck up to 15° produces rotation of the axis (but not head rotation). Beyond 15° of lateral flexion, more rotation occurs at the atlanto-axial joints and there is greater lateral displacement of the articular margin of the inferior facet on the lateral mass of the atlas as compared with the corresponding articular margin of the superior facet of the axis (Hohl and Baker, 1964).

C2–6

In the cervical spine, movement at a motion segment occurs simultaneously in the two lateral apophyseal joints, the interbody joints and the joints of Luschka. The C4/5 and C5/6 segments are the most mobile and, therefore, particularly susceptible to functional stress. Consequently, degenerative changes at these levels are common.

During *flexion*, the upper vertebral body tilts and slides anteriorly on the one beneath as the axis around which movement occurs lies within the subjacent vertebral body (Penning, 1968). This shearing effect is particularly pronounced in a child's neck. The intervertebral space is compressed anteriorly and the posterior annular fibres are stretched. The inferior articular facet of the superior vertebra slides upwards and anteriorly on the vertebra below and the interspace is opened posteriorly. The facets of the joints of Luschka slide relative to each other and 'guide' movement in the sagittal plane. Flexion is limited by tension in the posterior ligaments and contact of the chin on the sternum.

Cervical discs undergo more distortion during movements in the sagittal plane than discs in other spinal regions (Grieve, 1988). A lateral radiographic view of a normal cervical spine in full flexion shows that the line of the anterior vertebral body margins is broken in a series of steps. This is reversed when the neck is viewed in extension. If the interspinous spaces are palpated during sagittal movement, it can be felt that the spinous processes move apart in flexion and come closer in extension.

During *extension*, the upper vertebral body tilts and slides posteriorly. The intervertebral space is compressed posteriorly and the anterior annular fibres are stretched. The inferior articular facet of the superior vertebra slides downwards and posteriorly on the superior facet and tilts posteriorly, opening the interspace of the joints anteriorly.

Extension is limited by tension in the anterior longitudinal ligament, by the bony impact of the superior articular process of the lower vertebra on the transverse process of the upper vertebra, and by ligamentous bulk from the posterior arches.

Rotation at each level is approximately 8–10° in each direction. Due partly to the oblique inclination of the joints, this movement is not pure, but it is coupled with lateral flexion and slight extension. Rotation to the right is coupled with lateral flexion to the same side and extension: the right inferior articular facet of the vertebra above glides inferiorly, posteriorly and translates medially on the superior articular facet of the vertebra below, falling inside its margins; the left inferior facet of the vertebra above glides superiorly, anteriorly and translates laterally outside the margin of the opposing facet of the vertebra below (Fig. 5.5). The axis of rotation lies in the midline at the anterior part of the superior vertebral body. When the neck is rotated to the right, the right side of the spine is approximated while the left side becomes longer.

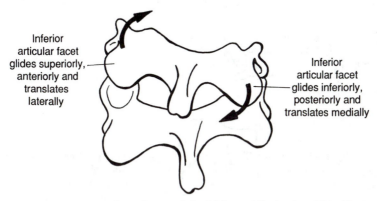

Inferior articular facet glides superiorly, anteriorly and translates laterally

Inferior articular facet glides inferiorly, posteriorly and translates medially

Fig. 5.5 Rotation to the right coupled with lateral flexion in mid and lower cervical region.

During *lateral flexion*, the facets on the concave side glide backwards, thereby inducing rotation to the same side. Therefore, lateral flexion is normally accompanied by rotation to the same side (Fig. 5.6). During this movement, the dimensions of the intervertebral foramina on the ipsilateral side are reduced (Fig. 5.7), potentially compromising the foraminal contents.

Compensatory movements in the cervical spine

Pure *rotation* of the head e.g. to the left, can only be achieved by intricate compensatory movements in the cervical spine which eliminate the unwanted components. As previously stated, in the lower cervical spine, rotation to the left is coupled with lateral flexion to the same side. In the suboccipital region, in addition to rotation to the left, there is a small degree of lateral flexion to the *right*, and some extension.

Pure *lateral flexion* of the head to the left is achieved by rotation to the right occurring in the sub-occipital region and the rotation to the left occurring in the lower cervical spine. Jirout (1971) examined 768 radiographic films taken of the neck in a position of lateral flexion. He observed that in 237 examples the lateral flexion was accompanied by

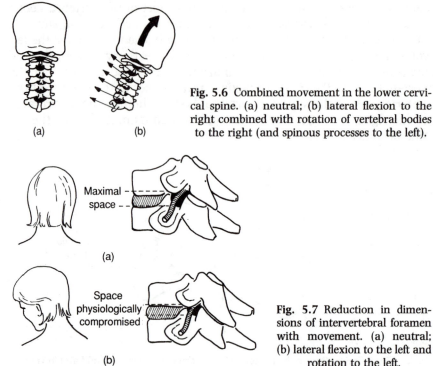

Fig. 5.6 Combined movement in the lower cervical spine. (a) neutral; (b) lateral flexion to the right combined with rotation of vertebral bodies to the right (and spinous processes to the left).

Fig. 5.7 Reduction in dimensions of intervertebral foramen with movement. (a) neutral; (b) lateral flexion to the left and rotation to the left.

flexion, in 118 it was combined with extension and in 413 there was no added forward or backward tilt. The lack of consistency in these findings suggests that a normal movement stereotype does not exist and it follows that any manipulation philosophy based on 'normal' movement patterns derived 'logically' from the plane of the facets may be fallacious (Grieve 1988). It is, therefore, essential that clinical assessment of individual movement takes precedence over biomechanical theories and theories of treatment techniques.

Cervico-thoracic Junction C6–T2

Motion at each segment at the cervico–thoracic junction reduces caudally, but not in a graduated manner. The amount of flexion and extension decreases, although it is not as restricted as lower in the thoracic spine.

Physiological movement combinations are the same as in the typical cervical spine, i.e. rotation is accompanied by lateral flexion to the same side.

This region, where the mobile cervical spine is adjacent to the relatively stiff thoracic spine, is a very common source of symptoms. A motion segment adjacent to a stiff segment is particularly susceptible to the stresses of movement of the cervical spine which are accentuated by transmission of the weight of the head (the approximate weight of the head is 5 kg).

In cervical spondylosis, the spinous processes of C7 and T1 often become very prominent and they are termed a 'bison's hump'. The paravertebral soft tissues become tight and thickened and the area is particularly tender to palpation. Movement abnormalities occur with these changes and all ranges quickly diminish. In addition, the lower cervical spine can become fixed in a flexed position, so consequently the upper cervical spine is extended to compensate and allow a normal visual field.

T3–10

The thoracic spine is the least mobile area of the spine. Protection of the viscera and internal organs is of prime importance and the thoracic spine and rib cage provide the necessary protection and stability at the expense of mobility. Reduced mobility is attributed to several factors: thin discs, facet planes, ligamentum flavum, attachments of the rib cage and sternum, configuration and proximity of the spinous processes, and an increased moment of inertia which stiffens the spine when rotatory forces are sustained. All movements are decreased in the thoracic spine although rotation the least so. Panjabi et al. (1976) showed that coupling patterns occur in all six degrees of freedom at thoracic segments while Hirsch and White (1971) noted that motion in the thoracic spine is frequently a combination of translation and rotation about each of three axes.

In addition to movements occurring at the interbody joints and apophyseal joints, movements of the ribs at the costovertebral, costotransverse and sternocostal joints will be considered.

During flexion, the interspace between two vertebrae opens out posteriorly. The inferior articular facets of the apophyseal joints slide superiorly and tend to overhang the superior articular process of the underlying vertebra. This movement is accompanied by only a small amount of forward translation of the superior vertebra, as the almost vertical disposition of the superior articular facets of the vertebra prohibits forward translation in the thoracic spine (Williams and Warwick, 1980). Although the dorsal musculature and soft tissues are under tension, the ligamentum flavum is the principal structure which restricts flexion (Akerblom, 1949). In some individuals, anterior rib overcrowding is as important a limiting factor as any (Grieve, 1986).

According to White and Panjabi (1978a), the instantaneous axis of rotation (IAR) in formally described conventional movement of a thoracic motion segment during flexion is placed just anterior to and a little above the centre of the subjacent vertebral body. Total sagittal range of movement in the thoracic spine is relatively small. The thoracic spine contributes 25% of total spinal flexion and extension

(Loebl, 1967). Between T3–6 there is the least amount of sagittal movement. Measurement of movement in the sagittal plane has shown that the median flexion/extension range between T1–6 is 4°, between T7–10 it is 6° and between T11–L1 it is 9–12° (White and Panjabi, 1978a). There is greater flexion than extension in the sagittal plane, and extension accounts for 30–42% of total sagittal movement.

During extension, the inferior facets of the superior vertebra descend on the superior facets of the vertebra below. Posteriorly, the vertebrae are approximated and the posterior annulus and posterior longitudinal ligament are compressed. If the interspinous space is palpated, the spinous processes can be felt to move closer together during extension. A tensile stress is placed on the anterior part of the disc and the anterior longitudinal ligament. During extension, the IAR is just anterior to and a little below the centre of the vertebra above (White and Panjabi, 1978a).

Extension is limited by contact of the inferior articular processes with the laminae below and by contact of the spinous processes. As the bony points approximate further, backward rotation is prevented, but some posterior translation may occur. This motion is limited by the articular capsule and the anterior structures (Valencia, 1988). In some mature 'normal' individuals, extension may also be limited, particularly in the upper thoracic spine, by soft tissue contracture of the intercostales, pectoral musculature, and clavipectoral fascia (Grieve, 1988).

As in other regions of the spine, axial rotation is coupled with lateral bending and vice versa. The extent to which this occurs varies – it is more distinct in the upper and lower parts of the thoracic spine and less distinct in the middle region. Only a small amount of this shearing motion occurs at each segment, but the cumulative effect is greater. Strong resistance to lateral shearing or horizontal translation is provided by the triangular arrangement of the annular fibres, their strong attachment to the end plate and the flat thoracic disc.

Analysis of the kinematic behaviour of autopsy specimens of the thoracic spine suggests that the upper and lower parts behave differently from the middle (White, 1969). In the upper thoracic spine, the direction of coupling is such that axial rotation of the vertebral body is into the concavity of the lateral curve, i.e. lateral bending to one side is coupled with axial rotation to the same side. White noted that this pattern existed in the middle and lower thoracic spine, but it was not as marked or as consistent. In some cases, the middle region showed the reverse behaviour, so that lateral bending was coupled with axial rotation to the opposite side. However, these experiments were carried out with the ribs and muscle mass dissected away and it is, therefore, unclear as to how accurately these findings truly represent in vivo motion.

The IAR on axial rotation is variable in that it may lie anywhere within the area of the nucleus pulposus or extend posteriorly to the anterior vertebral canal (White and Panjabi, 1978a). It lies more anteriorly in the upper and lower thirds of the thoracic spine than in the middle third (Davis, 1959). During lateral bending, the IAR passes centrally through the contralateral half of the subjacent vertebral body.

During lateral bending to the left, the inferior facets of the superior vertebra on the right slide superiorly and translate fractionally forward, while those on the left slide inferiorly and translate backwards. Hence, lateral bending is coupled with axial rotation. The movement is limited by the impact of the articular processes on the side of the movement and by the opposite ligamenta flava, outer annular fibres, intertransverse ligaments and antagonistic muscles. Rib overcrowding on the concave side is also a limiting factor. On the convex side, the intercostal spaces widen, the thorax is elevated, the thoracic cage is enlarged; on the concave side, the opposite occurs.

At each level, the median range of lateral bending is 6° at the segments between T1 and 10, while in the lower two segments the median range is 7–9°.

Rotation is the greatest movement in this region. The articular facets of the apophyseal joints slide relative to each other and the disc is twisted; only minimal shearing occurs here. Further rotation is prevented by the attachment of the ribs, which, in turn, are limited by their attachments to the sternum. The ribs, especially the cartilages, are distorted. The mean range of axial rotation at each segment is 8–9° in the upper segments and it reduces to 2° in the lowest three segments.

Movements of the Rib Cage in Respiration

The diaphragm is the main muscle of inspiration. It forms a musculotendinous dome concave towards the abdomen, the central part being tendinous and the peripheral part muscular.

During inspiration, the lowest ribs are fixed and, as the muscular fibres contract, the central tendon is at first drawn downwards pressing on the abdominal viscera and increasing the vertical diameter of the thorax. The extensibility of the abdominal wall allows this descent to a small extent, but the abdominal organs quickly limit this movement. The central tendon then becomes the fixed point for the action of the diaphragm, which then elevates the lower ribs. Elevation of the vertebrochondral ribs results in an outward and backward movement to produce an increase in the transverse diameter only. The anterior ends of the vertebrosternal ribs are pushed forwards and upwards, elevating the sternum and upper ribs, and increasing the anteroposterior dimension of the thorax. At the same time, these ribs are everted, thus increasing the transverse diameter.

Movements of the ribs at the costovertebral, costotransverse and sternocostal joints

Each rib has its own range and variety of movements. It can be seen as a lever, its fulcrum being immediately outside the costotransverse joint. Hence, if the shaft of the rib is elevated, the neck is depressed and vice versa. The lever arm of the shaft of the rib is much longer than that at the vertebral end, so small movements of the latter result in much greater movements at the anterior end. In general, the individual rib shafts are highly flexible, but together they contribute to the stiffness of the thorax (Schultz et al., 1974).

When a rib moves, it does so at the costovertebral, costotransverse and sternocostal joints. The costovertebral and costotransverse joints form a joint couple mechanically linked. The axis of movement, running through the centre of each joint, acts as a swivel for the rib. The direction of the axis varies in the upper and lower ribs, thus affecting the direction of movement of the ribs (Fig. 5.8). For the lower ribs, the axis lies more or less anteroposteriorly, whereas in the upper ribs it is more in a medial/lateral direction. Therefore, elevation of the lower ribs increases the transverse diameter of the lower thorax, and elevation of the upper ribs the anteroposterior diameter of the upper thorax. In the mid-thorax, the axis lies between the above two axes at an angle of 45° to the sagittal plane. Therefore, on elevation of these ribs, both diameters are increased. The shortest, higher ribs are stiffer than the longer, lower ribs. The orientation and shape of the articular surfaces varies at every rib and thus influences direction of movement.

The 1st and 2nd ribs take little part in quiet respiration, but are involved more in forced respiration. Although only relatively small amplitudes of motion occur at these levels, they are often affected by degenerative changes at the cervico-thoracic junction and are frequently a source of symptoms, in particular, unilateral suprascapular pain which may radiate to the shoulder.

As the articulating surfaces on the tubercles of the upper six ribs are convex from above downwards and the corresponding surfaces on the transverse processes are concave, elevation and depression of the ribs results in rotation of the rib neck about this axis. Elevation of the rib results in rotation upwards of the front of the neck of the rib, and depression results in rotation downwards. There is only very slight upwards and downwards movement of the neck of the rib itself.

The articulating surfaces of the 7th–10th tubercles of the ribs are flattened and face downward, medially and backwards. Corresponding articular surfaces are on the upper aspects of the transverse processes of the vertebrae. Movement of these ribs involves upward, backward and medial gliding of the rib tubercle during inspiration and downward, forward and lateral movement on expiration. The whole neck undergoes the same movement, and it is accompanied by a small degree of rotation.

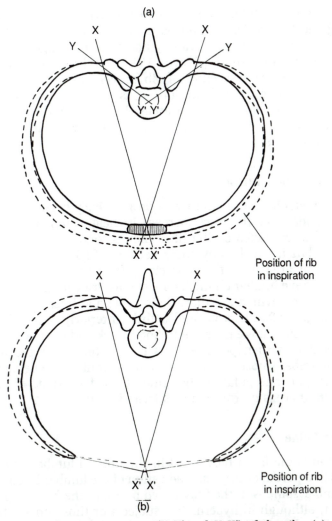

Fig. 5.8 Axes of movement (X–X′ and Y–Y′) of the ribs. (a) vertebrosternal ribs; (b) vertebrochondral ribs.

Movement occurs simultaneously at the sternocostal joints. The anterior ends of the ribs lie on a lower plane than the posterior, so that when the rib shaft is elevated, the anterior extremity is thrust forwards, taking the sternum with it. A gliding movement occurs at the sternocostal joints.

The 11th and 12th ribs are free at their anterior ends and do not have demifacets, intra-articular ligaments and costotransverse joints. Small movements can occur in all directions, but during respiration these ribs are depressed and fixed by quadratus lumborum, providing a fixed base for the action of the diaphragm.

The manubriosternal joint becomes ankylosed in 10% of people during the fourth decade and, later in life, the joints of the costal cartilages also ankylose, inevitably affecting the range of movement available for respiration (Grieve, 1986). It has been shown that although selective restriction of rib movement decreases the tidal volume of the restricted portion, it is associated with increased expansion of the non-restricted areas (Di Marco and Kelsen, 1981). Therefore, respiratory exchange may not be affected by localized rib lesions or corsets.

Thoraco-lumbar Junction

Movements in the sagittal plane progressively begin to increase in range caudally as the discs increase in height and the movements become less restricted by the ribs. There is one vertebral level, often T11/12, but it can be anywhere between T10 and L1, which is a transitional area from the thoracic type of vertebra to one which begins to have lumbar characteristics. This 'transitional' vertebra has superior facets which are thoracic in type, and inferior facets whose planes begin to face laterally and slightly anteriorly. When the spine is in full extension, there is a bone-to-bone block and no movement other than flexion is then possible. This is sometimes referred to as the thoracolumbar mortise joint. It is important to remember when mobilizing or manipulating the spine at this level that, when it is in *extension*, there is no rotation or lateral flexion.

Lumbar Spine

Flexion is the freest movement in the normal lumbar spine, and it results in a partial or general eradication of the lumbar lordosis. When the lumbar spine is in the fully flexed position, the bony alignment is straight, although in hypermobile subjects or those under the age of 30 (Allbrook, 1957) the lumbar spine might have a slight anterior concavity. Reversal of the lumbar curve occurs mainly above the L3 vertebra. There may be some reversal at the L4/5 segment, but not at the L5/S1 level (Pearcy *et al.*, 1984).

Flexion of the lumbar spine is a combination of anterior sagittal rotation and anterior translation of the lumbar vertebrae (Fig. 5.9). These two components are resisted and stabilized by different structures and in different ways by the apophyseal joints. On flexion, the superior vertebra rotates forward so that the inferior articular facets glide upwards and slightly backwards on the superior facets of the vertebra below. Thus, as anterior sagittal rotation occurs, there will be a small amount of gapping between the superior and inferior facets. As the body leans forwards, the effect of gravity or muscle contraction causes concomitant anterior translation of the superior vertebra, so

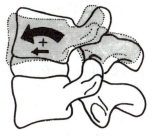

Flexion

Anterior sagittal
rotation and
anterior translation

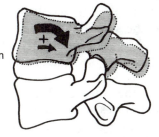

Extension

Posterior sagittal
rotation and
posterior translation

Fig. 5.9 Flexion and extension of a lumbar motion segment showing the two components of sagittal rotation and translation.

that the gap between the superior and inferior facet closes. Forward translation is resisted by impaction of the inferior articular facets of one vertebra with the superior articular facets of the vertebra below. The facets, therefore, have a major role in maintaining stability of the lumbar spine and preventing forward shear. The load is borne evenly across the entire articular surface of joints with flat articular surfaces (*see* pp. 50–1) but, in joints with curved articular surfaces, most of the load is borne by the anteromedial portion of the superior and inferior articular facets (Bogduk and Twomey, 1987). Experiments have shown that, on flexion, the highest pressures are recorded at the medial portion of the lumbar apophyseal joints (Dunlop *et al.*, 1984). These areas of stress are particularly vulnerable to degenerative changes.

The anterior sagittal rotation component of lumbar flexion is limited principally by the joint capsules, although the posterior ligaments and the interbody joints also resist the movement. The inferior articular facets glide upwards on the superior articular facets by 5–7 mm and in so do doing the joint capsule becomes tense. The supraspinous, interspinous, ligamenta flava and posterior annular fibres are also tensed.

Experimental studies investigating the relative importance of the structures of the lumbar motion segment in resisting flexion demonstrate that, when the posterior ligamentous structures and bony locking mechanism are sequentially severed, it is the intact apophyseal joints which have a greater restricting influence in flexion than the ligamentous structures (Twomey and Taylor, 1986). Intact apophyseal joints guide anterior sagittal rotation and resist forward slide so that, when the pedicles are cut, a greater degree of forward translation accompanies this rotation. Flexion is progressively braked by the supraspinous ligaments, interspinous ligaments, ligamenta flava and apophyseal joint capsules, but it ceases because of apposition of the superior and inferior articular facets (Twomey and Taylor, 1983). Experiments which investigate the effect of sequential severing of various structures on joint movement will not demonstrate the relative and simultaneous contributions of the different elements at different phases of movement.

The increase in movement observed in posterior release studies is much less in adults than in the young. This is due to the greater compliance of young discs. Age changes in the disc are mainly responsible for the observed decrease in lumbar range of movement with ageing.

As the lumbar spine flexes, the intervertebral disc is compressed anteriorly, the posterior annular fibres are stretched (*see* pp. 72–4) and the spinous processes can be felt to separate. Clinically, when flexion is examined, it should be considered that with increasing flexion, stress will be placed not only on the soft tissue structures, but also on the bony locking mechanism so that the end of the range of flexion may, therefore, be stressing the joints.

Lumbar spine extension is a combination of posterior sagittal rotation and a small amount of posterior translation of the vertebral bodies (*see* Fig. 5.9). The inferior articular facets glide downwards on the superior articular facets until the movement is limited by bony impaction of the tip of the inferior facets on the laminae of the vertebra below. The fat pads and loose areolar tissue of the inferior recesses of the apophyseal joints (Lewin, 1968; Bogduk and Engel, 1984) form a buffer between the hard, sharp inferior facets and the solid laminae, and help to attenuate the sudden jarring force of rapid full range extension. This loading in extension is concentrated in a localized area of each inferior recess, and the loading borne by the lamina at this point (the pars interarticularis) is attested by the sclerosis and thickening of compact bone observed in young adult spines (Twomey and Taylor, 1986).

Once the inferior facet has impacted on the lamina below, a continued increase in loading will cause axial rotation of the superior vertebra (Yang and King, 1984). The superior vertebra pivots on the impacted inferior articular process so that the opposite inferior articular process swings backwards. Its joint capsule becomes tense and severe forces may cause the capsule to rupture (Yang and King, 1984). Symptoms arising from an extension injury may, therefore, arise from strain or damage to the backwardly rotating apophyseal joint, trapping of the joint capsule between the inferior articular process and the lamina or erosion of the periosteum of the lamina at the site of impaction of the articular process.

Extension is associated with compression of the posterior annular fibres and stretching of the anterior annular fibres. Mechanical tests have shown that the anterior longitudinal ligament is much too weak to resist and limit extension of the lumbar spine. The spinous processes undoubtedly limit extension in rare cases of 'kissing spines'; more typically they may resist the movement by trapping the interspinous ligament between them. If the spinous processes are particularly widely spaced, then the apophyseal joints resist extension movements. The disc resists extension more strongly than flexion (Markolf, 1972) but, as the limit of movement is approached, it may be protected by the apophyseal joints as in other movements (Adams *et al.*, 1988). On palpation, the gap between the spinous processes is reduced or obliterated as the processes move closer together.

Rotation in the lumbar spine is approximately 3° to each side and is limited principally by apposition of the apophyseal joint surfaces. The axis of rotation of a lumbar vertebra passes through the posterior part of the vertebra so that, during axial rotation, the posterior elements of the moving vertebra swing round the axis. On axial rotation of a lumbar intervertebral joint to the right, the spinous process will swing to the left and the supraspinous and interspinous ligaments are placed under tension. The movement is limited by impaction of one of the inferior articular facets of the upper vertebra with the opposing superior articular facet of the vertebra below. Hence, on rotation to the right, the left inferior facet of the upper vertebra impacts against the superior facet of the vertebra below, and the apophyseal joint on the opposite side is gapped. Once impaction of the apophyseal joint occurs, any further rotation will take place about an axis located in the impacted joint.

The lumbar intervertebral discs also resist torsion. Annular fibres orientated in the direction of rotation are strained, while those in the opposite direction are relaxed. Collagen fibres can withstand 3–4% elongation, but sustain damage if stretched by more than 4% (Bogduk and Twomey, 1987). It has been calculated that the collagen fibres of the disc will allow 3° of movement, but if greater movement occurs the fibres undergo microinjury (Hickey and Hukins, 1980). Complete failure of the disc is thought to occur at 12° of rotation (Farfan *et al.*, 1970).

There is very little joint space at the lumbar apophyseal joints, so that the 3° of rotation that occurs is principally due to compression of the articular cartilages of the facets, which are able to sustain compression because their major constituents are proteoglycans and water. Water is squeezed out of the cartilages under compression and it is gradually reabsorbed when the load is released (Bogduk and Twomey, 1987).

Rotation is severely restricted by the apophyseal joints, and rotatory movement in excess of 3° places the annulus under considerable torsional stress. Rotation in excess of 3° occurs at the impacted joint and the vertebral body and opposite inferior articular process swing back around this axis. The vertebral body swings laterally and backwards and the opposite inferior articular process swings backwards and medially. As the vertebral body shifts laterally, it exerts a lateral shear on the subjacent disc which is in addition to any torsional stress of the disc that occurs during rotation. Backward movement of the opposite inferior articular process places the capsule of its apophyseal joint under great stress.

A very strong rotatory force may cause failure (1) of the impacted apophyseal joint, (2) the disc which is strained by torsion and shear, or (3) the tensed capsule of the opposite apophyseal joint. The posterior elements contribute 65%, to resisting torsion, while the disc contributes 35% (Farfan *et al.*, 1970). Axial rotation is always accompanied by a degree of lateral flexion. Axial rotation between L1–4 is accompanied by lateral flexion to the contralateral side, while at L5/S1 axial rotation is coupled with lateral flexion to the same side. Lateral flexion in the lumbar spine is a complex movement that is coupled with rotatory movements of the interbody joints and the apophyseal joints. On the side to which lateral flexion occurs, the inferior articular facet of the upper vertebra slides inferiorly on the superior articular facet of the vertebra below. The cross-sectional area of the intervertebral foramen is reduced on the side of the lateral flexion. Consequently, the inferior facet on the opposite side slides upwards on the superior facet on the vertebra below and the vertical diameter of the intervertebral foramen on that side is increased.

Between L1 and 4 lateral flexion to one side is accompanied by axial rotation to the opposite side. At the L5/S1 segment, lateral flexion to one side is accompanied by rotation to the same side. Lateral flexion is also most usually accompanied by a degree of extension (Bogduk and Twomey, 1987).

Axial distraction of the lumbar spine occurs during therapeutic traction. If the traction is applied with the intervertebral joints in a mid-position between flexion and extension, the facets of the apophyseal joints glide relative to each other and the annular fibres are tensed equally. Twomey (1985) observed that 40% of the lengthening of the spine occurred as a result of flattening of the lumbar spine, while 60% was due to separation of the vertebral bodies, and it was calculated that only approximately 0.9 mm distraction occurred at each joint. This amount of movement is insufficient to allow the 'sucking back' of a herniated disc and the beneficial effects of traction must occur through some other mechanism. The increase in length retained when traction is released is only 0.1 mm per intervertebral joint and this is obliterated as soon as the patient weight-bears through the spine.

Maintained lengthening of the lumbar spine is, therefore, not the mechanism by which therapeutic traction has its effect.

REFERENCES

Adams M.A., Dolan P., Hutton W.C. (1988). The lumbar spine in backward bending. *Spine*, **13**, 9, 1019.

Akerblom B. (1949). *Standing and Sitting Posture*. Thesis AB. Stockholm: Nordiska Bokhandeln.

Allbrook F.M. (1957). Movements of the lumbar spinal column. *J. Bone Jt. Surg.*, **39B**, 339.

Barnett C.H., Davies D.V., MacConaill M.A. (1961). *Synovial Joints – Their Structure and Mechanics*. London: Longman, Ch. 4, pp. 260–268.

Beighton P.H., Solomon L., Soskolne C.L. (1973). Articular mobility in an African population. *Ann. Rheum. Dis.*, **32**, 413.

Beighton P., Grahame R., Bird H. (1983). *Hypermobility of Joints*. Berlin, Heidelberg: Springer-Verlag, Ch. 5.

Bogduk N., Engel R. (1984). The menisci of the lumbar zygapophyseal joints: a review of their anatomy and clinical significance. *Spine*, **9**, 454.

Bogduk N., Twomey L.T. (1987). *Clinical Anatomy of the Lumbar Spine*. Edinburgh: Churchill Livingstone.

Campbell D.G., Parsons C.M. (1944). Referred head pain and its concomitants. *J. Nerv. Ment. Dis.*, **99**, 544.

Dalseth I. (1974). Anatomic studies of the osseous craniovertebral joint. *Man. Med.*, **12**, 130.

Davies P.R. (1959). The medical inclination of the human thoracic intervertebral articular facets. *J. Anat.*, **93**, 68.

Di Marco A.F., Kelsen S.G. (1981). Effects on breathing of selective restriction of movement of the rib cage and abdomen. *J. Physiol. Resp. Environ. Ex. Physiol.*, **50**, 412.

Dirheimer Y. (1977). *The Craniovertebral Region in Chronic Inflammatory Rheumatic Diseases*. Berlin: Springer-Verlag.

Dunlop R.B., Adams M.A., Hutton W.C. (1984). Disc space narrowing and the lumbar facet joints. *J. Bone Jt. Surg.*, **66B**, 706.

Farfan H.F., Cossette J.W., Robertson G.H. *et al.* (1970). The effects of torsion on the lumbar intervertebral joints: the role of torsion in the production of disc degeneration. *J. Bone Jt. Surg. Am.*, **52A**, 468.

Fielding J.W. (1954). Cineroentgenography of the normal cervical spine. *J. Bone Jt. Surg.*, **39A**, 1280.

Grieve G.P. (1986). Movements of the thoracic spine. In *Modern Manual Therapy of the Vertebral Column*. Edinburgh: Churchill Livingstone, Ch. 8, pp. 86–102.

Grieve G.P. (1988). *Common Vertebral Joint Problems*, 2nd edn. Edinburgh: Churchill Livingstone, p. 118.

Gutmann von G. (1970). X-ray diagnosis of spinal dysfunction. *Man. Med.*, **8**, 73.

Hickey D.S., Hukins D.W.L. (1980). Relation between the structure of the annulus fibrosus and the function and failure of the intervertebral disc. *Spine*, **5**, 100.

Hirsch C., White A.A. (1971). Characteristics in the thoracic spine motion. *Clin. Orthop. Rel. Res.*, **75**, 156.

Hohl M., Baker H.R. (1964). The atlanto-axial joint: roentgenographic and anatomical study of normal and abnormal motion. *J. Bone Jt. Surg.*, **46A**, 1739.

Jeffreys E. (1980). *Disorders of the Cervical Spine.* London: Butterworths.

Jirout J. (1971). Pattern of changes in the cervical spine in latero-flexion. *Neuroradiology*, **2**, 164.

Kapandji I.A. (1974). *The Physiology of the Joints. 3: The Trunk and the Vertebral Column.* Edinburgh: Churchill Livingstone.

Last R.J. (1972). *Anatomy: Regional and Applied*, 5th edn. Edinburgh: Churchill Livingstone.

Lewin T. (1968). Anatomical variation in lumbosacral synovial joints with particular reference to subluxation. *Acta Anatomica*, **71**, 229.

Loebl W.Y. (1967). Measurement of spine and range of spinal movement. *Ann. Phys. Med.*, **9**, 103.

Markolf K.L. (1972). Deformation of the thoracolumbar intervertebral joints in response to external loads. *J. Bone Jt. Surg.*, **54A**, 511.

Moll J.M.H., Wright V. (1971). Normal range of spinal mobility. *Ann. Rheum. Dis.*, **30**, 381.

Panjabi M.M., Brand R.A., White A.A. (1976). Three-dimensional flexibility and stiffness of the human thoracic spine. *J. Biomechan.*, **9**, 185.

Pearcy M., Portek I., Shepherd J. (1984). Three dimensional X-ray analysis of normal movement in the lumbar spine. *Spine*, **9**, 294.

Penning L. (1968). Functional pathology of the cervical spine. *Excerpta Medica*, Amsterdam, 167.

Penning L. (1978). Normal movements of the cervical spine. *Am. J. Roentgenol.*, **130**, 317.

Radin E.L., Paul I.L., Lowry M. (1970). A comparison of the dynamic force transmitting properties of subchondral bone and articular cartilage. *J. Bone Jt. Surg.*, **52A**, 444.

Schultz A.B., Benson D.R., Hirsch C. (1974). Force deformation properties of human ribs. *J. Biomechan.*, **7**, 303.

Steindler A. (1955). *Kinesiology of the Human Body.* Springfield, Illinois: Thomas, p. 147.

Stockwell (1979). Cited in Twomey L.T., Taylor J.R. (1987). Lumbar posture, movement and mechanics. In *Physical Therapy of the Low Back.* Edinburgh: Churchill Livingstone.

Stoddard A. (1962). *Manual of Osteopathic Technique*, 2nd edn. London: Hutchinson.

Sturrock R.D., Wojtulewski J.A., Dudley Hart F. (1973). Spondylometry in a normal population and in ankylosing spondylitis. *Rheumatol. Rehab.*, **12**, 135.

Twomey L. (1985). Sustained lumbar traction. An experimental study of long spine segments. *Spine*, **10**, 146.

Twomey L.T., Taylor J.R. (1983). Sagittal movements of the human vertebral column: a quantitative study of the role of the posterior vertebral elements. *Arch. Phys. Med. Rehab.*, **64**, 322.

Twomey L.T., Taylor J.R. (1986). Factors influencing ranges of movement in the lumbar spine. In *Modern Manual Therapy of the Vertebral Column* (Grieve G.P. ed.). Edinburgh: Churchill Livingstone.

Twomey L.T., Taylor J.R. (1987). Lumbar posture, movement and mechanics. In *Physical Therapy of the Low Back*. (Twomey L.T., Taylor J.R., eds.). Edinburgh: Churchill Livingstone, Ch. 2.

Valencia F. (1988). Biomechanics of the thoracic spine. In *Physical Therapy of the Cervical and Thoracic Spine*. (Grant R., ed.). Edinburgh: Churchill Livingstone.

White A.A. (1969). Analysis of the mechanics of the thoracic spine in man. *Acta Orthop. Scand.*, Suppl. 127.

White A.A., Panjabi M.M. (1978a). The basic kinematics of the human spine. *Spine*, **3**, 12.

White A.A., Panjabi M.M. (1978b). The clinical biomechanics of the occipito-atlantoaxial complex. *Orth. Clin. N. Am.*, **9**, 867.

Williams P.L., Warwick R. (1980). *Gray's Anatomy*, 36th edn., Edinburgh: Churchill Livingstone, p. 451.

Worth D.R. (1988). Biomechanics of the cervical spine. In *Physical Therapy of the Cervical and Thoracic Spine*. (Grant R., ed.). Edinburgh: Churchill Livingstone, Ch. 2, pp. 15–25.

Worth D.R., Selvik G. (1986). Movements of the craniovertebral joints. In *Modern Manual Therapy of the Vertebral Column* (Grieve G.P., ed.), Edinburgh: Churchill Livingstone, Ch. 5, pp. 53–63.

Yang K.H., King A.I. (1984). Mechanism of facet load transmission as a hypothesis for low-back pain. *Spine*, **9**, 557.

6

Sacroiliac Joints

An account of the functional anatomy of the sacroiliac joints is given because of their intimate association with spinal mechanics and pathology.

The pelvic girdle is massively constructed to withstand enormous stresses due to the weight of the body and powerful musculature. It comprises two innominate bones (Fig. 6.1) – each of which consists of an ilium superiorly, an ischium inferiorly and a pubis anteriorly – and the sacrum. The pubic bones are joined anteriorly at the pubic symphysis; posteriorly both ilia join the central sacrum (Fig. 6.2) at the sacroiliac joints. An osseocartilaginous ring is thus formed, which contains and protects the viscera. In adult life, the three parts of each innominate bone unite by bone and at this junction the acetabulum articulates with the head of the femur. The extensive surfaces of the pelvis afford attachments for the muscles of the trunk and lower limbs.

Due to the interdependence of the three pelvic joints (two sacroiliac and the pubis symphysis), a lesion occurring in any one of them will in

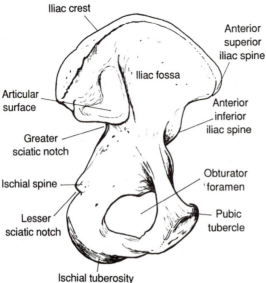

Iliac crest

Anterior
superior
iliac spine

Iliac fossa

Articular
surface

Anterior
inferior
iliac spine

Greater
sciatic notch

Ischial spine

Obturator
foramen

Lesser
sciatic notch

Pubic
tubercle

Ischial tuberosity

Fig. **6.1** Left innominate
bone.

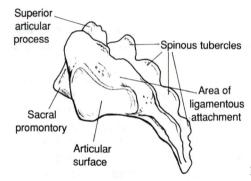

Superior articular process

Spinous tubercles

Area of ligamentous attachment

Sacral promontory

Articular surface

Fig. 6.2 Left lateral aspect of sacrum.

some way affect the other two. It will also inevitably result in abnormal stresses on the spine. Not uncommonly, a patient may present with signs and symptoms in both the spine and sacroiliac joint and the site of the original lesion is then more difficult to determine.

SHAPE AND ANGULATION OF THE SACRUM

The sacrum may be considered as an inverted keystone to the pelvic arch. When viewed from the front, sacra vary in shape, some being roughly rectangular and others more triangular. In the latter, the plane of the sacroiliac joints is more oblique; in the former, the joints are more vertical and, in consequence, more unstable (Brown, 1937).

The sacrum is angulated so that its base (superior surface) faces downwards and forwards. The size of the angle that the superior surface makes with the horizontal plane is approximately 42–45°, increasing by about 8° on standing (Hellems and Keates, 1971). To compensate for this angulation and to enable the spine to be upright, the lumbar spine assumes its lordotic curve.

Individuals show considerable differences in the degree of forward tilt of the sacrum, and this has an important effect on the mechanics of both the pelvic joints and the spine, in particular the lumbar region. When the sacrum is placed more in a horizontal position, it has rotated forwards on an axis, the centre of which is in the acetabulum or the heads of the femora (Brown, 1937). In this position, the sacroiliac joints are either above or anterior to the centre of the acetabulum or the heads of the femora. A sacrum with a markedly forward inclination will, therefore, increase the strains on the sacroiliac joints, and this will be even more marked in the presence of ligamentous laxity. Compensation has to occur in the remainder of the spine, and this is dependent on its particular anatomical structure. The compensatory position of the lumbar spine places the low lumbar apophyseal joints in an extreme position of extension causing strain and narrowing of the intervertebral foramina. Kapandji (1974) refers to this particular anatomical structure as the 'dynamic' type of vertebral column and shows, in addition, compensatory increased thoracic and cervical curves.

When the sacrum is more vertically placed, its base faces more upward and it can then act as a more effective keystone. In this position, the sacroiliac joints are above or posterior to the centre of the acetabulum and heads of the femora, and the low lumbar apophyseal joints are also above or posterior to the centre of rotation (Brown, 1937). The amount of movement possible in the sacroiliac joints with this type of sacrum is usually less than in the horizontal type. Kapandji (1974) depicts the associated spinal curvatures as being poorly developed, and refers to this anatomical structure as the 'static' type of vertebral column.

ARTICULAR SURFACES

The sacroiliac joint is synovial and often classified as a plane joint, although the articular surfaces in the adult are not flat. The auricular surfaces of the sacrum are more or less 'L'-shaped with the superior limb pointing vertically and the inferior limb pointing horizontally, which allows vertical load-bearing while preventing the sacrum from sliding upward between the ilia (Wilder et al., 1980). They articulate with those of the ilia which are of similar shape.

The articular surface of the sacrum is covered by hyaline cartilage, which is thicker than that covering the surface of the ilium – perhaps a factor in the higher incidence of sclerosis found on the iliac side of the joint than on the sacral side in osteitis condensans ilii. It was previously thought that the articular surface of the ilium was covered with fibrocartilage, but Paquin et al. (1983) concluded that it was, in fact, hyaline cartilage (i.e. it contains Type II collagen and not Type I collagen, which is characteristic of fibrocartilage).

An important fact to remember in spinal assessments is that the paired sacroiliac joints are normally asymmetrical to varying degrees. The paired posterior superior iliac spines are often, even in painfree subjects, not level. Each sacroiliac joint is unique in its structure, reflecting the forces that have been sustained by it and the individual's lifestyle. Although in the infant both articular surfaces are nearly flat, after puberty they become roughened and irregular, more so in the male. These irregularities vary so much in different individuals that almost every conceivable combination of grooves, ridges, eminences and depressions may occur (Schunke, 1938). They fit into one another to some extent, which increases the stability of the joint, yet allows small degrees of movement. The roughness of the depressions and humps is one of the factors determining the joint's mobility, in that flatter joint surfaces allow more movement but, at the same time, decrease the joint's stability. The planes of the upper, middle and lower part of each joint are slightly angulated to one another, but the overall plane of each joint may be roughly vertical (Solonen, 1957) or oblique (*see* Fig. 6.5).

The synovial membrane is surrounded by the fibrous capsule which is attached close to the margins of both articular surfaces and is reinforced by ligaments.

LIGAMENTOUS ATTACHMENTS (Figs. 6.3; 6.4; 6.5).

To a very large extent, the joint's integrity depends on the strength of its supporting ligaments, as virtually no muscles cross over and support the joint. The toughest ligaments in the body bind the ilia to sacrum: the interosseous sacroiliac, sacrotuberous and sacrospinous ligaments. Other ligaments – the ventral and dorsal sacroiliac and the iliolumbar ligaments – also contribute to the joint's stability.

Interosseous Sacroiliac Ligament (Fig. 6.5).

This is immensely strong, filling the irregular space above and

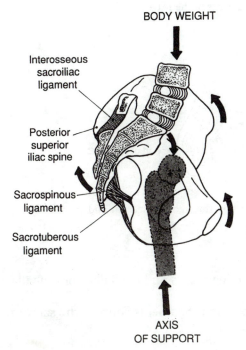

BODY WEIGHT

Interosseous
sacroiliac
ligament

Posterior
superior
iliac spine

Sacrospinous
ligament

Sacrotuberous
ligament

AXIS
OF SUPPORT

Fig. 6.3 Role of ligaments in weight bearing. Sagittal section showing inner aspect of left half of pelvis. In the erect posture, the interosseous sacroiliac ligament resists downward and forward movement of the sacral base. The sacrotuberous and sacrospinous ligaments resist the upward and backward tilting of the apex of the sacrum.

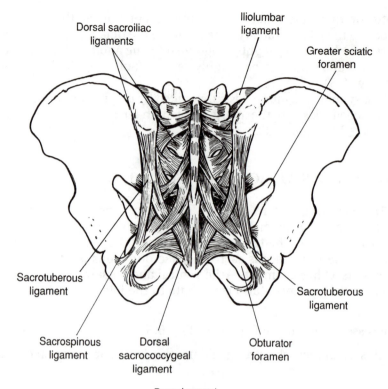

Dorsal aspect

Fig. 6.4 Ligaments of the pelvis.

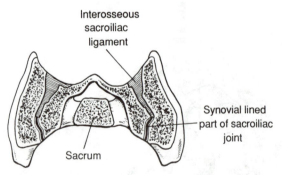

Fig. 6.5 Horizontal section through the sacrum and
sacroiliac joints.

behind the joint. Its fibres pass downwards and medially from the ilia
to the sacrum.

The sacrotuberous and sacrospinous ligaments connect the sacrum
to the ischium.

Sacrotuberous Ligament

This has a broad attachment superiorly from the posterior superior iliac spine to the upper part of the coccyx. Its fibres run obliquely downwards, anteriorly and laterally and narrow into a strong band which widens slightly to be inserted into the medial margin of the ischial tuberosity and ascending ramus of the ischium. This ligament is often found to be tense and tender in sacroiliac joint dysfunction.

Sacrospinous Ligament

This is attached to the ischial spine and passes superiorly, medially and posteriorly to attach to the lateral margins of the sacrum and coccyx, blending with the sacrotuberous ligament. Clinically, this ligament may be responsible for the secondary coccydynia experienced by patients with pelvic dysfunction (Lee, 1989).

EFFECT OF WEIGHT-BEARING ON PELVIC GIRDLE AND LIGAMENTS

When the spine is weight-bearing, there is a constant tendency for the sacral base to move downwards and forwards into the pelvic cavity. The fibres of the interosseous sacroiliac ligament are arranged so as to resist this movement. At the same time, the sacrospinous ligament and, in particular, the sacrotuberous ligament resist the upward and backward tilting of the apex of the sacrum (*see* Fig. 6.3).

As a result of the centre of gravity being located behind the transverse axis of the hip joints, the ilia tend to tilt backwards. This tendency is counterbalanced by the muscle activity of the back extensors and hip flexors.

Ventral Sacroiliac Ligament

This is a thickening of the anterior and inferior parts of the capsule. It is mostly thin, and is the weakest of the group. Clinically, when the sacroiliac joint is hypermobile, this ligament is invariably attenuated and often a source of pain.

Dorsal Sacroiliac Ligament

This covers the interosseous sacroiliac ligament, from which it is separated by the dorsal rami of the sacral spinal nerves and vessels. Its weak fasciculi pass from the intermediate and lateral crests of the sacrum to the posterior superior iliac spine and medial tip of the dorsal part of the iliac crest. The inferior fibres from the sacrum blend, laterally, with the sacrotuberous ligament and, medially, with the posterior layer of the thoracolumbar fascia, providing a direct anatomical link between the extensors of the hip joint and the supporting fascia of the lumbar spine via the sacrotuberous ligament. The skin overlying the dorsal sacroiliac ligament is a frequent area of pain in patients with lumbosacral and pelvic girdle dysfunction, but tenderness on palpation of the ligament does not necessarily incriminate this tissue given the nature of pain referral both from the lumbar spine and the sacroiliac joint (Lee, 1989).

Iliolumbar Ligament (Fig. 6.4)

This is a strong, complex structure which connects the transverse process of the 5th lumbar vertebra to the ilium. It has five parts and is described in more detail in the section on ligaments of the lumbar spine (pp. 47–8). The vertical fibres of the iliolumbar ligament pass anterior to the sacroiliac joint and contribute to its stability. Both iliolumbar ligaments sustain a great deal of tension in the upright posture when they play an important role in helping to prevent the 5th lumbar vertebra from sliding forwards on the sacrum. Together with the 5th lumbar vertebra, both ligaments are also said to prevent separation of the ilia on weight-bearing (Evans, 1955).

FUNCTIONS OF THE SACROILIAC JOINTS

Mechanically, the main function of the sacroiliac joints is the transmission of forces from the head, trunk and upper limbs to the lower limbs. Body weight from the vertebral column is transmitted via the 5th lumbar vertebra to the sacrum, through the sacroiliac joints, along the alae of the sacrum and through the ischial tuberosities towards the acetabulum. The structure of this bony route reflects its weight-bearing function. Part of the reaction of the ground to the body weight is transmitted to the acetabulum by the neck and head of the femur. The rest is transmitted across the horizontal pubic ramus and is counterbalanced at the symphysis by a similar force from the other side (Kapandji, 1974).

The sacroiliac joints may also have an important shock-absorbing function in relation to the lumbar spine, by virtue of energy absorbed in the ligamentous tissue on translatory movements. The increased incidence of the disc degeneration in the lumbar spine after deterioration of the sacroiliac joints is suggestive of this function (Wilder et al., 1980).

During pregnancy, laxity of the joints' ligaments allows an increase in the diameter of the pelvis to facilitate delivery of the baby.

MUSCLES ASSOCIATED WITH THE SACROILIAC JOINT

An unusual feature of the sacroiliac joint is that no muscles act as its prime movers. Movement is indirectly imposed on the joint by the actions of muscles which either pass over it or which attach the pelvis to the trunk or femora, e.g. the abdominal muscles.

The fact that the joint has no intrinsic muscles means that abnormal muscle tension cannot be specifically diagnostic of dysfunction. Spasm of the lower part of the erector spinae muscle is often present in sacroiliac lesions. This muscle is attached distally to the medial aspect of the iliac crest and the sacrum, i.e. in close proximity to the joint.

Other muscles associated with the joint are psoas major, the medial part of which passes anterior to the joint, and piriformis which originates in part from the capsule of the joint. Shortening or spasm of these muscles due either to a localized lesion or to one originating in the lumbar spine will influence the sacroiliac joint's mechanics.

The effect on the sacroiliac joints of the biarticular muscles of the thigh (Fig. 6.6) has been pointed out by Grieve (1980). For example, through its attachment to the ilium, the rectus femoris muscle indirectly causes anterior rotation of the ilium in the presence of hip extension with knee flexion. This occurs at the moment of push-off in the walking cycle when the line of gravity falls anterior to the stance

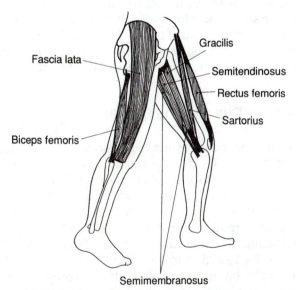

Fig. 6.6 The biarticular muscles of the thigh. (Adapted from E. Grieve, 1980. *The Biomechanical Characterization of Sacroiliac Joint Motion.* MSc Thesis, University of Strathclyde.)

leg. Eccentric contraction of rectus femoris, as in descending stairs, has the same effect on the ilium. Passive stretching of the hamstrings over the knee and hip joints, as occurs for example in rowing, causes posterior rotation of the ilia on the sacrum. For an account of the muscles controlling pelvic tilting, *see* pp. 132–5.

NERVE SUPPLY

Anteriorly, the joints are supplied by nerves derived from L3 to S2; posteriorly from L5 to S2. Variations may occur from one side to the other. This extensive nerve supply, and the proximity of major nerves to the joint's anterior aspect have important clinical implications. The obturator and femoral nerves and lumbosacral trunk pass anterior to the joints, while the superior gluteal nerve and vessels lie lateral and distal to them, leaving the pelvis above the piriformis through the greater sciatic foramen.

Inflammation of the joints or ligamentous laxity causing malalignment of the joints' surfaces can lead to irritation of these nerves, causing referred pain and other symptoms over wide and varied areas, e.g. in the lower trunk, buttock, groin and leg.

Patients with low back disorders often complain of pain over the area of one or other sacroiliac joint, but this does not necessarily vindicate the joint as the source of this pain.

Although the sacroiliac joint itself can be a primary source of pain, it is also the most common site of referred pain and tenderness from the lumbar spine. The examination of patients with pain in the sacroiliac area should, therefore, always include the lumbar spine.

MOVEMENTS OF THE SACROILIAC JOINTS

Much controversy has surrounded the question of whether or not movement of clinical significance occurs in normal sacroiliac joints, and this is largely due to the difficulty in analysing and measuring movement in them. One chief disagreement has been over the location of axes of movement. Studies (*see below*) show that there is, however, no doubt that in normal circumstances small, but definite, movements do occur in the joints. These small movements could perhaps be more accurately described as 'give' in the joints. Jackson (1934) was the first to recognize that because of mechanical leverage, the movement required to produce detrimental changes in the sacroiliac joint needs to be relatively small especially with the joint positioned in one of the extremes of its range.

Considerable variations have been shown between the degree of sacroiliac joint movement in different individuals, and also in both joints in one individual, because of anatomical variations in the articular surfaces of the joints, the prevailing degree of ligamentous laxity and any pathology that may be present. In addition, Pitkin and Pheasant (1936), on studying 144 male university students, found that positions of the ilia in normal stance, as well as their relative mobility, were affected by the dominant eye and hand.

The fact that these variations exist in 'normal' individuals has important clinical significance. All too easily, asymmetry can be mistakenly assumed to be of recent onset, and attempts to 'put the bones back into place' can prove futile.

Symmetrical Movements

Movements of both sacroiliac joints in the sagittal plane were examined by Weisl (1955) in subjects aged from 18 to 28 years. When the subjects moved from supine lying to standing, there was movement of the sacrum between the ilia such that the sacral promontory was displaced downwards and forwards from its 'dorsal' position to its 'ventral' position by as much as 5.6 mm (range 1.4 mm). The reverse movement occurred and was maximal when moving from standing to supine lying.

Similar movements occurred during flexion and extension of the trunk: during flexion, the sacral promontory moved downwards and forwards and, during extension, it moved upwards and backwards. In these instances the movements were smaller and less consistent.

This movement of the sacrum is not one of simple rotation about a fixed horizontal axis as had previously been thought, but is of an angular type (rotation combined with translation) with a dynamic axis generally lying 5–10 cm below the sacral promontory. A few subjects in Weisl's study demonstrated additional sliding movements. Wilder et al. (1980) also concluded that any rotatory movement would involve translation, and deduced from the specimens examined that the degree of movement permitted and the rotational axes would have varied considerably.

From a study on cadavers, Weisl found that with forward displacement of the sacral promontory, the iliac crests were approximated and the ischial tuberosities separated. The extent of this movement was not stated. Colachis et al's experiments on living subjects (1963) confirmed these findings. Using the posterior superior iliac spines as the bony landmarks, they recorded a maximal difference of 1.5 mm approximation in the sitting position and a maximal difference of 5 mm during trunk flexion in standing.

Other movements that have been demonstrated in the sacroiliac joints include both a gliding up and down and a slight anteriorposterior movement in specimens of cadavers under the age of 29 years (Sashin, 1930).

Asymmetrical Movements

Alternating torsion of the pelvis occurs during asymmetrical, every-day activities such as walking (Brooke, 1924), when one ilium is rotated on the sacrum in the opposite direction to the other. The right posterior superior iliac spine, for example, during hip extension in walking, shifts slightly downwards and backwards and hence becomes more prominent relative to that of the left which moves upwards and forwards. An axis of movement around which these movements of the ilia occur has not yet been clearly identified.

The effect of torsional stress on sacroiliac joint movements was examined by Colachis et al. (1963) and they found that such stress was greatest when subjects were in side-lying with one thigh flexed onto the chest and the other extended. This is a position that therapists often place their patients in to mobilize the sacroiliac joints.

A further investigation of movement from torsional stress was carried out by Frigerio et al. (1974) using both a cadaver and a living subject. In vivo movements of the ilia in relation to the sacrum, and between themselves, were demonstrated. In the cadaver, movements between points on the sacrum and ilium ranged up to 12 mm with an average of 2.7 mm. Between the ilia themselves, ranges were up to 15.5 mm. The in vivo ranges were considerably larger than those in the cadaver, movements of the ilia relative to the sacrum, for example, ranging up to 26 mm.

Movements of the sacroiliac joints were also assessed in one leg stance during alternate hip and knee flexion (Grieve, 1980) – a test procedure used in clinical practice.

Reciprocal movements at the symphysis must also occur in con-junction with sacroiliac joint movements, and the interdependence between the triad of pelvic joints is clearly demonstrated when there is abnormality or instability at the pubic symphysis, for example in athletes (Harris and Murray, 1974). Secondary stress lesions may develop in one or both sacroiliac joints; similarly instability in the sacroiliac joints may lead to a secondary stress reaction at the symphysis pubis.

EFFECTS ON THE SACROILIAC JOINTS OF LEG LENGTH INEQUALITY

Real Leg Length Inequality

Differences in relative leg lengths are common, the majority being minor and less than a quarter of an inch. Greater differences are not uncommon and may be congenital, or secondary to trauma or pathological changes in the lower limb.

Adaptation to a short leg takes place primarily in the sacroiliac joint where frequently a quarter of an inch is 'taken up', and secondarily in the lumbar spine (Stoddard, 1980).

Minor differences in leg lengths do not necessarily produce a lateral pelvic tilt and scoliosis. However, in people with more marked leg length inequality, the sacrum will be tilted and a compensatory scoliosis will occur in the lumbar spine, usually at the lower two levels. In these people, there is a natural tendency for the pelvis to adopt the twisted position which more nearly levels the anterosuperior surface of the sacrum. On the side of the longer leg, the ilium will be rotated posteriorly with respect to the sacrum, and the sacrum itself will be rotated about its long axis. The sacroiliac joints are then subjected to unequal stresses, and movements in them are correspondingly asymmetrical. There is a tendency for the joint on the side of the longer leg to stiffen in its posteriorly rotated position due to the stresses and strains of life (Bourdillon, 1982). Cyriax (1934) considered unequal leg length to be a primary cause of sacroiliac joint dysfunction, as did Durey and Rodineau (1976).

Apparent Leg Length Inequality

A state of pelvic torsion can also occur through an inadequacy of the interlocking mechanism, following trauma to the joint itself, during pregnancy, or postpartum when the ligaments are returning to their normal length (*see below*). The position of the posterior superior iliac spines relative to each other may be altered, e.g. the right PSIS may lie more posteriorly and caudally than the left, making the right one more prominent. Simultaneously, the right anterior superior iliac spine would be positioned slightly higher and more posteriorly. This pelvic asymmetry creates an apparent leg length inequality, and measurements taken from bony landmarks on the pelvis to estimate relative leg lengths are rendered seriously inaccurate.

HYPER/HYPOMOBILITY

Laxity of sacroiliac ligaments can occur as part of a generalized *hypermobility* syndrome (p. 169), during pregnancy and postpartum, or it can occur following trauma to the joint. It allows excess movement to occur in the sacroiliac joints. Together with a lack of muscles directly supporting them, the joints are then more prone to strain.

A state of apparent *hypomobility* can occur in these individuals, when the lax ligaments allow a joint to override and then become locked in an abnormal position. The affected joint may or may not be painful, but the consequence of this type of fixation is that it puts strain on the other pelvic joints as well as higher in the spine.

With age or degeneration, fibrous adhesions may form across the sacroiliac joints, with obliteration of the synovial cavity in both sexes, but more so in males. These changes have been demonstrated by Cohen *et al.* (1967) in 24% of individuals. Consequently, a state of true hypomobility then exists.

THE PUBIC SYMPHYSIS

The integrity of the pelvic ring depends not only upon the stability of the sacroiliac joints, but also on that of the pubic symphysis, a cartilaginous joint which holds the pelvic bones firmly together anteriorly. This acts as a compression strut, resisting the medial thrust of the femoral heads (Williams and Warwick, 1980). The adjacent surfaces of the joint are lined with hyaline cartilage and connected by an interpubic disc of fibrocartilage. It is supported by strong superior and inferior ligaments, which make it a strong joint not easily dislocated.

Clearly, movement cannot take place at one sacroiliac joint without affecting the symphysis pubis. Movement at the latter joint is normally minimal. Schunke (1938) demonstrated rotation at the sacroiliac joint causing forward displacement of the pubic bone at the symphysis on the side upon which an individual is bearing weight. In the abnormal joint, other movements may occur such as translation (upward on one side, downward on the other) and separation.

PREGNANCY

Effect on the Sacroiliac Joints

An increase in laxity of the pelvic ligaments is a normal and essential accompaniment of pregnancy. It renders the joints capable of more extensive movement, but it can make them susceptible to being strained. Overriding of a sacroiliac joint can then occur, rendering it apparently hypomobile. As the ligaments return to their normal condition postpartum, it is possible that the normal alignment of the joint may remain at fault and that overstretching of ligaments can give rise to symptoms. Some ligamentous laxity also occurs during the menstrual cycle, although to a lesser degree (Chamberlain, 1930).

Widening of the pubic symphyseal joint margins from the normal 4 mm to as much as 9 mm has been noted in some pregnancies (Young, 1940) and this, together with lax sacroiliac ligaments, may contribute to the instability which can develop and persist postpartum.

Ligamentous laxity begins in the first half of pregnancy and increases during the last 3 months with a subsequent return to normal that starts soon after delivery and is complete within 3–5 months (Abramson *et al.*, 1934). These changes correlate with levels of the hormone relaxin, which increases tenfold during pregnancy, reaching a maximum at 38–42 weeks (Zarrow *et al.*, 1955). It is possible that other hormones including progesterones and endogenous cortisol may also play a part (Calguneri *et al.*, 1982). In the second pregnancy, laxity is more marked than in the first. These mothers are, therefore, even more at risk from straining their sacroiliac joints, especially if they normally have hypermobile joints. Laxity does not continue to increase with third and subsequent pregnancies. Levels of the hormone in twin pregnancies are higher than in singleton pregnancies.

A comparison of the relaxin levels in pregnant women who complained of severe pelvic pain with a control group suggested that there was an association between high relaxin levels and pelvic pain and joint laxity during late pregnancy. The highest relaxin levels during pregnancy were found in patients who were the most incapacitated clinically (MacLennan *et al.*, 1986). However, not all patients with pelvic pain have obvious joint laxity and there are many other causes of this type of pain such as pressure from the gravid uterus, urinary tract infection, referred from higher in the spine, or nerve compression.

All pregnant women with moderately high relaxin levels do not have symptoms and it is thought that relaxin receptor levels in the connective tissues of the sacroiliac joints and pubic symphysis may be more significant than relaxin levels. It may be that some women are more susceptible to circulating or local concentrations of relaxin if a high level of receptors has been induced in these tissues. Induction of relaxin receptors is believed to be influenced by oestrogen (MacLennan *et al.*, 1986).

REFERENCES

Abramson V., Roberts S.M., Wilson P.D. (1934). Relaxation of the pelvic joints in pregnancy. *Surg. Gynecol. Obstet.*, **58**, 595.

Bourdillon J.F. (1982). *Spinal Manipulation*, 3rd edn. London: William Heinemann Medical Books.

Brooke R. (1924). The sacroiliac joint. *J. Anat.*, **58**, 299.

Brown L.T. (1937). The mechanics of the lumbosacral and sacroiliac joints. *J. Bone. Jt. Surg.*, **19**, 3, 770.

Calguneri M., Bird H.A., Wright V. (1982). Changes in joint laxity occurring during pregnancy. *Ann. Rheum. Dis.*, **41**, 126.

Chamberlain W.E. (1930). The symphysis pubis in the roentgen examination of the sacroiliac joint. *Am. J. Roentgenol.*, **24**, 621.

Cohen A.S., McNeill M., Calkins E. *et al.* (1967). The 'normal' sacroiliac joint: analysis of 88 sacroiliac roentgenograms. *Am. J. Roentg.*, **100**, 559.

Colachis S.C., Warden R.E., Bechtol C.O. *et al.* (1963). Movement of the sacroiliac in the adult male. *Arch. Phys. Med. Rehab.*, **44**, 490.

Cyriax E.F. (1934). Minor displacements of the sacroiliac joints. *Br. J. Phys. Med.*, **8**, 191.

Durey A., Rodineau J. (1976). Pubic lesions of athletes. *Ann. De. Med. Phys.*, **3**.

Evans F.G. (1955). Studies on pelvic deformation and fractures. *Anat. Rec.*, **121**, 141.

Frigerio N.A., Stowe R.R., Howe J.W. (1974). Movements of the sacro-iliac joint. *Clin. Orthop. Relat. Res.*, **100**, 370.

Grieve E. (1980). *The Biomechanical Characterization of Sacro-iliac Joint Motion* (Thesis, University of Strathclyde).

Harris N.H., Murray R.O. (1974). Lesions of the symphysis in athletes. *Br. Med. J.*, **4**, 211.

Hellems H.K., Keates T.E. (1971). Measurements of the normal lumbosacral angle. *Am. J. Roentgenol.*, **113**, 642.

Jackson R.H. (1934). Chronic sacro-iliac strain with attendant sciatica. *Am .J. Surg.*, **24**, 456.

Kapandji I.A. (1974). *The Physiology of the Joints, 3: The Trunk and the Vertebral Column*. Edinburgh: Churchill Livingstone.

Lee D. (1989). *The Pelvic Girdle. An Approach to the Examination and Treatment of the Lumbo-pelvic-hip Region*. Edinburgh: Churchill Livingstone, p. 25.

MacLennan A.H., Green R., Nicolson R. *et al.* (1986). Serum relaxin and pelvic pain of pregnancy. *Lancet* **ii**, 243.

Paquin J.D., Van der Rest M., Mort M.J. *et al.* (1983). Biochemical and morphological studies of cartilage from the adult human sacro-iliac joint. *Arthritis Rheum.*, **26**, 7, 887.

Pitkin H.C., Pheasant H.C. (1936). Sacrarthrogenetic tetalgia. *J. Bone. Jt. Surg.*, **18**, 365.

Sashin D. (1930). A critical analysis of the anatomy and pathological changes of the sacroiliac joints. *J. Bone Jt. Surg.*, **12**, 891.

Schunke G.B. (1938). The anatomy and development of the sacro-iliac joint in man. *Anat. Rec.*, **72**, 313.

Solonen K.A. (1957). The sacro-iliac joint in the light of anatomical, roentgenological and clinical studies. *Acta Orthopaed. Scand.*, Suppl. **27**, 1–127.

Stoddard A. (1980). *Manual of Osteopathic Technique*, 3rd edn. London: Hutchinson & Co. (Publishers) Ltd.

Weisl H. (1955). The movements of the sacro-iliac joint. *Acta Anatom.*, **23**, 80.

Wilder D.G., Pope M.H., Fromoyer J.W. (1980). The functional topography of the sacro-iliac joints. *Spine*, **5**, 575.

Williams P.L., Warwick R. (1980). *Gray's Anatomy*, 36th edn. Edinburgh: Churchhill Livingstone.

Young J. (1940). Relaxation of the pelvic joints in pregnancy. *J. Obstet. Gynaecol. Br. Emp.*, **47**, 493.

Zarrow M.X., Holmstrom E.G., Salhanick H.A. (1955). The concentration of relaxin in the blood serum and other tissues of women during pregnancy. *J. Clin. Endocrinol.*, **15**, 22.

FURTHER READING

Aitken G.S. (1986). Syndromes of lumbo-pelvic dysfunction. In *Modern Manual Therapy of the Vertebral Column*. (Grieve G.P., ed.) Edinburgh: Churchill Livingstone, Ch. 43.

Luk K.D.K., Ho H.C., Leong J.C.Y. (1986). The iliolumbar ligament: a study of its anatomy, development and clinical significance. *J. Bone Jt. Surg.*, **68B**, 197.

7

Innervation of the Vertebral Column

A knowledge of the neurology of spinal tissues is essential for the treatment of spinal disorders and aids a better understanding of the clinical features of degenerative disease. In particular the therapist should have a knowledge of:

- The possible level of origin of pain resulting from tissue changes
- Areas to which pain is commonly referred
- Concomitant signs and symptoms (other than pain) which are due to malfunction of the nervous system
- Abnormalities of posture, and changes in range and quality of movement associated with neurological signs and symptoms

SPINAL NERVES

Thirty-one pairs of spinal nerves attach to the spinal column. They are short nerves which lie within the intervertebral foramina. Each spinal nerve divides into an anterior and posterior portion and connects with the spinal cord via ventral and dorsal nerve roots (Fig. 7.1). The ventral roots attach on each side in a longitudinal series to the anterolateral aspect of the cord, while the dorsal roots pass bilaterally to the posterolateral aspect of the cord. Each ventral and dorsal root then divides into a number of small branches called rootlets (*see* Fig. 8.3, p. 246) which form the junction with the spinal cord.

The dorsal roots carry only sensory fibres from the spinal nerves to the spinal cord, whereas the ventral nerve roots transport mostly motor and some sensory fibres. Near the junction of the dorsal and ventral roots, the dorsal root has a swelling known as the *dorsal root ganglion*. It is a collection of cell bodies of all the sensory fibres that run in the related spinal nerve. Dorsal root ganglia are usually situated in the intervertebral foramina, but the ganglia of the 1st and 2nd nerves lie on the vertebral arches of the atlas and axis, the ganglia of the sacral nerves are within the vertebral canal and that of the coccygeal is within the dura.

Degenerative changes may affect the dorsal and ventral roots

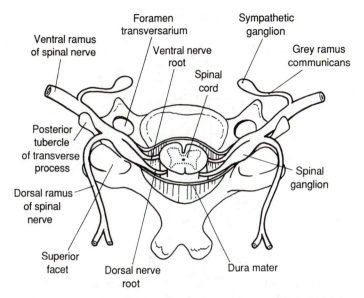

Fig. 7.1 Formation of a spinal nerve – cervical region. (Adapted from P.L. Williams and R. Warwick, 1980. In *Gray's Anatomy*, 36th edn. Edinburgh: Churchill Livingstone, p. 1088.)

separately and irritation of the separate roots has been shown to produce different symptoms, Frykholm (1971) stimulated the ventral and dorsal roots in subjects with existing cervical spine disorders. Stimulation of the cervical dorsal root gave pain within a dermatomal distribution, but stimulation of the ventral root produced a more diffuse pain in the neck, shoulder and upper arm.

The thirty-one pairs of spinal nerves are named according to the vertebra to which they are related. There are eight cervical, twelve thoracic, five lumbar, five sacral and one coccygeal pairs of spinal nerves. The first cervical nerve (suboccipital nerve) passes out from the vertebral canal between the occipital bone and the atlas and, consequently, the cervical spinal nerves lie above the cervical vertebra with the same number. The exception to this is the 8th cervical nerve which emerges *below* the 7th cervical vertebra. Caudal to this level the remaining spinal nerves lie below the correspondingly numbered vertebra. Through its connections with the ventral and dorsal roots and their branches, each nerve attaches to a discrete part of the spinal cord and, hence, the spinal cord is divided into a series of imaginary segments numbered according to the spinal nerve which attaches to it (Fig. 7.2).

Each nerve is covered by pia mater and loosely invested with arachnoid mater up to the point where the roots pierce the dura. The two roots pierce the dura separately and receive a sheath from it. The

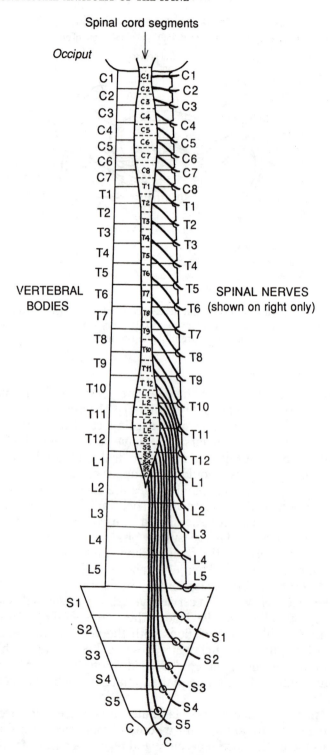

Spinal cord segments

Occiput

VERTEBRAL
BODIES

SPINAL NERVES
(shown on right only)

ganglia receive a covering from the dura and the dura then becomes continuous with the epineurium of the spinal nerve.

Direction of the Nerve Roots

Direction and length of the nerve roots varies at each segmental level. In the early development of the central nervous system, the spinal cord and bony vertebral column are the same length. At this stage, each spinal nerve runs transversely to its corresponding intervertebral foramen. However, due to the disproportionate growth of the bony and neural elements, in the adult, the spinal cord ends at the level of the L1/2 disc. Consequently, for the spinal nerves to remain attached to their respective cord segments and emerge through the corresponding intervertebral foramen, the length and obliquity of the nerve roots increases caudally (see Fig. 7.2). The 1st and 2nd cervical nerve roots are almost horizontal as they exit from the canal. The 3rd–8th roots are directed obliquely downwards. The obliquity and length of the roots successively increases. The distance of the roots from their attachment to the spinal cord to their exit from the vertebral canal is not greater than one vertebra in this region.

In the lower cervical and upper thoracic spine, the rootlets descend for a variable distance within the dura and, on piercing it, they are angled upwards in their course to the intervertebral foramen (Fig. 7.3). At the cervico-thoracic junction, the roots may descend intradurally for several millimetres below the margin of the intervertebral foramen and then become sharply angulated to pass upwards in order to emerge through it (Nathan and Fuerstein, 1974). The spinal nerve emerges through the intervertebral foramen to pass downwards again. Some roots may undergo two marked angulations, particularly those at vertebral junction regions. The degree of angulation may be as much as 30–45°, with the roots of C6–T9 being most often affected and those of T2 and 3 having the greatest degree of angulation. Roots may be further distorted by degenerative changes.

The thoracic roots are small and increase in length caudally. Upper thoracic nerve roots travel about one segmental level to emerge through their respective intervertebral foramina but, in the lower thoracic spine, they descend in contact with the spinal cord for approximately two vertebral levels before leaving the vertebral canal.

The lumbar, sacral and coccygeal nerve roots descend with increasing obliquity. The spinal cord ends at the level of the L1/2 disc, so that the upper lumbar roots travel 9 cm and the lower lumbar roots 16 cm

Fig. 7.2 Diagrammatic representation of spinal nerves in relation to vertebral levels. (Adapted from G.P. Grieve, 1988. *Common Vertebral Joint Problems*, 2nd edn. Edinburgh: Churchill Livingstone.)

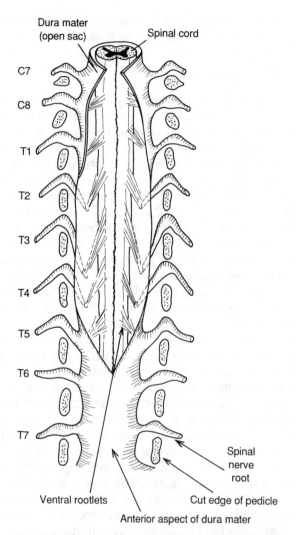

Dura mater
(open sac)

Spinal cord

C7

C8

T1

T2

T3

T4

T5

T6

T7

Spinal
nerve
root

Ventral rootlets

Cut edge of pedicle

Anterior aspect of dura mater

Fig. 7.3 Schematic drawing of the angulated cervicothoracic nerve roots. (From H. Nathan and M.
Feuerstein, 1970. Angulated course of spinal nerve
roots. *J. Neurosurg.*, **32**, 349–352, with permission.)

before emerging through the intervertebral foramina. The collection of
nerve roots below the 1st lumbar vertebra is called the *cauda equina*.

In the cervical spine, the nerve root is anterior and superior to the
apophyseal joint; in the thoracic spine, it is directly anterior to the
joint. In the lumbar spine, the nerve root is anterior and inferior to
the apophyseal joint and also in close proximity to the posterior and
posterolateral aspect of the numerically corresponding intervertebral
disc. Consequently, spinal nerve roots are vulnerable to trespass or
irritation from degenerative changes at the apophyseal joints and,

particularly in the lumbar spine, bulging or prolapse of the intervertebral discs. The spinal nerves may be compressed or irritated at any point in their course from the spinal cord to their exit through the intervertebral foramina.

The nerve roots have a degree of inherent elasticity which allows them to accommodate for changes in vertebral movement. Disease of the vertebral column may adversely affect the mobility of the nerve roots and this is a feature of many spinal pain syndromes (*see* pp. 256, 285).

Components and Branches of the Spinal Nerves

A typical spinal nerve contains both somatic and visceral fibres. The somatic components are both afferent and efferent fibres. The somatic efferent fibres innervate skeletal muscle, while the somatic afferent fibres carry impulses to the spinal cord from receptors in the skin, subcutaneous tissue, muscle, joints, ligaments and fascia. The visceral components of the spinal nerves are afferent and efferent autonomic fibres. They include sympathetic and parasympathetic fibres at different levels (*see* pp. 236–9).

The paravertebral plexus (Stillwell, 1956) is a dense network of fibres in the region of the somatic nerve roots and sympathetic ganglia. Fibres interconnect between the grey rami comunicantes, the sympathetic ganglia and the anterior and posterior primary rami. Mixed branches of this plexus pass externally to supply the periosteum and ligaments at the front, sides and backs of the vertebral bodies. Some fibres join the medial branch of the posterior primary rami of each spinal nerve root to supply the receptors of the apophyseal joints.

The sinuvertebral nerve (also known as the meningeal or recurrent meningeal nerve) is derived from the paravertebral plexus. It has two or more branches on either side, contains mixed efferent autonomic fibres and afferent somatic fibres, and is present at all vertebral levels. The sinuvertebral nerve re-enters the spinal canal through the intervertebral foramen, passing anterior to the dorsal root ganglion. On entering the canal, it divides into mixed ascending, descending and transverse fibres which supply the dura mater, the walls of the blood vessels, the periosteum of the vertebral bodies, the ligaments and the external annular fibres (*see* p. 79).

In the cervical region, the branches may wander up and down the canal for two or three segments before terminating in receptor endings. The ascending branches of the upper three cervical meningeal nerves are relatively large and supply the cerebral dura mater of the posterior cranial fossa and, if irritated, as in a whiplash injury, they may cause cervical headaches.

In the thoracic and lumbar spine, the sinuvertebral nerve may wander up and down the spinal canal for four or five segments before terminating. An example of this are the fibres from the L2 segment which descend along the posterior longitudinal ligament to L5, and it is thought that irritation of this nerve in the upper lumbar spine may give rise to pain in the lower lumbar spine (Brodal, 1981).

Cervical dorsal rami

The dorsal (posterior primary) rami of all the cervical spinal nerves, with the exception of the first, divide into medial and lateral branches. All these branches innervate muscles, but only the medial branches of C2–4 and sometimes C5 supply cutaneous areas.

The 1st cervical dorsal ramus (suboccipital nerve) arises from the C1 spinal nerve and emerges superior to the posterior arch of the atlas and inferior to the vertebral artery. It pierces the suboccipital triangle and supplies the muscles which bound this region.

The 2nd cervical dorsal ramus arises from the C2 spinal nerve dorsal to the atlanto-axial joint and deep to the inferior oblique muscle. It divides into medial, lateral, superior communicating and inferior communicating branches. The medial branch is called the *greater occipital nerve* and, with a branch of the C3 spinal nerve, it ascends into the occipital area where it divides into branches which communicate with the lesser occipital nerve to supply the skin of the scalp as far as the vertex of the skull. The lateral branch supplies the posterior neck muscles.

The 3rd cervical dorsal ramus arises from the C3 spinal nerve in the C2/3 intervertebral foramen. It passes posteriorly around the articular pillar of the 3rd cervical vertebra and divides into medial, lateral and communicating branches. There are two medial branches; the larger is called the *3rd occipital nerve* which ends in the skin of the lower part of the occipital region. The 3rd occipital nerve has been implicated in headache syndromes. Trevor-Jones (1964) found the nerve trapped by osteophytes of the C2/3 joint in three patients with severe headaches. Surgical release of the entrapment relieved the symptoms.

The dorsal rami of C4–8 arise from their respective spinal nerves just outside the intervertebral foramina. The nerves pass backwards around the articular pillar and divide into medial and lateral branches. The medial branches of C4 and 5 supply the skin, while the lateral branches of C4–8 supply the posterior neck muscles.

The atlanto-occipital and lateral atlanto–axial joints are innervated by branches of the ventral rami of C1 and 2. The C2/3 apophyseal joint receives an articular branch from the C3 *dorsal* ramus. Articular branches to the C3/4 apophyseal joint arise from the medial branch of the C3 dorsal ramus.

The medial branches of C4–8 dorsal rami supply articular branches to the apophyseal joints above and below them. Articular branches from adjacent segmental levels may communicate with one another to form a communicating loop posterior to the apophyseal joints (Bogduk, 1982).

Thoracic dorsal rami

The thoracic dorsal (posterior primary) rami arise from their respective spinal nerves just outside the intervertebral foramina. The dorsal rami pass backwards in close proximity to the apophyseal joints and divide into medial and lateral branches.

The *medial branches* emerge between the apophyseal joint, the medial section of the costotransverse ligament and the intertransverse muscle. The medial branches of T1–6 run between semispinalis thoracis and multifidus which they supply. They pierce rhomboids and trapezius, and the cutaneous branches descend for some distance before reaching the skin by the sides of the vertebral spines.

The medial branches of T7–12 dorsal rami supply multifidus and longissimus thoracis and only occasionally supply the skin.

The lateral branches run between the superior costotransverse ligament and the intertransverse muscle before inclining posteriorly on the medial side of levator scapulae. They supply longissimus thoracis, iliocostalis thoracis and levatores costarum. The lateral branches of the upper thoracic dorsal rami give a variable supply to the skin, but those of T6–12 give off cutaneous branches that reach the skin in line with the angle of the ribs. The lateral cutaneous branches may descend the breadth of four ribs before becoming superficial.

The costovertebral and costotransverse joints are both innervated by the thoracic dorsal rami as well as the related intercostal nerves (Wyke, 1975).

The course of two thoracic dorsal rami are of particular importance. The dorsal rami of the 2nd thoracic nerve descend paravertebrally until they emerge at the level of T6. The nerve then ascends over the posterior chest wall and scapula to the acromion. Irritation of this nerve can produce pain over the posterior chest wall and shoulder area. The lateral branches of the dorsal rami of the 12th thoracic nerve descend paravertebrally in the lumbar spine to the postero-lateral iliac crest. They then run laterally and supply the skin over the buttock area. Vertebral disease that causes irritation or compression of this nerve can, therefore, give pain in the low lumbar and buttock area.

Lumbar dorsal rami

The L1–4 dorsal rami of the lumbar spinal nerves pass backwards and medially to divide into medial and lateral branches at every level.

Intermediate branches are sometimes present. The L5 dorsal ramus is longer and passes over the alar of the sacrum (Bogduk *et al.*, 1982).

The lateral branches supply the erector spinae. The lateral branches of the L1–3 give off cutaneous nerves which supply the skin of the gluteal region, and may extend as far as the level of the greater trochanter.

Intermediate branches supply the lumbar fibres of the longissimus muscle. Medial branches of the upper four lumbar dorsal rami pass along the top of their respective transverse processes, piercing the intertransverse ligament at the base of the transverse process. The nerve passes around the base of the superior articular process, crosses the lamina and then divides into multiple branches, which supply the multifidus muscle, interspinous muscles and ligaments, and two apophyseal joints. Each medial branch supplies the apophyseal joints above and below its course (Bogduk, 1982). The L5 dorsal rami supply the lumbosacral apophyseal joints.

The muscular supply of the medial branches is very specific. Each medial branch supplies only those muscles attached to the laminae and spinous process of the vertebra with the same segmental number as the nerve. Therefore, the L1 medial branch supplies only those fibres arising from the 1st lumbar vertebra. This indicates that the muscles which move a particular segment are innervated by the nerve of that segment (Bogduk and Twomey, 1987).

Sacral and coccygeal dorsal rami

The sacral dorsal rami are small and, with the exception of the 5th sacral nerve, they emerge through the dorsal sacral foramina.

The medial branches of S1–3 end in multifidus. The lateral branches join together and with branches of L4 and 5 dorsal rami form loops on the dorsal surface of the sacrum. These loops join with a second series of loops under gluteus maximus, which give cutaneous branches to supply the skin over the posterior gluteal area.

The dorsal rami of S4 and 5 do not divide into medial and lateral branches, but unit together and, with the dorsal ramus of the coccygeal nerve, form loops on the dorsal surface of the sacrum. Cutaneous branches from these loops supply the skin over the coccyx.

INTERVERTEBRAL FORAMINA

The intervertebral foramina are oval, ellipsoid spaces that are bound inferiorly by the pedicles, anteriorly by the intervertebral disc and adjacent vertebral bodies and posteriorly by the apophyseal joints (Fig. 7.4). The foramina contain:

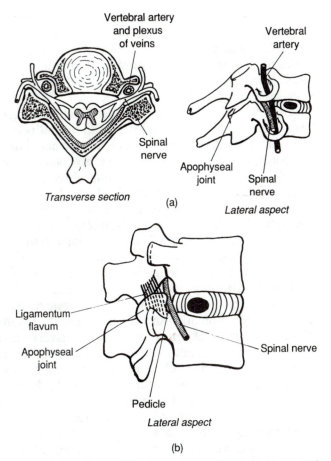

Fig. 7.4 Boundaries of the intervertebral foramen. (a) cervical
spine; (b) lumbar spine.

Areolar tissue
Adipose tissue
The spinal nerve
Spinal artery
A plexus of small veins
Lymphatic vessel
Branches of the sinuvertebral nerve

The nerve and its sheath occupy between one-third and one-half of
the cross-sectional area of the foramen. The foraminal contents are
partially protected by the surrounding fat, and the cerebrospinal fluid
protects the nerve root in the subarachnoid space.

The vertical height of the foramen is greater than the anteroposterior measurement. In the cervical spine, the pedicle and posterior

tubercle of the transverse process form the inferior boundary of the foramina to make a gutter for the spinal nerve. This gutter may exceed 1 cm in length. The foramina of the thoracic spine have the smallest anteroposterior measurement. In the lumbar spine, the vertical height of the foramina varies between 12–19 mm, while the anteroposterior measurement varies from 7–10 mm.

In the lumbar spine, the spinal nerve lies in the lateral recess of the foramina. The lateral recess is bounded by the medial portion of the superior articular facet and lamina above, the pedicle laterally and the vertebral body and adjacent intervertebral disc below. The nerve is most vulnerable in its course through the lateral recess.

The dimensions of the foramina may be reduced developmentally or by degenerative changes. Developmental factors such as short pedicles, shallow lateral recess or shorter interfacetal distance will result in a narrow canal (spinal stenosis). The dimensions of the canal may be further reduced if degenerative changes are superimposed and the foraminal contents become particularly vulnerable to trespass.

The foramina are naturally smaller in the lower cervical and lower lumbar spine; these regions are also particularly prone to degenerative disease. A simple reduction in disc height is usually insufficient to embarrass the nerve root. Diminution of the transverse diameter is more likely to trespass the foraminal contents. Posterior protrusion or herniation of the intervertebral disc, osteoarthritis of the apophyseal joints with thickening and exostosis and a retrolisthesis may all give rise to acquired spinal stenosis with resultant nerve root compression.

The dimensions of the foramina alter with vertebral movement. The height of the foramina will tend to decrease in extension and increase in flexion. Side-flexion will tend to reduce the height of the foramina on the side to which movement occurs and increase the height of the foramina on the opposite side.

VERTEBRAL ARTICULAR RECEPTOR SYSTEMS

Four types of receptor nerve endings have been identified in synovial joints (Wyke, 1967). They each have individual characteristic behavioural properties and their distribution varies in different joints and in different regions of each joint capsule. Types I, II and III are corpuscular mechanoreceptors and Type IV are non-corpuscular nociceptive (pain) receptors.

Type I

These are small globular mechanoreceptors which are located in the peripheral layers of the fibrous apophyseal joint capsule. They are particularly numerous in the cervical spine. These receptors are low threshold, slowly adapting and are sensitive to mechanical stress. The pressure differences inside and outside joint capsules and the capsular stress produced by surrounding muscles and ligaments causes some Type I receptors to discharge continuously at a low frequency. They contribute to awareness of joint position in active and static joints. These receptors are most numerous in the areas subjected to the greatest stress. Other receptors are sensitive to direction, speed and degree of active and passive joint movement. They also monitor atmospheric pressure changes. Type I receptors have an inhibitory effect on the transynaptic centripetal flow of nociceptive afferent activity from Type IV receptors and are, therefore, important in pain suppression.

Type II

These are larger and found mainly in the deeper layers of the capsule and on the surface of intra-articular fat pads, where they often lie in close association with blood vessels. These receptors are also more numerous in the cervical apophyseal joint capsules. They are low threshold, rapidly adapting and do not discharge at rest. They discharge at the beginning and end of movement and are sensitive to acceleration and deceleration. They are reflexogenic and do not respond to changes in joint position or movement.

Type II discharge in response to vibratory stimulation and have transient inhibitory effects on the centripetal nociceptive afferent activity, thereby aiding pain suppression.

Types I and II receptor systems are operative in normal and abnormal circumstances. The reduction in pain achieved by some physiotherapy techniques, e.g. passive oscillatory mobilization, traction, massage, is thought to be in part due to stimulation of Types I and II mechanoreceptors which then have an inhibitory effect on afferent nociceptive activity (see pp. 224–5).

Type III

These occur only in intra- and extra-articular ligaments of peripheral joints, and are not present in the capsules or ligaments of the vertebral joints.

Nociceptive System

The Type IV receptor system is a three-dimensional plexus of unmyelinated nerve fibres. It is nociceptive (pain provoking), high threshold and non-adaptive. The system is activated when its nerve fibres are depolarized by high mechanical stress (e.g. abnormal postures, fractures, disclocations) or exposure to chemical irritants (e.g. histamine, lactic acid) which accumulate in the tissue fluid of acutely and chronically inflamed joints. The Type IV receptors are distributed throughout the tissues of the spine (Table 1).

There are no nerve endings in the synovial membrane, articular cartilage or menisci.

Degenerative Disease Affecting Articular Receptor Systems

Afferent impulses from the Type I mechanoreceptors in periarticular tissue influence efferent impulses which control the tone of the skeletal muscles. Maintainance of normal posture and performance of voluntary movement is dependent on the normal afferent activity of Type I receptors. Damage or irritation of the periarticular tissues in degenerative disease affect the impulses from the Type I receptors so

Table 1
Distribution of Type IV Receptors

Tissue	Type IV receptors
Cancellous bone of vertebral bodies and arches	Blood vessels of cancellous bone are accompanied by perivascular nociceptive plexuses. The small diameter fibres are poorly myelinated or unmyelinated
Periosteum of vertebrae, tendons, fasciae, aponeuroses	Unmyelinated plexiform endings
Periarticular arteries, arterioles, epidural and paravertebral veins and venules	Plexuses of unmyelinated nociceptive nerve filaments
Deep and superficial capsule and fat pads	Plexiform nociceptive receptors Fat pads have a very rich supply
Ligaments – longitudinal, flaval, ligamentum nuchae and inter-transverse	Unmyelinated free nerve endings Particularly numerous in the posterior longitudinal ligament
Dura mater – anterior and dural sleeves only Posterior aspect is not innervated	Unmyelinated plexiform endings
Cervical epidural adipose tissue	Unmyelinated plexiform endings

that postural and kinaesthetic sensations are impaired. Afferent (non-sensory) activity of the Type I and Type II mechanoreceptors exerts powerful tonic reflexogenic influences on facilitatory and inhibitory patterns in the motorneurone pools of the cervical, limb and jaw musculature (Wyke, 1979), and these underlie the functional groupings of muscles during postural control and voluntary activity. Dee (1978) suggests that these reflexes are important in maintaining articular congruity and assist in distributing the load on the joint.

Degenerative disease, which alters afferent input from Type I and II mechanoreceptors, impairs these arthrokinetic reflexes, thereby making the joints more susceptible to damage through stresses and strains. These arthrokinetic reflexes are also disturbed when joints are immobilized, e.g. splints, corsets, collars and, consequently, postural and kinaesthetic sense may be affected. The upper cervical apophyseal joints are particularly rich in mechanoreceptors. The latter become defective in degenerative disease and can give rise to symptoms of dysequilibrium. If the cervical spine is immobilized in a collar, the altered afferent input from the Types I and II mechanoreceptors influences postural and kinaesthetic sense, so that the subject may find control of balance more difficult. Postural sensation is not totally dependent on joint mechanoreceptors – cutaneous and myotatic (muscle spindle) mechanoreceptors also have a role in maintenance of posture (Wyke, 1981).

Degenerative disease that affects Type IV mechanoreceptors will produce pain, abnormal patterns of muscle reflexes and also have reflexogenic effects on the respiratory and cardiovascular system.

During the ageing process, in the peripheral nerves there is a greater degeneration of the myelinated large diameter afferent mechanoreceptor neurones than the smaller pain fibres. Elderly people have a decreased pain tolerance, and it has been suggested that this may be due to the decrease in inhibitory effect of the large fibre mechanoreceptors on the dorsal horn gate mechanism (*see* pp. 224–5). Afferent impulses from touch and pressure receptors are conveyed by Group II large diameter fibres. These fast conducting fibres are also affected by degenerative disease. Wyke (1976) states that mechanoreceptor depletion occurs in paravertebral zones of increased sensitivity. This may be a mechanism through which such local areas of tenderness occur.

SOURCES OF PAIN

The International Association for the Study of Pain has defined pain as 'an unpleasant sensory and emotional experience associated with actual or potential tissue damage, or described in terms of such damage'.

Pain arising from the different structures in the spine varies in quality, distribution and behaviour. When assessing a patient, skilful questioning and careful listening are essential if the therapist is to understand and interpret the nature of the patient's pain.

Joint Pain

Pain arising from degenerate spinal joints is frequently unilateral and described as a deep diffuse ache. It is probably caused by irritation of mechanical and chemical nociceptors in the synovial joint capsules and the innervated connective tissue of the interbody joints concurrently involved (Grieve, 1988). Joint pain is often made worse by sustained postures and positions in which the joint surfaces are approximated, e.g. prolonged standing with a lordotic posture. Small myelinated and unmyelinated nerve fibres have been described in the epiphyseal and metaphyseal regions – they wind round the trabeculae and spread out on the under-surface of the articular cartilage. Compressive forces causing impingement of these plexuses may be a factor in the production of joint pain, as may engorgement of vessels in the subchondral bone.

Ligamentous Pain

Ligaments are rich in nociceptors and they may become irritated by mechanical and chemical changes in degenerate joints or if they are subjected to sustained tension. Ligamentous pain has been described as a deep diffuse ache which may be referred proximally or distally (*see* p. 226). Typically, the pain is aggravated by sustained tension, particularly by the stresses of poor posture, when it may be related to the patient's working positions. It is also made worse by prolonged periods of inactivity.

Muscle Pain

Nociceptors of skeletal muscle are distributed in a plexiform network around all vessels except capillaries and respond to mechanical and chemical irritants (Mills *et al.*, 1984). The build-up of metabolites, in particular lactic acid, 5-hydroxytryptamine, bradykinin and histamine, may give rise to local pain. Mechanical distortion of enlarged vessels in a muscle will also irritate the nociceptors of the vessel walls.

Pain may result from the chemical irritants of ischaemia, prolonged tension between muscle attachments or an increase in tone of a muscle overlying a joint problem.

In a normal individual, prolonged isometric contraction or repeated contractions of a muscle may cause pain, and it will be more readily felt if the person is untrained or elderly (Wyke, 1987; *see* p. 90). Muscles subjected to prolonged postural stress fatigue so that a deep diffuse ache often develops. Once metabolites have built up in the tissues, it may take some time for them to disperse, even in a supported antigravity position e.g. in bed.

Muscle pain and tenderness may be felt in lesions involving segmentally related viscera (*see* pp. 230–1).

The relationship between pain, spasm and tenderness is very complex. Pain may arise from local joint pathology rather than the muscle overlying the lesion. Both pain and muscle tenderness may be referred, and hypertonus of a muscle does not always cause pain.

When assessing a patient with a spinal disorder, it is essential that the relevant muscle groups are considered and that examination is not confined to the joints alone, as muscles will not infrequently contribute to the pain.

Vascular Pain

Two types of vascular pain are recognized: arterial pressure and venous congestion.

Pain that is rhythmical, surging, pounding or beating is associated with arterial pressure. Mechanoreceptors in the plexiform nervous network around the vessel walls are stimulated by vascular pulsation. They fire at the beginning or ending of movement, thereby giving rise to a throbbing sensation rather than continuous pain.

Inflammation of the soft tissues of the vertebral column is associated with venous congestion and pain may develop due to mechanical or chemical irritants. Mechanical stress of mechanoreceptors in the joint capsule or ligaments may cause pain as will the formation of metabolites during tissue breakdown.

Nerve Root (Radicular) Pain

Compression of a spinal nerve does not necessarily cause pain (Lindahl, 1966). Radicular pain may be due to a combination of compression and inflammation (Howe, 1979). Kibler and Nathan (1960) demonstrated that radicular pain could be relieved by local anaesthesia of the nerves a long way distal to the site of damage of a nerve root. Hence, nerve impulses of undamaged tissue are necessary for pain to be felt, and damage to a nerve root may block impulses which normally inhibit pain excitation rather than the nerve root producing increased excitation at the point of damage.

Acute nerve root pain is severe and is often described as sickening, lancinating, burning. It is generally worse distally and its distribution is clearly demarcated within the dermatome of the affected nerve root (*see* Figs. 7.9 and 7.10). The pain may be accompanied by paraesthesiae, neurological signs of altered skin sensation, reduced muscle power and absent or diminished reflexes.

There may be a latent period to the pain so that pain surges into the affected limb some seconds after the causative movement has been performed. These symptoms are usually highly irritable and great care must be taken when handling a patient with nerve root pain to ensure that the pain is not exacerbated. Two theories have been proposed to explain latency (Grieve, 1988):

1. Compression of a nerve selectively affects fibres of different diameters, thereby influencing their rates of conduction recovery and nociceptor impulse reactivity.
2. Spinal or limb movements may displace tissue exudate into surrounding tissues, thereby causing more mechanical or chemical irritation.

Bone Pain

Bone pain is often described as having an unpleasant deep throbbing quality. It may be due to:

1. Neoplasm – primary or secondary
2. Intrinsic bone disease, e.g. Paget's disease
3. Fractures – particularly stress fractures of the spine secondary to osteoporosis
4. Venous engorgement of the vertebral veins
5. Osteomyelitis

There is no evidence that osteophytosis or bone cysts can by themselves create pain (Harkness *et al.*, 1984).

PAIN PATHWAYS

Pain is perceived as a result of a complex convergence, summation and modulation of different temporal and spatial stimuli. A damaging stimulus is a noxious stimulus. A noxious stimulus of a single receptor or single type of receptor alone will not result in the perception of pain. Noxious stimuli must reach a certain intensity before pain is felt. The *pain threshold* is the *least* intensity of noxious stimulation at which a subject perceives pain. Experiments using stimuli such as radiant heat, electric shock and mechanical pressure have demonstrated that the pain perception threshold is fairly constant from person to person (Bowsher, 1988a). The *pain tolerance level* is the greatest intensity of noxious stimulation an individual can bear, and it varies widely from person to person. Many factors influence the pain tolerance level – cultural background, previous experience of pain, mental state, drugs. Motivation and emotional significance of pain can also alter the pain tolerance level. Clinically, patients seek help when their pain has gone beyond their tolerance level.

There are three types of nerve fibres: A, B and C. The velocity of impulses conducted in nerve fibres is directly related to the fibre diameter; the thicker the fibre, the faster the conduction velocity. Group A fibres are myelinated and subdivided into four groups – alpha, beta, gamma, delta – with decreasing diameters and conduction velocities. Group B fibres are unmyelinated postganglionic autonomic fibres. Group C fibres are unmyelinated postganglionic efferent autonomic fibres and somatic and visceral afferent fibres.

Fibres involved in the perception of pain are A delta, C, and A beta fibres.

A Delta Nociceptors

These unmyelinated neurones are distributed mainly in the skin, although small numbers have been located in joints and muscle. They are sensitive to high intensity mechanical stimuli and noxious temperatures. They carry impulses at an average speed of 15 m/s and produce sharp, pricking localized pain.

C Polymodal Nociceptors

These are unmyelinated and found in the deep layers of the skin and most tissues of the body. They remain silent unless activated by noxious stimuli and are sensitive to mechanical, thermal and chemical stimuli. They are not sensitive to different forms of energy, but to a factor common to damaged tissue, however the damage is caused. Impulses are conducted along the polymodal nociceptors at a rate of 1 m/s and reproduce a dull, aching, diffuse pain.

Following a noxious stimulus, e.g. pinching, two types of pain are normally experienced. The initial sharp pain is due to stimulation of the faster conducting A delta fibres, and the aching which develops a few seconds later is transmitted by the slower conducting C fibres.

Cell bodies of the A delta and C nociceptors are in the spinal dorsal root of trigeminal nerve ganglia. The proximal ends of the A delta axons and 70% of the C polymodal axons enter the central nervous system through the dorsal roots. The remaining 30% of C polymodal nociceptors double back to the mixed nerve and enter the spinal cord through the ventral root. This arrangement partly explains why dorsal rhyzotomy (cutting of the dorsal root) does not relieve pain completely.

A delta and C fibres are facilitatory to the input of pain transmission at the substantia gelatinosa.

A Beta Neurones

These are large fibre low threshold cutaneous mechanoreceptors. They carry impulses at 30 m/s and have a low threshold to noxious stimuli, a low threshold to electrical stimulation and a high threshold to chemicals. They are inhibitory to the input transmission at the substantia gelatinosa.

Melzack and Wall (1965) proposed the Gate Control Theory of Pain. Details of the theory are still being disputed, but it has increased the understanding of pain mechanisms and modulation. It is proposed that there are mechanisms at spinal cord level that 'open the gate' to noxious stimuli, so pain is perceived, or 'close the gate', so we are less aware of pain. Cells in the outer laminae of the spinal grey matter receive afferent impulses from the A delta and C nociceptors, which tend to facilitate onward transmission, and afferent impulses from A beta fibres which tend to inhibit transmission; when the input from the A delta and C nociceptors reaches a critical level, reflexes associated with noxious input occur and pain is experienced.

Pain can be modulated in a number of ways (Fig. 7.5). The A beta fibres are known to have a modulatory effect on impulses travelling along the C fibres. The C nociceptors excite cells in Lamina II and III (substantia gelatinosa) which converge onto spinoreticular cells in deeper layers. The main axons of the A beta fibres pass up the dorsal columns of the spinal cord, but on entering the cord, they give off segmental collateral axons which terminate on the terminals of the C fibres in the substantia gelatinosa.

When A beta fibres are activated, e.g. by rubbing, the collaterals partially excite the nociceptor terminals. When impulses then come along the nociceptor fibres, the terminals are in a refractory state (reduced excitability) so the quantity of transmitter substance released from the nociceptor terminals in response to the impulses is decreased or abolished. This is termed *presynaptic inhibition*. This mechanism is the basis of pain relief of some therapeutic treatments, i.e. massage, rocking, passive movement, manual mobilizations, vibration, transcutaneous electrical nerve stimulation (TENS).

It is thought that there are several different 'gate control mechanisms' within the spinal cord and at higher levels within the nervous system (Bowsher, 1988b).

Chemical modulation occurs at the substantia gelatinosa. Opiate receptor sites have been identified on the membrane and dendrites of some nerve cells. *Enkephalin* is a naturally occurring opiate that acts at the receptor sites to inhibit the neurone. Acupuncture is known to affect pain by stimulating enkephalinergic neurones. A delta fibres end on marginal cells in lamina I and also on spinothalamic cells in lamina V. They have collateral axons which reach inhibitory enkephalinergic interneurones in the substantia gelatinosa. The inhibitory neurones are driven by primary A delta afferents which are activated by pinprick (Acupuncture). It is thought that acupuncture points are where small bundles of A delta afferents and sympathetic efferents pierce the deep fascia. This theory only applies to acupuncture applied within the

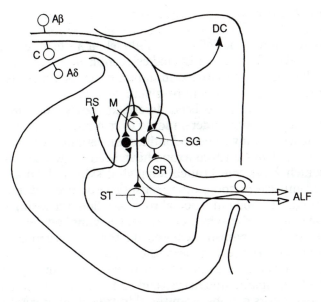

Fig. 7.5 Spinal cord circuitry. C polymodal nociceptors excite cells in the substantia gelatinosa (SG), which converges onto spinoreticular cells (SR) in deeper layers. Acting on the C terminals are terminals of collateral axons of A-beta fibres, whose main fibres pass up the dorsal columns (DC). Thus TENS stimulation applied to peripheral A-beta fibres or anti-dromic stimulation of DC fibres in the spinal cord will presynaptically inhibit C terminals. A-delta fibres end on marginal layer (M) cells in lamina I, as well as on deeper (lamina V) spinothalamic (ST) cells; but they also have collaterals reaching inhibitory enkephalinergic interneurons (solid black) in the substantia gelatinosa, which inhibit relay cells (SG) in the substantia gelatinosa. Since the inhibitory interneurons are driven by A-delta primary afferents, the effective stimulus will be pinprick (i.e. acupuncture); fibres descending from the brainstem (RS) also reach these inhibitory interneurons; since they are enkephalinergic, their action is reversible by nalox-one. ALF = anterolateral funiculus. (From Peter E. Wells, Victoria Frampton and David Bowsher, 1987. *Pain: Management and Control in Physiotherapy*. London: Heinemann Medical Books, with permission.)

same segment of pain, as the mechanism of acupuncture applied at a site distant to the pain segment must be different.

Pain modulation described above occurs within the central nervous system. Aspirin raises the peripheral threshold of primary nociceptor afferents (Mense, 1982) and it is the only known example of peripheral modulation of pain (Bowsher, 1988c).

REFERRED PAIN

Referred pain may be defined as: 'Pain felt at a site other than that of tissue damage'. It frequently makes identification of the damaged tissues difficult, and careful examination of the patient is necessary if accurate local treatment is to be given.

Two mechanisms have been described (Bowsher, 1988b) which provide a basis for the understanding of referred pain (Figs. 7.6; 7.7). Bifurcated axons have been identified in peripheral sensory nerves (Taylor *et al.*, 1984). These axons have been shown to have sensory units, which have one branch supplying skin and another branch supplying muscle or some other sensory structure. Bifurcated axons have a single cell body in a dorsal root ganglion and a single proximal axon travelling to the spinal cord from the ganglion cell.

The second mechanism is based on the convergence of separate peripheral sensory nerves onto the same cell in the spinal cord. Therefore, nociceptors from viscera travelling to the spinal cord in sympathetic or splanchnic nerves end on the same dorsal horn cells as do the nociceptors coming from the skin travelling in somatic nerves. The central cell may be more used to receiving input via one of the peripheral neurones and it may interpret input from the normally less active neurone as coming from the normally more active neurone (Fig. 7.7).

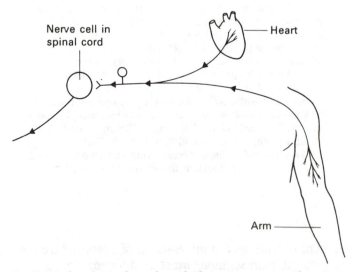

Fig. 7.6 Referred pain due to branched sensory neurons. The primary afferent shown has branches supplying both heart and arm. (From Peter E. Wells, Victoria Frampton and David Bowsher, 1987. *Pain: Management and Control in Physiotherapy.* London: Heinemann Medical Books, with permission.)

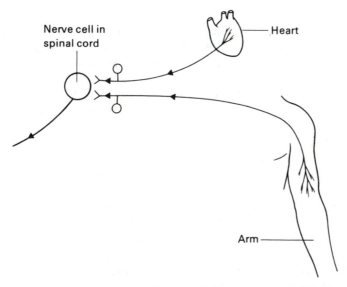

Fig. 7.7 Referred pain due to convergence. The nerve cell in the spinal cord receives input from two different peripheral neurons, one supplying the arm, the other the heart. Since the central cell is more 'used' to getting input from the arm, input from the heart may be interpreted as coming from the arm. (From Peter E. Wells, Victoria Frampton and David Bowsher, 1987. *Pain: Management and Control in Physiotherapy*. London: Heinemann Medical Books, with permission.)

Three types of referred pain are commonly recognized – somatic referred, visceral referred and radicular pain.

Somatic Referred Pain

A lesion in a somatic structure may cause pain to be felt at a location distant to the site of the lesion; this is termed somatic referred pain. There is now considerable evidence to show that noxious stimulation of the non-nervous tissues in the spine may give rise to referred pain which may be felt around the chest wall or radiating into the limbs.

Lumbar somatic referred pain

By injecting saline into the tissues, Kellgren (1938) showed that noxious stimulation of the interspinous structures and back muscles reproduced not only low back pain, but also referred pain and tenderness in the lower limbs. Similar experiments by other investigators have confirmed these findings (Feinstein *et al.*, 1954; Hockaday and Whitty, 1967).

Attempts have been made to define specific areas of segmentally referred somatic pain, similar to the dermatomes used in the diagnosis of segmental level of nerve root compression. Segmental areas of somatic innervation have been termed sclerotomes (Inman and Saunders, 1944). Clinically, it would be useful if such charts could be established, but their value in determining the level of a lesion is strictly limited. In each individual, there is considerable overlap in the area of referred pain from specific segments. Between different individuals, there is considerable variation in the segmental pattern of referred pain (Bogduk, 1980). However, in a single subject, when the same segment is repeatedly stimulated, the area of referral of pain is consistently the same.

Somatic referred pain from the lumbar spine is most commonly distributed over the buttock area, but it may extend as far as the foot (Kellgren, 1939; Mooney and Robertson, 1976). It has been reported that the intensity of the stimulus is proportional to the distance of referral of pain into the leg (Mooney and Robertson, 1976). An important feature of somatic referred pain is its quality, which is often described as a deep, diffuse ache. It differs from radicular pain which has a sharper, lancinating quality, and which is clearly demarcated within the dermatome of the affected nerve.

Experimental evidence has also shown that the lumbar apophyseal joints may also be implicated in the production of referred pain. Noxious stimulation of the lumbar apophyseal joints has been shown to refer pain to the buttocks, groin and lower limbs (McCall et al., 1979; Fig. 7.8). Equally, in some patients the introduction of an anaesthetizing injection into a local symptomatic apophyseal joint lesion relieves referred pain (Carrera, 1980).

The anterior part of the dura mater is innervated and hence pain sensitive. Traction of the dura mater can produce buttock and thigh pain (Smyth and Wright, 1958).

Thoracic somatic referred pain

Diagnosis of referred pain to the chest wall can be difficult as many viscera refer pain to the chest wall. Chest pain can be caused by pleurisy, cardiac ischaemia, disorders of the gallbladder, pancreas, oesophagus and diaphragm. Pain referred around the thorax can also arise from a spinal or rib lesion, and it may mimic visceral disease. Diseases of the viscera are frequently potentially serious, and it is essential that they are excluded as a source of pain, but the therapist must also be aware that chest wall pain may be skeletal or somatic in origin.

Experiments have shown that noxious stimulation of the thoracic interspinous structures can produce somatic referred pain to the anterior, lateral and posterior aspects of the chest wall (Kellgren, 1939; Feinstein et al., 1954). Although there is no consistent area for

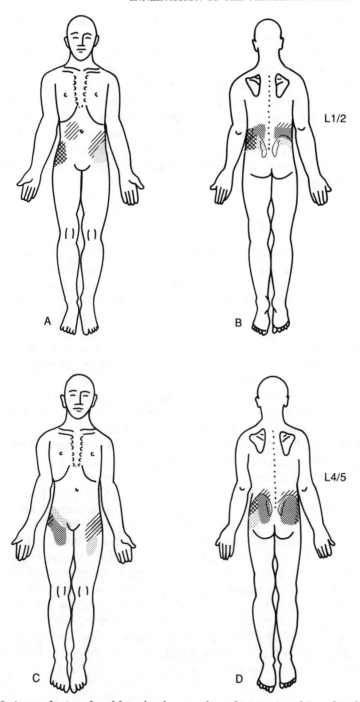

Fig. 7.8 Areas of pain referral from lumbar apophyseal joints. A and B = distribution of pain referral from intracapsular injections of saline solution at L1/2; C and D = distribution of pain referral from intracapsular injections of saline solution at L4/5. (Adapted from I.W. McCall, W.M. Park and J.P. O'Brien, 1979. Induced pain referral from posterior lumbar elements in normal subjects. *Spine*, **4**, 5, 441.)

referred pain from a particular segment, stimulation of the higher thoracic levels tends to refer pain to the higher parts of the chest wall. However, stimulation of a particular level may produce referred pain above or below that particular segment and segmental level of a lesion cannot be identified from the area of referred pain.

Unlike the cervical and lumbar regions, the role of the apophyseal and costotransverse joints in the production of referred pain has not been studied. It is likely that the same mechanism occurs in the thoracic spine as in other areas, and future experiments on the joints of this region may demonstrate that they also cause referred pain (Bogduk, 1988a).

Cervical somatic referred pain

Somatic referred pain from the cervical spine may be distributed in the head, chest wall or upper limb. Noxious stimulation of the interspinous ligaments and muscles in the cervical spine produces referred pain. Stimulation of the upper cervical levels (C1–3) can produce referred pain in the head and occipital area (Bogduk, 1988b). Stimulation of structures innervated by C4 can cause pain in the occipital region, but stimulation of C4 and below have not been reported as causing pain in the forehead. Pain in the upper limb has been produced by stimulation of the lower cervical levels (C5–T1), while shoulder pain can be produced by stimulation of any level from C1 to C8 (Feinstein et al., 1954; Kellgren, 1939). Pain referred to the chest wall from the cervical spine may mimic angina.

Similar to the other spinal regions, there is considerable overlap in the area of segmental referral and inconsistency in the location of referred pain in different subjects so that the area of referred pain is not diagnostic of the affected level. Nevertheless, as shoulder pain can arise from any level in the cervical spine, the neck should be carefully examined in those patients presenting with shoulder pain.

In patients with local apophyseal joint lesions, the introduction of a local anaesthetic into the joint relieves both neck and referred pain (Bogduk and Marsland, 1986; Hildebrandt and Argyrakis, 1986). This suggests that the apophyseal joints are also a source of referred pain.

Noxious stimulation of the cervical discs (Cloward, 1959) by electrical and mechanical means produced pain over the posterior chest wall and scapular region. This evidence, together with studies on disc innervation (see p. 79) indicates that the discs can be a primary source of both local and referred pain.

Visceral Referred Pain

Visceral disease can produce pain that mimics a vertebral joint disorder. This phenomenon of referred pain is thought to be due to somatovisceral convergence, where separate nociceptors from skin and viscera converge on the same dorsal horn cells in the spinal cord (Hinsey and Phillips, 1949). Distension, traction and, in some instances, strong contractions of a viscus, may produce pain. True visceral pain from pathological conditions affecting a viscus is often difficult for a patient to localize due to the relative paucity of nerve endings, and may be dull, vague, cramping or stabbing, overlying the general area of the viscus.

Noxious stimulation of a viscus may produce an area of cutaneous pain that is tender to touch. This may be accompanied by cutaneous vasoconstriction and increased tone in the overlying muscles (Keele and Neil, 1971). The areas of skin on the chest wall which have the same segmental innervation as a particular viscus are termed *zones of secondary hyperalgesia*. These zones are more commonly found in acute or subacute visceral disease than in the chronic stage of visceral disease (Kunert, 1965).

Experimental stimulation of a viscus produced spasm of spinal muscles in two or three segments on the same side of the vertebral column and innervated by the same segments (Elbe, 1960). The extent of increased tone in vertebral segments is proportional to the intensity of the stimulus, and this irritability may spread to the contralateral side.

Although there is no evidence that lesions of the spinal column can cause visceral disease, Kunert (1965) comments that the state of the vertebral column has a bearing on the functional status of the internal organs. The philosophy of many osteopaths and chiropractors is based on a good understanding of the neurophysiology of the autonomic nervous system and segmental innervation of the viscera, as they believe that certain visceral conditions may be influenced by spinal treatment. The osteopathic concept is that the 'facilitated spinal cord segment(s) is the focus of viscerosomatic and somatovisceral activity' and that manual treatment to the segmental level breaks down the disease-producing pattern (Stoddard, 1983). In clinical practice, the prime reason for manual treatment of the vertebral column must, of course, be for the treatment of a musculoskeletal disorder and not visceral disease.

Radicular Pain

Compression of the spinal nerve roots has long been acknowledged as a source of referred pain. Indeed, the emphasis on nerve root pain has been so great that it has been largely overlooked that somatic referred pain is an integral part of some spinal pain syndromes. Grieve (1981) states that 'all root pain is referred pain, but not all referred pain is root pain', and this is vital to our understanding of spinal pain syndromes.

Certain experimental studies have identified critical features concerning nerve root pain. Experimental compression of *normal* nerve roots in the intervertebral foramen produces paraesthesiae and numbness, but not pain (MacNab, 1972). Experiments on animals have shown that mechanical stimulation increases the activity of the nociceptive afferent fibres of previously damaged nerve roots, but not normal nerve roots (Howe *et al.*, 1977). Smyth and Wright (1958) demonstrated that pulling on nerve roots previously damaged by disc herniation produced pain. These studies indicate that although clinically damaged nerve roots will give rise to pain, normal nerve roots do not. Mechanical compression alone is unlikely to account for root pain and inflammation probably plays an important role (Grieve, 1988). Stimulation of the dorsal root ganglia may increase nociceptor activity whether they are normal or damaged. The dorsal root ganglia, therefore, appear to be more susceptible to mechanical stimulation than the axons (Howe *et al.*, 1977).

Bogduk (1987) states that there is no known mechanism whereby compression of a nerve root selectively affects the nociceptive fibres alone. The large diameter fibres that convey touch, vibration and proprioception will simultaneously be affected and give rise to the signs and symptoms of large diameter fibre compression. Compression blocks conduction in the axons, so that true radicular pain is accompanied by particular clinical features: numbness and paraesthesiae, muscle weakness and altered reflexes. Referred pain that is not accompanied by objective neurological signs is unlikely to be due to nerve root compression.

Experiments on peripheral nerves have shown that paraesthesiae occurs as a result of ischaemia of nerves. Paraesthesiae in the presence of nerve root compression is likely to be due to compression of radicular vessels rather than compression of the nerve root itself.

Nerve root compression cannot selectively affect only those axons that innervate the vertebral column and not those supplying the limbs. Therefore, root compression is unlikely to be the pathological mechanism in patients who have local spinal pain with no area of referred pain and in the absence of neurological signs.

The 1st and 2nd cervical spinal nerve roots do not run in intervertebral foramina and do not have any structural relations that make them susceptible to trespass (Bogduk 1988b), so that compression of these roots is unlikely to be a source of upper cervical pain. At all other levels of the spine, the nerve roots lie within the intervertebral foramen and are vulnerable to compression and subsequent radicular pain with associated neurological signs. Radicular pain has a definite quality. It is described as sharp, lancinating, throbbing and follows the area innervated by the particular nerve root (Figs. 7.9; 7.10). In this way, it differs from the diffuse aching of somatic referred pain.

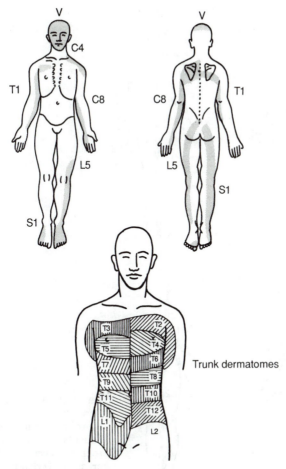

Fig. 7.9 Areas of referred pain. Dermatome charts based on areas of referred pain found in most patients who present with nerve root involvement. Variations of areas of overlap may occur when there are anomalies of the nerve supply.

Combined States

In many instances, particularly in the more degenerate spine, a patient's symptoms may be due to two or more lesions coexisting so that both referred somatic pain and radicular pain may be present. For example, osteoarthritic changes in an apophyseal joint may be intrinsically painful and, with overriding facets or growth of osteophytes, the nerve root in front of the joint may also be compressed. The patient may then present with a combination of local spinal pain, referred somatic pain, radicular pain and neurological signs.

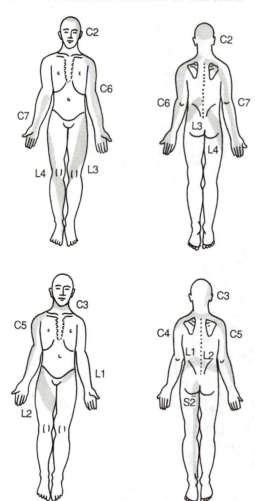

Fig. 7.10 Areas of referred pain. Dermatome charts based on areas of referred pain found in most patients who present with nerve root involvement. Variations of areas of overlap may occur when there are anomalies of the nerve supply.

AUTONOMIC NERVOUS SYSTEM

The peripheral nervous system consists of two nervous systems which function as an integrated whole: the autonomic (visceral) and the somatic. The autonomic nervous system is generally concerned with the innervation of viscera, glands, the muscular walls of blood vessels and unstriated muscle, and the somatic nervous system with the innervation of skin, skeletal muscle and their tendons, joints and connective tissue. However, the distinction is not as clear-cut as this, as autonomic fibres have been found in the intervertebral discs (Bogduk *et al.*, 1981; O'Brien, 1984). Both systems have nerve tracts within the spinal cord that run to and from the brain, and each spinal nerve contains both autonomic and somatic fibres.

The autonomic nervous system can be subdivided into the sympathetic and parasympathetic nervous systems. Both these systems are connected to the central nervous system by two neurones in series. Axons leave the central nervous system and synapse with a second neurone. Ganglia are collections of cell bodies of the second neurones. Axons conveying information from the central nervous system to the ganglia are called *preganglionic axons*, and axons from the ganglia which travel to the peripheral target organ are called *postganglionic axons*. A major difference between the two systems is that the parasympathetic ganglia lie close to the target organ, while sympathetic ganglia lie at some distance away. Hence, parasympathetic postganglionic fibres are short, while sympathetic postganglionic fibres are longer.

In both systems the transmission of impulses at the *synapses* between the pre- and postganglionic neurones is accomplished by the liberation of acetylcholine. At the *terminals* of postganglionic fibres in the sympathetic nervous system, the transmitter substance is usually noradrenaline; in the parasympathetic nervous system it is acetylcholine.

The sympathetic nervous system is the larger subdivision of the autonomic nervous system. It can have the following effects:

- Stimulation of the sinuatrial node of the heart, thereby increasing heart rate
- Direct stimulation of cardiac muscle to increase the power of cardiac contraction
- Relaxation of smooth muscle of the alimentary tract
- Stimulation of sphincters to contract
- Relaxation of smooth muscle of the bronchi
- Acting on α-receptors, it contracts smooth muscles of arterioles resulting in vasoconstriction
- Acting on β-receptors, sympathetic nerves cause vasodilatation
- Dilation of the pupil
- Erection of the hairs on the skin and sweating

Broadly, the functions of the sympathetic nervous system are concerned with preparing the body for 'fight, flight, fright' and diverting blood supply to essential areas. An increase in sympathetic activity also occurs during physiological stress e.g. pain, fear, extreme temperature, severe muscle work.

The parasympathetic nervous system has the opposite effects:

- Slowing sinuatrial node, thereby reducing heart rate
- Contraction of bronchial smooth muscle
- Contraction of smooth muscle of the alimentary canal
- Relaxation of sphincters
- Increase in secretion of salivary and lacrimal glands
- Constriction of pupil and accommodation of the lens

- Increase in mucus secretion in respiratory system
- Acid secretion in alimentary canal
- Vasodilatation of the internal and external carotid circulation

The parasympathetic system helps to conserve energy resources of the body and it is the effector for visceral motor systems.

Sympathetic Nervous System

Two chains of nerve fibres called the sympathetic trunks run longitudinally on either side of the vertebral column. These trunks are formed by preganglionic and postganglionic neurones of the sympathetic nervous system. At the site of synapse of the pre- and postganglionic neurones are swellings called sympathetic ganglia. The sympathetic trunks are situated in front of the transverse processes in the neck, anterior to the heads of the ribs, on the anterolateral aspects of the lumbar vertebral bodies, on the front of the sacrum medial to the anterior sacral foramina, and on the front of the coccyx.

There are a variable number of ganglia – approximately 2 cervical, 11 thoracic, 4 lumbar, 4 sacral, 1 coccygeal. The superior cervical ganglion lies between C1–3 and there is a star-shaped ganglion at the cervico-thoracic junction called the stellate ganglion. An intermediate ganglion is sometimes present at C6.

Sympathetic nerves travel to the viscera in the splanchnic nerves. Preganglionic fibres leave the spinal cord in the ventral nerve roots between the 1st thoracic and 2nd lumbar segments (Fig. 7.11). Then in the white ramus communicans, they enter a ganglion in the sympathetic trunk. They may ascend or descend in the chain to synapse with the cells of origin of many postganglionic fibres, which travel via grey rami communicans in the splanchnic nerves to the target organ. An exception to this are the sympathetic nerves supplying the abdominal viscera which are innervated by the greater, lesser and least splanchnic nerves. The nerves are formed by preganglionic sympathetic axons which pass through the sympathetic trunk without synapsing. They synapse with ganglia surrounding the arteries, which supply the abdominal viscera and then travel with the artery to the organ.

Classical accounts of the sympathetic nervous system describe sympathetic fibres leaving the central nervous system as having a thoracolumbar outflow. Some European anatomists have reported the presence of preganglionic sympathetic fibres in the ventral rami of C5–8 (Laruelle, 1940; Guerrier, 1944). Cinquegrana (1968) suggested that irritation of such sympathetic elements within the cervical nerve roots could cause vasoconstriction of the blood supply to the shoulder and periarticular structures, resulting in locally-induced changes occurring intrinsically within the shoulder. This may be a mechanism by which a 'frozen shoulder' develops (Middleditch and Jarman, 1984).

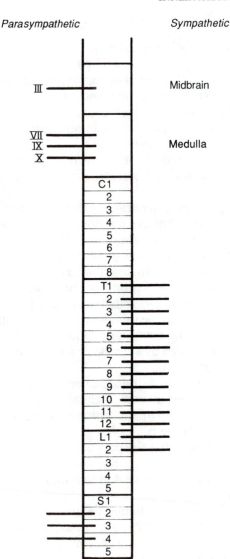

Parasympathetic   *Sympathetic*

III — Midbrain

VII
IX   Medulla
X

C1
2
3
4
5
6
7
8
T1
2
3
4
5
6
7
8
9
10
11
12
L1
2
3
4
5
S1
2
3
4
5

Fig. 7.11 Schematic representation of parasympathetic and sympathetic outflow of autonomic nervous system.

Parasympathetic Nervous System

The cell bodies of preganglionic parasympathetic neurones are located in the nuclei of the III, VII, IX and X cranial nerves. Efferent fibres leave the central nervous system at (1) the base of the brain with cranial nerves III (oculomotor), VII (facial), IX (glossopharyngeal) and X (vagus), and (2) with somatic nerves S2, 3 and 4 to supply the rectum with visceromotor fibres; the bladder with visceromotor, and its sphincter with inhibitory fibres; and the sexual organs with vasodilator fibres (*see* Fig. 7.11).

Visceral Afferent Fibres

The autonomic nervous system is entirely *efferent*. Visceral *afferent* fibres share the same pathways as sympathetic and parasympathetic fibres except that they do not synapse in autonomic ganglia. The cells of origin of visceral afferent fibres lie in cranial and posterior root ganglia. Although pain evoked by visceral afferents may have a quality that distinguishes it from somatic pain, it is not autonomic pain and is more correctly described as visceral pain.

Afferent impulses initiate visceral reflexes and are thought to be concerned with visceral sensations such as hunger, rectal distension and pain.

The concept of autonomic pain as a separate entity is probably fallacious. Investigators have shown that stimulation of autonomic elements produces pain. Gross (1974) stimulated the cervical sympathetic trunk during surgery under local anaesthetic and produced pain that did not correspond to a dermatomal distribution and, under conditions of lumbar anaesthesiae, cutting of the splanchnic nerves produced severe pain in a patient. Nevertheless, Grieve (1988) states that 'pure autonomic pain' is a meaningless term. Somatic nerve roots carry autonomic efferent neurones and 'autonomic pain' produced by experiments is accompanied by somatic changes such as muscle spasm and cutaneous hyperalgesia.

In all spinal conditions, the somatic and autonomic nervous systems are activated in varying degrees, so that musculoskeletal pain cannot be considered in isolation from changes in the autonomic nervous system or the phenomenon of visceral pain.

Some of the more obscure symptoms that the patients complain of – such as throbbing or burning pain, formication, numbness, hyperaesthesia, tingling, fullness and puffiness – may be due to malfunction of the autonomic nervous system.

Certain spinal syndromes have been attributed to involvement of the autonomic nervous system. Ebbetts (1971) recommended spinal manipulation in the early stages of the following syndromes, to correct the altered autonomic mechanism that he believed caused them: shoulder-hand syndrome; scapulo–humeral capsulitis (frozen shoulder); cervico–brachial pain and carpal tunnel syndrome. In his view, local pathological changes such as increased fibrosis stimulated further increase in sympathetic tone, establishing a self-perpetuating and usually progressive cycle.

Abnormal vasomotor responses caused by irritation of sympathetic fibres in cervical nerve roots can result in *vascular* pain, the mechanism being similar to that when spasm occurs in the smooth muscles in a viscus. Tinel (1937) showed that irritation of the 5th, 6th and 7th cervical nerve roots, with subsequent vasoconstriction of vasodilatation, produced vascular pain in the head, neck, chest and arm.

The headache phase of classical migraine has been attributed to dilatation of the arteries of the scalp and an increase in cerebral blood flow.

The 'cold sciatic leg' is another example of increased sympathetic activity reflexly excited by pain, causing vasoconstriction in cutaneous blood vessels.

The peripheral autonomic nervous system is influenced by higher centres including the hypothalamus, which itself is under the inhibitory influence of the cortex of the frontal lobe. There is, therefore, a close link between mental states and somatic and visceral activities. Pain or anxiety induce overactivity in the sympathetic nervous system.

REFERENCES

Bogduk N. (1980). Lumbar dorsal ramus syndrome. *Med. J. Aust.*, **2**, 537.

Bogduk N. (1982). The clinical anatomy of the cervical dorsal rami. *Spine*, **7**, 319.

Bogduk N. (1987). Innervation, pain, patterns and mechanisms of pain production. In *Physical Therapy of the Low Back*. (Twomey L.T., Taylor J.R., eds.) Edinburgh: Churchill Livingstone, p. 94.

Bogduk N. (1988a). Innervation and pain patterns of the thoracic spine. In *Physical Therapy of the Cervical and Thoracic Spines*. (Grant R., ed.) Edinburgh: Churchill Livingstone, p. 34.

Bogduk N. (1988b). Innervation and pain patterns of the cervical spine. In *Physical Therapy of the Cervical and Thoracic Spines*. (Grant R., ed.) Edinburgh: Churchill Livingstone, p. 10.

Bogduk N., Tynan W., Wilson A.J. (1981). The nerve supply to the human lumbar intervertebral disc. *J. Anat.*, **132**, 39.

Bogduk N., Wilson A.J., Tynan W. (1982). The human lumbar dorsal rami. *J. Anat.*, **134**, 383.

Bogduk N., Marsland A. (1986). On the concept of third occipital headache. *J. Neurol. Neurosurg. Psychiatr.*, **49**, 775.

Bogduk N., Twomey L. (1987). *Clinical Anatomy of the Lumbar Spine*. Edinburgh: Churchill Livingstone, p. 99.

Bowsher D. (1988a). Acute and chronic pain assessment. In *Pain: Management and Control in Physiotherapy*. (Wells P.E., Frampton V., Bowsher D., eds.) London: Heinemann Medical Books.

Bowsher D. (1988b). Nociceptors and peripheral nerve fibres. In *Pain: Management and Control in Physiotherapy*. (Wells P.E., Frampton V., Bowsher D., eds.) London: Heinemann Medical Books, pp. 20–21.

Bowsher D. (1988c). Central pain mechanisms. In *Pain: Management and Control in Physiotherapy*. (Wells P.E., Frampton V., Bowsher D., eds.) London: Heinemann, pp. 22–29.

Brodal A. (1981). *Neurological Anatomy in Relation to Clinical Medicine*. 3rd edn. Oxford: University Press.

Carrera G.F. (1980). Lumbar facet joint injection in low back pain and sciatica. *Radiology*, **137**, 665.

Cinquegrana O.D. (1968). Chronic cervical radiculitis and its relationship to chronic bursitis. *Am. J. Phys. Med.*, **47**, 1, 23.

Cloward R.B. (1959). Cervical discography. *Ann. Surg.*, **150**, 1052.

Dee R. (1978). The innervation of joints. In *The Joints and Synovial Fluid I.* (Sokoloff L., ed.) London: Academic Press.

Ebbetts J. (1971). Autonomic pain in the upper limb. *Physiotherapy*, **57**, 270.

Elbe J.N. (1960). Pattern of responses of the paravertebral musculature to visceral stimulation. *Am. J. Physiol.*, **198**, 429.

Feinstein B., Langton J.B.K., Jameson R.M. *et al.* (1954). Experiments on referred pain from deep somatic structures with charts of segmental pain areas. *Clin. Sci.*, **4**, 35.

Frykholm R. (1971). The clinical picture. In *Cervical Pain* (Hirsch C., Zotterman Y., eds.) Oxford: Pergamon Press, p. 5.

Grieve G.P. (1981). *Common Vertebral Joint Problems*. Edinburgh: Churchill Livingstone, p. 175.

Grieve G.P. (1988). *Common Vertebral Joint Problems*. 2nd edn. Edinburgh: Churchill Livingstone, pp. 314, 324.

Gross D. (1974). Pain and the autonomic nervous system. In *Advances in Neurology* (Bonica J.J., ed.) New York: Raven Press, p. 92.

Guerrier Y. (1944). Le sympathetique cervical. *Impremière de la Charitie*, Montpelier.

Harkness J.A.L., Higges E.R., Dieppe P.A. (1984). Osteoarthritis. In *Textbook of Pain* (Wall P.D., Melzack R., eds.) Edinburgh: Churchill Livingstone, p. 215.

Hildebrandt J., Argyrakis A. (1986). Percutaneous nerve block of the cervical facets – a relatively new method in the treatment of chronic headache and neck pain. *Man. Med.*, **2**, 4.

Hinsey J.C., Phillips R.A. (1949). Observations in diaphragmatic sensation. *J. Neurophysiol.*, **3**, 175.

Hockaday J.M., Whitty C.W.M. (1967). Patterns of referred pain in the normal subject. *Brain*, **90**, 481.

Howe J.F. (1979). A neurophysiological basis for the radicular pain of nerve root compression. In *Advances in Pain Research and Therapy.* (Bonica J.J., ed.) New York: Raven Press, p. 547.

Howe J.F., Loeser J.D., Calvin W.H. (1977). Mechano-sensitivity of dorsal root ganglia and chronically injured axons: a physiological basis for the radicular pain of nerve root compression. *Pain*, **3**, 25.

Inman V.T., Saunders J.B., De C.M. (1944). Referred pain from skeletal structures. *J. Nerve Ment. Dis.*, **90**, 666.

Keele A.C., Neil E. (eds.) (1971). *Samson Wright's Applied Physiology*. 12th edn. Oxford: Oxford University Press.

Kellgren J.H. (1939). On the distribution of pain arising from deep somatic structures with charts of segmental pain areas. *Clin. Sci.*, **4**, 35.

Kibler R.F., Nathan P.W. (1960). Relief of pain and paraesthesiae by nerve block distal to the lesion. *J. Neurol. Neurosurg. Psychiatr.*, **23**, 91.

Kunert W. (1965). Functional disorders of internal organs due to vertebral lesions. *Ciba Symp.*, **13**, 85.

Laruelle N.L. (1940). Les bases anatomiques du système autonome cortical et bulbo-spinal. *Rev. Neurol.*, **72**, 349.

Lindahl O. (1966). Hyperalgesia of the lumbar nerve roots in sciatica. *Acta Orthop. Scand.*, **37**, 367.

Macnab I. (1972). The mechanism of spondylogenic pain. In *Cervical Pain.* (Hirsch C., Zotterman Y. eds.) Oxford: Pergamon, p. 89.

McCall I.W., Park W.M., O'Brien J.P. (1979). Induced pain referral from posterior lumbar elements in normal subjects. *Spine*, **4**, 441.

Melzack R., Wall P.D. (1965). Pain mechanisms: a new theory. *Science*, **150**, 971.

Mense S. (1982). Reduction of bradykinin-induced activation of feline group III and IV muscle receptors by acetysalicyclic acid. *J. Physiol.*, **326**, 269.

Middleditch A., Jarman P. (1984). An investigation of frozen shoulders using thermography. *Physiotherapy*, **70**, 11, 433.

Mills K.R., Newham D.J., Edwards R.H.T. (1984). Muscle pain. In *Textbook of Pain.* (Wall P.D., Melzack R., eds.) Edinburgh: Churchill Livingstone, p. 319.

Mooney V., Robertson J. (1976). The facet syndrome. *Clin. Orthop. Rel. Res.*, **115**, 149.

Nathan H., Feuerstein M. (1974). Angulated course of spinal nerve roots. *J. Neurosurg.*, **32**, 349.

O'Brien J.P. (1984). Mechanisms of spinal pain. In *Textbook of Pain.* (Wall P.D., Melzack R., eds.) Edinburgh: Churchill Livingstone, p. 240.

Smyth M.J., Wright V. (1958). Sciatica and the intervertebral disc: an experimental study. *J. Bone Jt. Surg.*, **40A**, 1401.

Stillwell D.L. (1956). Nerve supply of the vertebral column and its associated structures in the monkey. *Anat. Rec.*, **125**, 129.

Stoddard A. (1983). *Manual of Osteopathic Practice.* 2nd edn. London: Hutchison. Appendix 3, p. 242.

Taylor D.C.M., Pierau Fr-K., Mizutani M. (1984). Possible bases for referred pain. In *The Neurobiology of Pain.* (Holden A.V., Winslow W., eds.) Manchester: Manchester University Press, pp. 143–156.

Tinel J. (1937). *Le Système Nerveux Vegetatif.* Paris: Masson.

Trevor Jones R. (1964). Osteoarthritis of the paravertebral joints of the second and third cervical vertebra as a cause of occipital headaches. *SA Med. J.*, **38**, 392.

Wyke B.D. (1967). The neurology of joints. *Ann. Roy. Coll. Surg. Engl.*, **41**, 25.

Wyke B.D. (1975). Morphological and functional features of the innervation of costovertebral joints. *Folia Morph.*, **23**, 296.

Wyke B.D. (1976). Neurological aspects of low back pain. In *The Lumbar Spine and Back Pain.* (Jayson M., ed.) London: Sector, p. 189.

Wyke B.D. (1979). Neurology of the cervical spinal joints. *Physiotherapy*, **65**, 72.

Wyke B.D. (1981). The neurology of the joints: a review of general principles. *Clin. Rheum. Dis.*, **7**, 23.

Wyke B.D. (1987). The neurology of low back pain. In *The Lumbar Spine and Back Pain*, 3rd edn. (Jayson M.I.V., ed.) Edinburgh: Churchill Livingstone, p. 56.

8

Biomechanics of the Spinal Cord and Meninges

During normal movement, the spinal cord and nerve roots are able to adapt to changes that occur within the vertebral canal. The connective tissues (meninges) surrounding the spinal cord protect the neural tissue, while allowing impulses to travel along the axons during movement or in any desired posture. The meninges also afford some protection against compressive forces.

Sclerotic or fibrotic lesions may restrict mobility or extensibility of the nervous tissues or meninges, giving rise to signs and symptoms of adverse mechanical tension. Examination of the response to movement of these pain-sensitive structures within the vertebral canal is an inherent part of the assessment of all patients with spinal disorders.

SPINAL CORD (Fig. 7.2, p. 208)

The spinal cord lies within the bony vertebral canal. It is almost cylindrical in shape, although slightly flattened anteroposteriorly. As a continuation of the medulla oblongata, the spinal cord extends from the foramen magnum to the level of the L1/2 disc. Below this level, the lumbar and sacral nerve roots occupy the spinal canal, and they form the collection of nerve roots known as the cauda equina. Caudally, the spinal cord is cone-shaped, and it is attached to the coccyx by the filum terminale. This is a fibrous, non-nervous structure which is an extension of the pia mater and is covered by dura mater.

SPINAL MENINGES (Fig. 8.1)

Three membranes surround the spinal cord: the dura mater, the arachnoid and the pia mater.

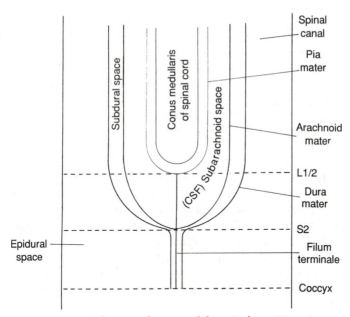

Fig. 8.1 Schematic diagram of the spinal meninges.

Dura Mater

The dura mater is the outermost layer of the spinal meninges. The outer endosteal layer of the cranial dura mater is continued as the periosteum of the vertebral canal, whereas the inner meningeal layer of the cerebral dura becomes continuous with the dura mater of the spinal cord. The spinal dura mater extends from the foramen magnum to the 2nd sacral segment and then continues caudally, covering the filum terminale, eventually blending with the periosteum on the dorsal surface of the coccyx. It is attached superiorly to the foramen magnum and the posterior surface of the 2nd and 3rd cervical vertebral bodies. As the dura is connected to the bony skeleton, movement of the vertebral canal will result in forces being transmitted to the meninges (Troup, 1986). Small fibrous slips attach the dura to the posterior longitudinal ligament, particularly in the lumbar spine. Laterally, the dura mater envelops the nerve roots as they pass through the intervertebral foramen. In the upper spine, the dural sheaths are short, but they increase in length caudally because of the obliquity of the nerve roots. At the dorsal root ganglion or slightly distal to the intervertebral foramen, the dura is continued as the perineurium of the spinal nerve. Hence, traction forces on the spinal nerve are transmitted directly to the spinal dura and arachnoid mater and then via dentate ligaments to the spinal cord (*see* pp. 246–7). The epidural tissue of the spinal cord and nerve roots is continued as the epineurium of the spinal nerve (Sunderland, 1974).

In the cervical spine, the paired root sleeves of dura and arachnoid are attached loosely to the cervical foramina. Nerve roots of C4–6 are stabilized in the gutter of the transverse process by myofascial slips and fusion with the adventitia of the vertebral artery (Sunderland, 1974). These attachments become firmer with increasing age and degenerative change.

Throughout the rest of the spine, with the possible exception of S1, the nerve roots are not attached to the intervertebral foramina, thereby allowing the nerve roots to move in and out of them (Sunderland, 1974). Attachment of the 1st sacral nerve to the wall of the foramen was described by Hollinshead (1969).

The dura consists mainly of white fibrous tissue with a fine network of elastic fibres. Collagenous fibres lie in longitudinal bundles which are straight when stretched and wavy when unstretched. Experiments on dogs have shown that the dura is under longitudinal strain due to attachment of the dural sheaths (Tunturi, 1977). It was also observed that the elastic network was stretched almost to the limit and that it was the collagenous fibres that contributed to the elasticity of the spinal dura.

Anteriorly, the dura is innervated by free nerve-endings from the sinuvertebral nerve (Edgar and Nundy, 1966).

Epidural (or extradural) space

This lies between the vertebral canal and dura. It contains fat, areolar tissue, lymphatic vessels, the internal vertebral venous plexus and the spinal arteries.

Veins forming the venous plexus are large and valveless (see pp. 155–6). They are easily compressed and their volume changes with spinal movement (Dommisse, 1975).

Subdural space

This is a potential space between the dura mater and the arachnoid, containing serous fluid.

Arachnoid

The arachnoid is a thin, delicate membrane lying between the dura and pia. It is continuous above with the intracranial arachnoid membrane and ends caudally at the base of the subdural cavity at the 2nd sacral segment. Laterally, the arachnoid lines the dural sleeves but, unlike the dura mater, it does not become continuous with the peripheral nerve covering. Between the ventral and dorsal nerve roots, the arachnoid links the adjacent dural layers, thereby contributing to the interradicular septum (Fig. 8.2).

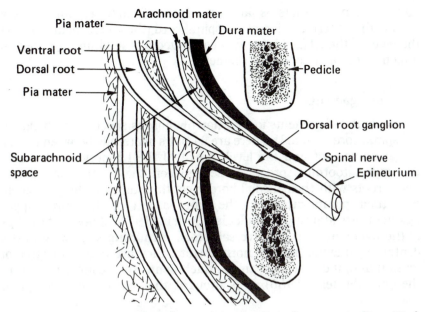

Fig. 8.2 The disposition of the meningeal sheaths of spinal nerve roots. (From Nigel Palastanga, Derek Field and Roger Soames, 1989. *Anatomy and Human Movement: Structure and Function.* Oxford: Heinemann Medical Books, with permission.)

Structurally, it is a loose, irregular connective tissue network made up of collagen, elastin and reticulum fibres. The fibres are arranged in a lattice pattern which permits lengthening and shortening (Breig, 1978). The arachnoid is relatively avascular, but provides support for blood vessels passing from pia to dura. Tight cells within its structure form a mechanical barrier to diffusion into the central nervous system from the subarachnoid and subdural spaces. A network of delicate trabeculae cross the subarachnoid space, connecting the arachnoid and pia mater and providing support for small vessels.

Subarachnoid space

This lies between the arachnoid and pia and contains the cerebro-spinal fluid (CSF). This fluid supports the meninges and helps to disperse forces acting through it.

Pia Mater

The pia mater is the innermost layer which adheres closely to the spinal cord. It has an outer layer, the epipia which supports large blood vessels, and an inner layer, the pia intima, which is continuous with nervous tissue of the spinal cord. It forms a sheath for the ventral and dorsal nerve roots as far as the interradicular septum. The pia ends with the termination of the spinal cord (the conus medullaris) at the level of the L1/2 disc, and is continued as the filum terminale to attach to the first coccygeal segment.

Dentate Ligaments

The dentate ligaments form a narrow fibrous sheet on each side of the spinal cord (Fig. 8.3). There are 21 pairs bilaterally between the C1 spinal nerve root and the level of exit of the L1 nerve root. These triangular, toothlike processes lie between the ventral and dorsal nerve roots with their medial border continuous with the pia. Laterally, their points attach to the inner aspect of the dura. Upper ligaments are almost perpendicular. Epstein (1976) states that the tips of the ligaments act as universal joints, permitting swivelling of the dentate ligaments. In their normal state, they are under a degree of tension and, if cut at their dural attachments, they contract down to the cord (Epstein, 1966). It is thought that tension on the spinal

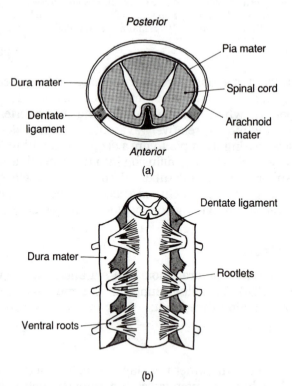

Fig. 8.3 The dentate ligaments. (a) horizontal section through spinal cord and meninges; (b) anterior aspect of spinal cord.

nerves is conveyed from the dura via the dentate ligaments to the spinal cord. Equally, movement of the cord is quickly transmitted to the dura so that the spinal cord and its meninges are biomechanically interdependent.

BIOMECHANICS OF THE VERTEBRAL CANAL AND THE PAIN-SENSITIVE STRUCTURES

In the normal spine, the spinal cord, meninges and nerve roots will freely adapt to changes of vertebral movement, postures and pressure differences (Breig, 1960). As the dura mater has bony fixations, both cephalad and caudad, any change in the vertebral canal is auto-matically accommodated by the spinal cord and meninges. Breig referred to the nervous tissue and its supporting connective structures, which extend from the brain to the conus medullaris as the pons-cord tract. He demonstrated that the tract is highly plastic and, during normal movement, it may change in length, diameter, shape and direction. Breig disputed that the cord and dura move up and down the canal on flexion and extension, and proposed that the necessary osteoneuromeningeal relations are maintained due to the tract's inherent plasticity. He further suggested that the collagen rhomboid network in the pia mater allowed this shortening and lengthening and that the dentate ligaments via their direct attachments with the pia and dura transmitted tension uniformly along the length and across the cord.

However, there is some evidence that slight up and down movement of the cord may occur. O'Connell (1946) noted that movement of either the head or lower limbs induced longitudinal tension in the cord and dura and also caused up and down movement of the tract. Experiments on monkeys (Smith, 1956) showed that during head and trunk flexion there was elongation of each cord segment proportional to the increase in the bony canal length. These changes were accompanied by forward displacement of the cord.

Anterior displacement of the cord has been observed by other investigators (Adams and Logue, 1971; Louis, 1981) and the anterior component of force exerted by the cord and dura was found to reach 30–40 lbs per square inch in flexion as opposed to 2 lbs per square inch in the neutral position (Reid, 1960). Accommodation of the cord during flexion has been calculated as roughly two-thirds axial shift and one-third increase in length (Adams and Logue, 1971).

Flexion

On forward flexion of the spine, there is an increase in the length of the vertebral canal and the elongation of the posterior border of the canal is greater than that of the anterior canal border. Extensive cadaveric experiments have shown that the cervical and lumbar spines lengthen by 28 mm, but the thoracic spine only increases in length by 3 mm (Louis, 1981). A major function of the tissues of the cord and meninges is to adapt to the increase in length of the vertebral canal as it moves from a neutral to a flexed position. In the neutral position the cord and dura are under slight tension and, as the spine flexes, they become drawn out and smooth, so that there is a small decrease in the cross-sectional area of the cord. As tension in the cord increases, it moves anteriorly due to its elasticity. Gravity will also tend to displace the cord anteriorly, when flexion occurs in a sitting or standing position. As the cord moves anteriorly, it may become stretched over any spondylotic ridges or protusions that are present.

Louis observed in flexion and extension studies that most movement of the cord and dura occurred in the cervical and lumbar regions, and that very little movement occurred in the thoracic spine. He also noted that at the C6, T6 and L4 intervertebral levels no neuromeningeal movement occurred relative to the bony canal, so that at these levels neuromeningeal and spinal canal relationships remain constant (Fig. 8.4). These levels or 'tension points' often show abnormalities in patients with adverse mechanical tension signs. Treatment of the joints at these levels by mobilization or manipulation can produce impressive changes to abnormalities of tension test range (Butler and Gifford, 1989).

Analysis of changes in the lumbar dural sac during movements showed that changes in dural length were smaller than length changes of the bony canal (Penning and Wilmink, 1981). They suggested that this is due firstly to anchorage of the root sheaths and secondly to the limited elasticity of the dura.

Flexion of the spine places tension on the nerve roots and their sleeves. Thoracic roots above T6 tend to follow a more vertical course,

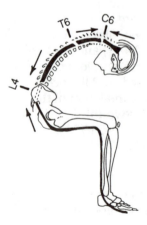

Fig. 8.4 Movement of the dura mater and nerve roots in relation to the spinal canal during flexion. There is no movement in the regions of C6, T6 and L4. (From *Proceedings of the Fifth Biennial Conference of the Manipulative Therapists Association of Australia*, Melbourne 1987, with permission.)

while those between T6 and 12 become more horizontal. In the lumbar region, the nerve roots above L3 become lax during flexion and follow a more wavy course. Their direction becomes more horizontal and they move away from the pedicle. The L3 nerve roots remain the same length during flexion, while those below L3 are stretched by up to 16% and become more vertical in direction, so that they move into contact with the medial border of the superior pedicle (Louis, 1981).

Flexion of the cervical spine alone causes elongation of the cord and dura. Tension is transmitted throughout the spine, so that there is very slight upwards movement of the thoracic cord and cauda equina, and a decrease in the cross-sectional area of the sacral cone. Cervical flexion affects the lumbar nerve roots causing them to become more vertical, so that they move into contact with the pedicles.

Extension

In general, the opposite effects occur when the vertebral column is extended. In extension, the vertical height of the column is shortened and there is a decrease in the anteroposterior dimensions of the canal. Ligamenta flava may bulge anteriorly into the canal, further reducing the available space (Breig, 1960). Tension in the cord and dura is reduced, and they form transverse folds within the canal, so that there is an increase in the transverse diameter of the cord. There is posterior movement of the dural sac and the lower part of the dura moves caudally by up to 2 mm. The nerve roots follow a more wavy course, moving away from the pedicles.

Extension of the cervical spine alone will create slight slackening of the thoracic and lumbar dura. The lumbar and sacral nerve roots also slacken and move out of contact with the pedicles.

Lateral Flexion

Lateral flexion of the vertebral column in standing causes a lengthening of the canal on the convex side and a shortening of the canal on the concave side. Likewise, in this position, the dura on the convex side is elongated, while the dura on the concave side forms transverse folds (Breig, 1978). For example, in right lateral flexion, the dura on the left side of the cord is lengthened, becoming smooth, but the dura on the right side of the cord forms transverse folds. Lumbosacral nerves on the concave side follow a more wavy course, those on the convex side are stretched and have a more vertical pathway.

In the side-lying position, the changes in the dura vary according to which side the trunk is laterally flexed, rather than being directly influenced by the side on which the subject lies. For example, in right side-lying, if the trunk is laterally flexed to the *left*, the dura on the underside (right) is elongated and that on the left slackens. The caudal sac is held close to the centre of the canal by the dentate ligaments, but the nerve roots of the cauda equina sag towards the dura on the right. Nerve roots of the cauda equina on the left are relaxed. Alternatively, if the trunk is laterally flexed to the *right*, in the right side-lying position, the dura, dentate ligaments and nerve roots on the left become stretched, and the lumbosacral cord moves towards the centre of the canal. The left lumbosacral nerves are stretched in this position (Massey, 1986).

Rotation

There is no significant alteration in length of the vertebral column during rotation. In the cervical spine, dorsal roots on the side to which rotation occurs are stretched and anterior roots are relaxed, and opposite effects occur on the opposite side (Grieve, 1988).

Limb Movements

The nervous tissues of the body are continuous from the skull to the distal areas of the limbs. Movement of the limbs will, therefore, increase tension within the nerve roots and this is transmitted to the dura and cord.

Neuromeningeal responses to movement of an arm or leg are considered in the sections below under upper limb tension test (pp. 254–6) and straight-leg raising test (p. 251).

Tension Tests

The importance of examining the neuromeningeal structures was emphasized by Maitland (1978). A range of tests have been developed to assess the state of the nervous tissues and their connective tissue coverings. Tension tests are no longer used for purely diagnostic purposes. Passive mobilizing techniques applied to the nervous tissues can be successfully used to treat adverse mechanical tension in the nervous system. Butler and Gifford (1989) comment that these tests should not be thought of as 'dural', because of the effects they have on many other structures, and they now need to be considered in a broader context of the nervous system as a whole. They state that the following structures must therefore be considered:

1. The nerve and its relationship with the surrounding tissues – bone, muscle, ligaments, etc.
2. Connective tissue covering of the nerve – epineurium, perineurium and endoneurium. These have their own nerve supply and can therefore produce symptoms.

3. Connective tissues covering the spinal cord – dura, arachnoid and pia mater.
4. The neurones of the nervous tissue.
5. Intrinsic blood supply of the nervous system.

Movements of the body which are components of particular tension tests not only increase tension within the nerve, but also move the nerve relative to its surrounding tissues. The tissues anatomically adjacent to the nervous tissues that can move independently of the nervous system have been termed the *mechanical interface* (Butler, 1987).

Pathology at the mechanical interface at any point along the length of a nerve can produce abnormalities in nerve movement and increase tension in the nerve. Adverse mechanical tension at any one point in the nervous system will inevitably have mechanical repercussions elsewhere along the tract.

Biomechanics of tension tests

1. **Passive neck flexion** is used as a tension test for the thoracic and lumbosacral nerve roots. As the neck is passively flexed in supine-lying, minor shifts occur in the lumbar dura, tension increases in the lumbosacral nerve roots and they become slightly elongated. This is the least sensitive test for the lumbar nerve roots and, if it is positive, (i.e. reproduces the patient's low back or distal leg symptoms), it is often indicative of a major lesion.

2. **Straight-leg raising test (SLR – Laségue's sign).** Classically, the straight-leg raising test has been used in the assessment of patients with a suspected lumbar disc protrusion, but this test used in isolation is insufficient for diagnostic purposes. The real value of this test as an examination procedure for testing the mobility of the lumbosacral nerve roots is now well recognized.

Nervous tissue and the meninges have different properties. The nervous tissue of the sciatic nerve is elastic and it can, therefore, sustain a slow stretch, although sudden stretching of the nervous structures may be injurious to the tissues. The circumferential arrangement of the fibres of the meninges limits stretching along the long axis of the tract and the meninges become taut within 5% of their normal length.

During the straight-leg raising test, the leg is passively raised in supine-lying, so that the hip flexes and the knee remains extended.

Goddard and Reid (1965) extensively examined the effects of this test on the lumbosacral nerve roots. The greatest amount of movement induced is more distally in the sciatic nerve at the greater sciatic notch and it commences when the heel is elevated 5–15 cm from the horizontal. As elevation continues, this movement is transmitted proximally and almost immediately affects the lumbosacral cord as it passes over the ala of the sacrum. At 20–30°, movement occurs in the intervertebral foramina and the lumbosacral nerve roots and dura are pulled downwards; after 70° there is little additional movement, but an increase in tension.

The course of the individual nerve roots varies, thereby influencing the amount of movement that occurs within them. L4 and 5 run a tortuous course through the intervertebral foramina, so that there is slack to be taken up. S2 and 3 curve in a marked manner and also have slack to be taken up. S1 runs in a direct and vertical course and moves the greatest distance (4–5 mm) on straight-leg raising. No downward movement of L3 has been noted during this test (Fig. 8.5).

Additions which increase the sensitivity of the straight-leg raising test are:

1. Ankle dorsiflexion (Breig and Troup, 1979);
2. Medial rotation of hip (Breig and Troup, 1979);
3. Passive neck flexion (Breig, 1960);
4. Hip adduction (Sutton, 1979);
5. Ankle plantar flexion with inversion (Butler and Gifford, 1989);
6. Alteration of lumbar spine position e.g. left SLR with lumbar spine lateral flexion to the right (Butler and Gifford, 1989).

Distal movements of the sciatic nerve during straight-leg raising have been studied in monkeys (Smith, 1956). Proximal to the knee, the tibial nerve moves caudad in relation to its mechanical interface, while distal to the knee, the tibial nerve moves cranially in relation to its surrounding tissues. Hence, there is a point behind the knee where the nerve and its surrounding tissues remain constant during straight-

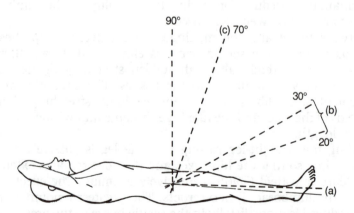

Fig. 8.5 Effects of straight-leg raising. (a) movement of sciatic nerve begins at greater sciatic notch; (b) movement of roots begins at intervertebral foramen; (c) minimal movement only, but increase in tension.

leg raising, so that this is a 'tension point'. Attachment of the common peroneal nerve to the head of the fibula is also a tension point (Butler and Gifford, 1989).

Components of the sciatic nerve are subject to pressure at various points, in particular against the greater sciatic notch, but also over the convexity of the ala of the sacrum and, to a lesser extent, in the intervertebral foramina of L4 and 5. Many slips of tissue connect the sciatic nerve and its roots to underlying fascia and bone. Development of adhesions (see pp. 256–8) at any point along the sciatic nerve or its roots will adversely affect their mobility.

Studies suggest that it is the neural structures which are primarily responsible for finally limiting the movement of straight-leg raising in a normal population (Lew and Puendetura, 1985). Many people have a normal discrepancy of 5–10° between limits of right and left straight-leg raising and a normal healthy range may vary between 50° and 120° (Troup, 1986).

It should be remembered that straight-leg raising also affects many other structures. Soft tissues such as the hamstrings, buttock tissues, lumbosacral muscles and ligaments may all be placed under a varying amount of tension. In addition, the hip joint is flexed, the pelvis is rotated backwards and it is also rotated slightly towards the opposite side. The lumbar spine apophyseal joints are also flexed. A lesion, adhesions or irritation of any of these soft tissues or joints will inevitably affect the clinical findings of the straight-leg raising test.

3. **Well-leg raising test** (Cross-over Laségue).   On straight-leg raising the nerve roots on the opposite side emerge from their respective foramina and move towards the side of the straight-leg raise. Likewise, the spinal cord shifts towards the side of the limb being raised (Woodhall and Hayes, 1950). Hence, testing of the straight-leg raise – on the symptom-free side may produce the patient's symptoms on the side affected by pathology.

4. **Slump test.**   This is a sensitive test which stretches the dura, cord, nerve roots and the sciatic nerve to its distal termination in the foot (Maitland, 1978). The test consists of thoracic and lumbar flexion in the sitting position, followed by cervical flexion, extension of the knee/s, ankle dorsiflexion and hip flexion.

The response to this test has been observed in normal subjects aged from 19 to 24 (Maitland, 1978). He concluded that it was unusual to find full painfree range of movement in the test subjects. The following responses were recorded:

1. Pain/discomfort in the mid thoracic spine to T9 on trunk and cervical flexion;
2. Pain/discomfort behind the knee on trunk and cervical flexion with knee extension, increased by ankle dorsiflexion;
3. Bilateral reduction in range of ankle dorsiflexion in cervical and trunk flexion with knee extension;

4. Reduction of pain/discomfort with release of the neck flexion component;
5. Increase in range of knee extension or ankle dorsiflexion with release of neck flexion.

The slump test is positive if it reproduces the patient's symptoms or if asymmetry of range is observed. This test has been shown to be more effective in reproducing symptoms than passive neck flexion, straight-leg raising or dorsiflexion added to straight-leg raising in patients with low back pain, with or without referred pain (Massey, 1982).

5. **Prone knee bend** (femoral nerve stretch test). This test is used with the patient in prone-lying – the hip and thigh are stabilized and the knee is passively flexed.

Flexion of the knee moves and increases tension in nerves and roots related to the L2, 3 and 4 spinal segments (O'Connell, 1951).

Sensitizing additions of this test are:

1. Cervical flexion;
2. Slump in side-lying (Davidson, 1987) (Neck, trunk flexion and hip extension);
3. Alterations in hip abduction, adduction and rotation (Butler and Gifford, 1989).

6. **Upper limb tension tests.** The aim of the upper limb tension tests is to place tension on the roots of the brachial plexus and distally on the major nerve trunks in the arm as far as their terminations in the hand.

Depression of the shoulder girdle causes the neurovascular bundle to become taut at this point (Frykholm, 1955). As this happens, movement occurs in the C4–8 and T1 nerve roots. The 4th cervical nerve is involved due to its relationship with the shoulder girdle as the nerve leaves the C3/4 foramen and travels to the shoulder as the supraclavicular nerve. Roots from C5–T1 are affected because of their relationship with the brachial plexus. An increase in tension occurs throughout the length of the neural tissues between the shoulder and the cervical spine. The subclavian artery and vein also move and sustain tension during shoulder girdle depression (Elvey, 1988).

When the shoulder is fixed and the cervical spine is laterally flexed to the opposite side, tension increases in the C4–8 nerve roots and the T1 root. Greater movement occurs at C4–7 and there is minimal movement at C8 and T1. No alteration in movement of the subclavian artery or vein occurs, because there is no direct attachment of these vessels to the cervical spine.

Elvey (1988) observed that abduction of the arm at the glenohu-meral joint with the shoulder girdle fixed caused most movement of the C5, 6 and 7 nerve roots, less movement of the C8 and T1 roots and no movement of the subclavian artery or vein.

The upper limb tension test has been researched and developed by

Elvey (1979). He stresses that there is not a standard brachial plexus tension test for the upper quarter, but a concept of testing that involves many techniques. The ulnar, median and radial nerve have different pathways within the upper limb, so that one particular test would not put all the nerves under tension at the same time.

The basic upper limb tension test consists of the following movements (Keneally *et al.*, 1988):

1. Abduction, extension and lateral rotation of the glenohumeral joint;
2. Forearm supination and elbow extension;
3. Wrist and finger extension.

The major nerve trunks will be affected distally by the upper limb tension test as follows (Keneally *et al.*, 1988):

1. The *median nerve* (C5–T1) runs slightly medial to lateral in the upper arm, anteriorly across the elbow, down the forearm to the wrist and hand. This trunk is stretched by abduction and lateral rotation of the glenohumeral joint and extension of the elbow, wrist and hand.
2. The *musculocutaneous nerve* (C5–7) runs medial to lateral in the upper arm and across the anterior aspect of the elbow to become the lateral cutaneous nerve of the forearm. It is stretched by abduction and lateral rotation of the glenohumeral joint and elbow extension.
3. The *ulnar nerve* (C7–T1) runs posterior to the medial epicondyle of the elbow and passes into the anterior forearm through the two heads of flexor carpi ulnaris. In its upper part, it will be stretched by abduction and lateral rotation of the glenohumeral joint, while in the forearm the ulnar nerve will be elongated by elbow flexion, forearm supination, wrist and finger extension.
4. The *radial* (C5–T1) and *axillary nerve* (C5 and 6) have a posterior course in the arm, and are unlikely to be stretched by shoulder abduction and lateral rotation. Abduction and medial rotation of the glenohumeral joint may elongate these nerves (Keneally *et al.*, 1988).

Sensitizing additions of the upper limb tension test are:

1. Cervical movements – flexion, lateral flexion to the opposite side, rotation to the opposite side;
2. Upper limb tension of the opposite arm;
3. Straight-leg raising.

The normal responses to the upper limb tension test have been assessed in 100 normal subjects (Keneally, 1983):

1. Extension, abduction and lateral rotation of the glenohumeral joint – mild stretch across anterior aspect of shoulder joint.

2. Addition of supination and elbow extension – deep painful stretch extending down forearm and stretch across anterior shoulder.
3. Final test position of extension, abduction, lateral rotation of shoulder, forearm supination, wrist and finger extension – deep stretch or ache in cubital fossa extending down anterior and radial aspects of forearm and occasionally on to dorsum of hand.
4. Tingling of the thumb and first three fingers.

Apart from a minor stretch across the anterior shoulder, the upper limb tension test does not reproduce shoulder pain in a normal subject. Any shoulder pains produced are considered abnormal and likely to be of cervical origin.

A second upper limb tension test has been developed by Butler (1987), which aims to mirror the work posture used in many upper limb repetition disorders. The most sensitive position is depression of the shoulder girdle, medial rotation of the glenohumeral joint, elbow extension and forearm pronation (Butler and Gifford, 1989).

FACTORS AFFECTING MOBILITY OF THE SPINAL CORD AND NERVES

Any pathological changes affecting the spinal cord, meninges, nerve roots or tissues in close relationship to them are likely to alter the mobility and tension in these structures.

The pain-sensitive structures may be subjected to compressive, tensile or bending stresses. They may be subjected to mechanical or chemical irritation or become adherent at any point along their length.

There is a decrease in the inherent plasticity of the meningeal tissues with ageing, when they are then less able to sustain tension stresses. As degenerative changes occur, the intervertebral discs lose height and the vertebral bodies approximate so that the neural canal becomes shorter. Folds develop within the dura to accommodate the decrease in vertical height. Degenerative changes may also lead to a decrease in the size of the bony canal. Spondylotic ridges and osteophytes may intrude into the canal, reducing the available space for the cord and meninges.

Within the body there are many sites where pathological processes may affect the mobility and elasticity of the nervous system (Sunderland, 1978; Dawson et al., 1983). Fibro-osseous (e.g. carpal tunnel) or osseous (e.g. intervertebral foramen) tunnels are sites where such pathological changes commonly occur.

Sunderland (1976) describes a pressure gradient which must exist in the intervertebral foramen for normal neural function:

- Pressure in the epineurium of the nutrient artery →
- Pressure in endoneurial capillaries →
- Pressure in veins in epineurium →
- Intrafunicular pressure →
- Intraforaminal pressure

Increase in the intraforaminal pressure could lead to venous congestion and stasis. Sunderland (1976) identifies three stages that may occur with persistent pressure in the carpal tunnel – hypoxia, oedema and fibrosis – and considers that similar events could occur in other tunnel sites. In the hypoxic state, the decreased intrafunicular circulation impairs nerve fibre nutrition and may lead to local pain. Continuation of this situation will lead to damage of the capillary endothelium so that leakage of protein rich oedema occurs. This oedema is unable to disperse because the perineurium is not crossed by lymphatics (Lundborg, 1975) and there is a subsequent increase in intrafunicular pressure.

The protein-rich oedema enhances fibroblast formation so that intraneural fibrosis develops. Such increases in connective tissue raise the intraneural pressure so that a self-perpetuating cycle is established. At this stage, axonal transmission properties are affected and the situation is no longer reversible. The affected area becomes a 'fibrous cord' and 'friction fibrosis' may then occur at other vulnerable sites along the tract (Sunderland, 1976). The fibrosis that occurs is also known as 'adhesions' or 'tethering'.

Movement disorders of the nervous system have been categorized into:

1. Extraneural – lesions which affect movement and tension from outside the nerve (mechanical interface);
2. Intraneural – lesions affecting movement and tension within the nerve (Butler, 1987).

The intraneural and extraneural components may be examined by passive movement (Fig. 8.6).

Prolonged adverse mechanical tension at any point within the nerve tracts is likely to have mechanical repercussions elsewhere (Butler and Gifford, 1989). Upton and McComas (1973) studied 115 patients with carpal tunnel syndrome or lesions of the ulnar nerve at the elbow and found that 70% had electrophysiological and clinical evidence of neural lesions in the cervical spine.

They termed these dual pathologies as 'double crush phenomenon' and believed that altered 'axioplasmic flow' was the cause of the disorder. Other authors have also observed similar occurrences (Crymble, 1968; Dyro, 1983) in other clinical disorders. Clinically, these studies highlight the importance of examining the mobility of the whole length of the nervous system in both spinal and peripheral disorders.

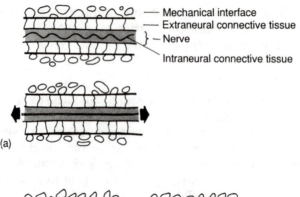

— Mechanical interface
— Extraneural connective tissue
} — Nerve
Intraneural connective tissue

(a)

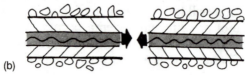

(b)

(c)

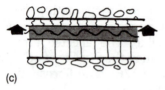

Fig. 8.6 Diagrammatic representation of passive movements of the nervous system available to examination and treatment. (a) increased tension in the intraneural component, i.e. 'tension from both ends' as in the slump test; (b) increased tension in the extraneural component, i.e. maximal movement of the nerve in relation to the mechanical interface as in straight-leg raising; (c) movement in another plane, i.e. tension in part of the extraneural component. (From *Proceedings of the Fifth Biennial Conference of the Manipulative Therapists Association of Australia*, Melbourne 1987, with permission.)

REFERENCES

Adams C., Logue V. (1971). Studies in cervical spondylotic myelopathy. *Brain*, **94**, 557.

Breig A. (1960). *Biomechanics of the Central Nervous System: Some Basic Normal and Pathological Phenomena*. Stockholm: Almquist and Wiksell, pp. 31–34, 60–61, 94.

Breig A. (1978). *Adverse Mechanical Tension in the Central Nervous System*. Stockholm: Almquist and Wiksell, pp. 15, 154–155, 160–161.

Breig A., Troup J.D.G. (1979). Biomechanical considerations in the straight-leg raising test, cadaveric and clinical studies of the effects of medial hip rotation. *Spine*, **4**, 242.

Butler D.S. (1987). Adverse mechanical tensions in the nervous system. Application to repetition strain injury. In *Proceedings of the Manipulative Therapists Association of Australia*, 5th Biennial Conference, Melbourne.

Butler D.S., Gifford L. (1989). The concept of adverse mechanical tension in the nervous system. Part 1. Testing for dural tension. *Physiotherapy*, **75**, 11, 622.

Crymble B. (1968). Brachial neuralgia and the carpal tunnel syndrome. *Br. Med. J.*, **3**, 470.

Davidson S. (1987). Prone knee bend – a normative study and investigation into the effect of cervical flexion and extension. In *Proceedings of the Manipulative Therapists Association of Australia*. 5th Biennial Conference, Melbourne.

Dawson D.M., Hallett M., Millender L.H. (1983). *Entrapment Neuropathies*. Boston: Little, Brown.

Dommisse G. (1975). Morphological aspects of the lumbar spine and lumbo-sacral region. *Clin. Orthop. Rel. Res.*, **115**, 22.

Dyro F.T. (1983). Peripheral entrapments following brachial plexus lesions. *Electromyog. Clin. Neurophysiol.*, **23**, 251.

Edgar M.A., Nundy S. (1966). Innervation of the spinal dura mater. *J. Neurol. Neurosurg. Psychiatr.*, **29**, 530.

Elvey R.L. (1979). Painful restriction of shoulder movement – a clinical observational study. *Proc. Disord. Knee, Ankle, Shoulder*. Western Australia Institute of Technology, Perth.

Elvey R.L. (1988). The clinical relevance of signs of adverse brachial plexus tension. In *Proceedings of the International Federation of Orthopaedic Manipulative Therapists Congress*, Cambridge.

Epstein B.S. (1966). An anatomic, myelographic and cinemyelographic study of the dentate ligaments. *Am. J. Roentgenol.*, **98**, 704.

Epstein B.S. (1976). *The Spine – a Radiological Text and Atlas*. 4th edn. Philadelphia: Lea & Febiger, pp. 44–47.

Frykholm R. (1955). Cervical nerve root compression resulting from disc degeneration and root sleeve fibrosis. A clinical investigation. *Acta Chir. Scand.*, Suppl. 160.

Goddard M.D., Reid D.J. (1965). Movements induced by straight-leg raising in the lumbosacral roots, nerves and plexus, and in the intrapelvic portion of the sciatic nerve. *J. Neurol. Neurosurg. Psychiatr.*, **28**, 12.

Grieve G.P. (1988). *Common Vertebral Joint Problems*, 2nd edn. Edinburgh: Churchill Livingstone, pp. 314, 324.

Hollinshead, W.H. (1969), *Anatomy for Surgeons*. 2nd edn. Vol. 3. New York: Harper and Row, p. 176.

Keneally M. (1983). The upper limb tension test. An investigation of responses amongst normal, asymptomatic subjects. Unpublished thesis cited in *Physical Therapy of the Cervical and Thoracic Spines* (Grant, R., ed.) 1988. Edinburgh: Churchill Livingstone, p. 188.

Keneally M., Robenach H., Elvey R. (1988). The upper limb tension test: the SLR test of the arm. In *Physical Therapy of the Cervical and Thoracic Spines* (Grant R., ed.). Edinburgh: Churchill Livingston, p. 10.

Lew P.C., Puentedura E.J. (1985). The straight-leg raise test and spinal posture: a tension test or a hamstring measure in normals? In *Proceedings of the Manipulative Therapists Association of Australia*. 4th Biennial Conference, Brisbane, 183.

Louis R. (1981). Vertebroradicular and vertebromedullar dynamics. *Anatomica Clinica*, **3**, 1.

Lundborg G. (1975). Structure and function of the intraneural microvessels as related to trauma, oedema formation and nerve function. *J. Bone Jt. Surg.*, **57A**, 938.

Maitland G.D. (1978). Movement of pain-sensitive structures in the vertebral canal in a group of physiotherapy students. *Proceedings, Inaugural Congress of Manipulative Therapists Association of Australia*, Sydney.

Massey, A.E. (1982). The slump test – an investigation of the movement of the pain-sensitive structures in the vertebral canal in subjects with low back pain. Unpublished thesis, South Australian Institute of Technology.

Massey A.E. (1986). Movement of pain-sensitive structures in the neural canal. In *Modern Manual Therapy of the Vertebral Column*. (Grieve G.P., ed.). Edinburgh: Churchill Livingstone, pp. 182–193.

O'Connell J.E.A. (1946). Clinical signs of meningeal irritation. *Brain*, **69**, 9.

O'Connell J.E.A. (1951). Protrusions of the lumbar intervertebral discs. *J. Bone Jt. Surg.*, **33B**, 8.

Penning L., Wilmink J.T. (1981). Biomechanics of the lumbosacral dural sac: a study of flexion-extension myelography. *Spine*, **6**, 398.

Reid J. (1960). Effects of flexion-extension movements of the head and spine upon the spinal cord and nerve roots. *J. Neurol. Neurosurg. Psychiatr.*, **23**, 214.

Smith C.G. (1956). Changes in length and posture of the segments of the spinal cord with changes in posture in the monkey. *Radiology*, **66**, 259.

Sunderland S. (1974). Meningeal–neural relations in the intervertebral foramen. *J. Neurosurg.*, **40**, 756.

Sunderland S. (1976). The nerve lesion in carpal tunnel syndrome. *J. Neurol. Neurosurg. Psychiatr.*, **39**, 615.

Sunderland S. (1978). *Nerves and Nerve Injuries*. Edinburgh: Churchill Livingstone.

Sutton J.L. (1979). The 'straight-leg raising test'. Unpublished thesis. South Australian Institute of Technology, Adelaide.

Tunturi A. (1977). Elasticity of spinal cord dura in the dog. *J. Neurosurg.*, **47**, 391.

Troup J.D.G. (1986). Biomechanics of the lumbar spinal canal. *Clin. Biomechan.*, **1**, 31.

Upton A.R.M., McComas A.J. (1973). The double crush in nerve entrapment syndromes. *Lancet*, **ii**, 359.

Woodhall B., Hayes G.H. (1950). The well-leg raising test of Fajersztajn in the diagnosis of ruptured lumbar intevertebral disc. *J. Bone Jt. Surg.*, **32A**, 786.

9

Embryology, Development, Ageing and Degeneration

EMBRYOLOGY AND DEVELOPMENT

Prenatal life is divided into embryonic and fetal periods, the embryonic period comprising the first eight postovulatory weeks and the fetal period extending to birth.

The embryo, by the third week of development, is in the form of a flat disc consisting of two layers of cells: the ectoderm and the endoderm. Cells from the ectoderm give rise to a third layer, the mesoderm. At the end of the fourth week, a solid rod of cells called the notochord grows in the midline and forms a framework around which the primitive vertebral column will develop. Notochordal cells induce the ectoderm posterior to it to initiate formation of the neural plate, from which develops the brain, spinal cord and most of the remainder of the nervous system.

Segmentation of the Mesoderm

On both sides of the axis formed by the notochord and neural plate, the mesoderm forms three columns: a medial, thickened paraxial mesoderm, an intermediate mesoderm and a lateral plate.

The paraxial mesoderm becomes segmented into a longitudinal series of blocks or somites, commencing in the region of what will be the head and proceeding distally. By 30 days of development, 42–44 pairs of somites can be identified in the embryo, 11–12 pairs of which regress or participate in the formation of the occipital region of the skull. Variations in the number of somites may occur such as an additional or a missing one, which is often compensated for by a variation in an adjacent region.

The cells in each somite gradually change into loosely arranged tissue called mesenchyme. Cells in the anteromedial part of the somite constitute the sclerotome; those in the posterolateral part constitute the dermomyotome.

Development of the Vertebral Column

The development of the vertebral column occurs in three stages: the mesenchymal stage, the cartilaginous stage and the ossification stage. These stages are not entirely distinct, rather they merge into one another.

1. Mesenchymal stage

During this stage, changes occur in the mesenchyme that result in the formation of a primitive model of the vertebral column. Differentiation occurs in each somite into a dense caudal band and a loose cranial band. The aorta, lying anterior to the notochord, sends intersegmental branches around the middle of each loose band.

In the sclerotome, the developing spinal nerve grows laterally into the dermomyotome and, in time, is surrounded by perineural tissue formed from the cranial half of somite.

The remainder of the somite participates in the formation of the vertebral column. Two processes develop in the caudal half of each somite: a dorsal process, which grows to form the neural arch, and a ventrolateral process, which forms the costal element. Less dense condensations of mesenchyme join the neural arches of adjacent segments and eventually give rise to ligaments.

Meanwhile, multiplying and surrounding the notochord is a continuous column of cells called the axial mesenchyme. This forms the centrum, which is the greater part of the vertebral body, the remainder of it being formed by a third process from the sclerotome. A zone of increased density in the lower end of the cranial part of the axial mesenchyme forms the predecessor to the future intervertebral disc (Verbout, 1985).

The dermomyotome divides into the myotome, which is the forerunner of striated muscle, and the dermatome, which gives rise to the skin and subcutaneous tissues.

At about the 40th day of development, the spinal nerve divides into a ventral and dorsal ramus. The myotome splits into two portions, the posterior of which is innervated by the posterior ramus, and the anterior, the anterior ramus.

2. Cartilaginous stage

The cartilaginous stage is a short one, commencing at about the sixth week of development in the cranial end of the column and proceeding caudally. Two centres of chondrification appear in each vertebral centrum and one in each half of the neural arch. The latter expand posteriorly to complete the neural arch and a cartilaginous spinous process develops at their union. Expansion also occurs laterally into the transverse process and anteriorly to blend with the chondrifying centrum.

3. Ossification stage

Primary ossification centres begin to appear by the ninth fetal week at the sites where blood vessels grow into the cartilaginous vertebrae.

An ossification centre first appears in each half of the neural arch, the earliest centres being in the cervicothoracic region. In the vertebral body, the most common pattern is for it to have a single ossification centre (Bagnall *et al.*, 1984). Ossification starts at different times in the vertebral arches and bodies in different areas of the spine, but, by the seventh month, centres have been established in all areas.

As the primary ossification centre in the vertebral body expands, it does not extend to its superior and inferior surfaces, which remain cartilaginous to ensure continuing growth. The laminae and the bulk of the spinous process become fully ossified during the first year after birth.

Certain areas remain cartilaginous until secondary ossification centres appear during puberty in the cartilaginous tips of the spinous process, the tips of the transverse processes and in the cartilaginous mamillary processes (Carpenter, 1961; Warwick and Williams, 1980). These are separated from the rest of the vertebra by a narrow interval of cartilage, and remain so during the final periods of spinal growth. This cartilage is gradually replaced by bone by the 25th year of life.

Formation of the Intervertebral Disc

In the mesenchymal intervertebral disc, central cells are loosely arranged around the notochord and peripheral cells are arranged in a radial pattern. Gradually, the cells closer to the notochord transform into embryonic cartilage (Peacock, 1951). Towards the end of the second month of embryonic life, the notochord enlarges between the developing vertebrae. Collagen fibres formed from the peripheral cells become laminated at a very early stage and insert into the cartilage plates covering the superior and inferior parts of the vertebral bodies. The cartilage cells closer to the annulus undergo transition to fibrocartilage. At this stage, therefore, the disc has three zonal compartments: the notochord centrally, the collagenous annulus peripherally and fibrocartilage in between. The nucleus pulposus is formed from the notochord and fibrocartilage.

At birth, some of the notochord cells may persist in the disc, but these eventually atrophy and disappear during infancy.

Growth of the Vertebral Body

The vertebral body grows horizontally by periosteal ossification, and longitudinally by proliferation of the cartilages on the whole of its superior and inferior surfaces. The cells nearest to the vertebral body become ossified and are replaced by cells from the cartilage plate.

The shape of the vertebral bodies changes through an increase in their anteroposterior growth rate, with the assumption of the erect posture in infants and corresponding increase in lordosis. There are related changes in the shapes of the intervertebral discs and vertebral end plates, and the position of the nuclei pulposi. The end plates are convex in fetal and infant vertebrae, and become concave in children, adolescents and adults. During adolescence, the dimensions of the vertebral bodies in females are somewhat smaller than in males, but by adulthood they approach male dimensions more closely (Bogduk and Twomey, 1987).

Ossification ceases by the age of 25 and the growth plates become thinner. They become sealed off from the vertebral body by a calcified layer of cartilage and a subchondral bone plate. The other part of each cartilage plate, which becomes the end plate of the intervertebral disc, remains unossified throughout life except for an outer bony rim or apophysis which is apparent by the age of 12 years. This fuses with the vertebral body when longitudinal growth ceases, although it does not itself contribute to growth. The ring apophysis provides a bony attachment for the peripheral annular fibres.

Development of the Apophyseal Joints

The dorsal processes of the mesenchymal neural arches in adjacent somites blend with one another at the sites of the future apophyseal joints. As chondrification of the articular processes proceeds, the mesenchyme recedes to form the articular capsule, any intra-articular structures and a joint space (Bogduk and Twomey, 1987). The articular processes are not completely ossified at birth.

There is a change in the orientation of the lumbar apophyseal joints which is of particular importance. At birth all the lumbar apophyseal joints are orientated in the coronal plane but, by the age of 11 years, this has changed to the adult orientation (Odgers, 1933). Several reasons have been suggested as to the cause of this change, but it remains unclear. It is possible that there may be a genetic determination, but another theory is that the multifidus muscle by pulling on the mamillary process swings the lateral part of the superior articular process dorsally, thereby rotating the plane of the joint or imparting a curvature to it (Bogduk and Twomey, 1987).

Developmental Anomalies

Most congenital anomalies appear during the embryonic period (Bradford and Hensinger, 1985). The main cause of many of these anomalies has been attributed to genetic transmission (Jeffreys, 1980), other factors being metabolic, the use of drugs, irradiation, infections, and maternal alcoholism (Tredwell *et al.*, 1982).

Bony and soft tissue anomalies in the vertebral column are common; indeed, it is rarer to find true structural symmetry. Attempts to 'put bones back into place' often prove to be futile, since they are usually not out of place to start with.

While some anomalies are purely of academic interest, others may have a marked influence on the biomechanics of the spine and symptomatology due to the abnormal stresses they impose on joints and ligaments. Otherwise quiescent anomalies can have serious repercussions in traumatic incidents.

While structural anomalies can occur anywhere in the spine, it is the transitional regions that are most prone (Schmorl and Junghanns, 1971), in particular the craniovertebral region, where asymmetry is common and, therefore, of particular relevance to manipulators. Here the most common anomaly is posterior spina bifida of the atlas (Spillane *et al.*, 1957). There is also a high incidence of asymmetry of the superior articular facets of the atlas; Singh (1965) found that this occurred in over one-tenth of spines. The relationship between developmental anomalies of the craniovertebral region and headaches has been pointed out by McRae (1953). Congenital absence of the odontoid peg (os odontoideum) is a rare finding; loss of the odontoid is usually caused by trauma.

The lumbosacral region is also prone to anomalies. One of particular relevance to therapists is articular tropism, or asymmetrical orientation of the apophyseal joints, so that at one vertebral level the plane of one apophyseal joint is more inclined in the frontal or sagittal plane than the plane of the contralateral apophyseal joint. It is most common at the lowest two lumbar levels (Cyron and Hutton, 1980) and occurs to a varying degree in approximately one-quarter of spines (Grieve, 1989).

Tropism has been linked with a rotation instability which puts the ligaments of the apophyseal joint under strain (Cyron and Hutton, 1980). This may also lead to a rotation strain of the disc as more stress is placed on the intervertebral disc on the side of the more obliquely orientated apophyseal joint.

When flexion occurs in the presence of tropism, it will usually do so about some oblique axis x–x' (*see* Fig. 1.26, p. 53), so that the capsular ligaments will be equidistant from the axis of rotation. Flexion about x–x' causes maximum stretching of the posterolateral annulus, hence posterolateral tears will usually be at the side of the more oblique facet.

In studies done by Farfan and Sullivan (1967), there was a high correlation between the side of the more oblique facet and the side of sciatica.

It is not within the scope of this book to describe every anomaly that can occur. The commonest causes of most bony anomalies are: failure of development of a vertebra, non-union of parts of a vertebra, and failure of segmentation. Anomalies in the intersegmental branches of the dorsal aorta may result in anomalies of segmentation. In the mesenchymal stage, these vessels normally run around the centres of the loose bands and provide nutrition for the primitive vertebrae. It is conceivable that absence of a vessel could mar development in part of a vertebra.

Block vertebrae

Defective development of the loose bands in the mesenchymal stage may give rise to block vertebrae (so-called fused vertebrae). Compensatory movement and stress usually occur above and below the fused segment/s, predisposing these levels to spondylotic changes in later life (Brain and Wilkinson, 1967).

Wedge and hemivertebrae

Interference with vertebral development can be caused by failure of condensation in the early mesenchymal stage. If partial, this can give rise to vertebral wedging, the amount of failure of formation varying and, with it, the degree of vertebral wedging, or if there is complete failure of development on one side, a hemivertebra may develop (James, 1976). These abnormal vertebrae lead to an increasing scoliosis during growth and predispose to early degenerative change (McMaster and David, 1986).

Asymmetric growth of the right and left halves of the vertebral arches commonly occurs and results in pedicles of unequal lengths. This has the effect of rotating the vertebral body towards the side of the shorter pedicle.

Schmorl's nodes (Fig. 9.1)

During segmentation of the mesoderm, weak areas or 'dimples' may be left in the centre of the nuclear aspect of each end plate, which remain until adolescence. These are the points at which failure occurs first on experimental compression (Brown *et al.*, 1957).

A second mechanism may occur which leads to other areas of reduced resistance. During fetal life, the annulus and end plates receive a blood supply from peripheral intersegmental vessels which grow radially towards the nucleus. These vessels involute during childhood and are replaced by connective tissue, constituting channels

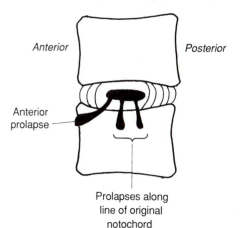

Anterior

Posterior

Anterior
prolapse

Prolapses along
line of original
notochord

Fig. 9.1 Two types of intravertebral
disc prolapses (Schmorl's nodes).

which are weaker than the surrounding cartilage, and compressed disc material may rupture along them in adolescents or young adults (Taylor and Twomey, 1984).

Schmorl's nodes, or intravertebral disc prolapses, most common in the lower thoracic and thoracolumbar spine, can occur through the above two mechanisms. Usually less than 2% of disc volume is involved. These prolapses are more commonly seen along the line of the original notochord, but sometimes more peripheral nodes occur along the radially directed channels as described above, to the anterior aspect of the vertebra (Fig. 9.1). These anterior prolapses are usually larger and could be a source of pain by irritation of nociceptive endings in the periosteum or anterior longitudinal ligament. 'Scheuermann's kyphosis' occurs when the nodes are more extensive, leading to a reduction in height of the anterior vertebral bodies (Schmorl and Junghanns, 1971). In this condition, defective anterior endochondral ossification has also been implicated (*see* Further Reading).

Spinal stenosis

Congenital narrowing (stenosis) of the spinal canal predisposes to a higher incidence of symptoms from degenerative changes later in life. Payne and Spillane (1957) noted that in patients with myelopathy secondary to cervical spondylosis, the average sagittal diameter of the cervical spinal canal was around 3 mm less than normal.

Spina bifida is the commonest form of non-union. It ranges from failure of the laminae to unite dorsally behind the cauda equina (spina bifida occulta), which is minor and common, to complete splitting of the skin, vertebral arch and underlying neural tube with associated neurologic deficits. Some forms of spina bifida appear during the embryonic period, while others such as spina bifida occulta develop during the fetal period.

Sacralization and lumbarization

The lowest lumbar vertebra may become incorporated into the sacrum (sacralization) so that, in effect, there are only four mobile lumbar vertebrae. Conversely, the first sacral vertebra may be mobile (lumbarization). The effects that sacralization has on degeneration in the spine are discussed on p. 277.

Congenital scoliosis

Scoliosis is a lateral curvature of the spine, the causes of which are many. The congenital type of scoliosis is due to vertebral anomalies varying from a single hemivertebra to multiple, complex defects throughout the vertebral column.

Congenital scoliosis is structural so that, in addition to a lateral curvature, there is vertebral rotation. In the individual vertebra, the bony elements on the concave side have not grown as much as on the convexity. The body is wedged on the concave side, the pedicle is shorter and narrower, and the lamina smaller than on the convex side. The spinous process is directed away from the midline towards the concavity of the curve. Ligamentous structures between the vertebrae are adapted in length. Often the posterior joints are abnormal, being compressed on the concave side, where they show earlier than normal osteophytosis.

An irregular pattern of structural curves may be seen in congenital scoliosis. Usually, there is one single curve, but two or even three structural curves may be visible. Thoracic curves are the most common. The ribs on the convexity are carried backwards with the vertebral body rotation and are, therefore, more prominent, whereas the ribs on the concavity are crowded together and carried forward, so that there may be an anterior protrusion of the chest wall on this side. Usually there are missing, deformed or fused ribs or a combination of all three, usually – but not always – on the concave side.

The curve is nearly always progressive, because the irregular ossific centres and growth plates increase the asymmetry as growth proceeds. The scoliosis can be combined with lordosis or kyphosis depending on the site of the defect. Congenital thoracolumbar and lumbar curves tend to increase considerably; in part this is related to the difficulty of developing compensation below and the association of congenital pelvic obliquity (James, 1976).

Minor degrees of skeletal asymmetry occur in up to 20% of adolescents (Taylor, 1983). There is a greater likelihood of progression in females compared with males for several reasons. The vertebral body shape in females is slimmer from 8 years onwards due to greater growth in vertebral height in females and greater growth in vertebral girth in males. Coupled with weaker muscular support in the female, any slight curvature is more likely to buckle under axial loading (Taylor and Twomey, 1984).

Commonly associated with spinal curvature is a dropping of one shoulder, a prominent scapula, forward protrusion of the anterior chest wall on one side and prominence of one iliac crest.

Congenital kyphosis

Congenital kyphosis is a spinal deformity occurring exclusively or primarily in the sagittal plane, developing from one or more vertebral body malformations. The defect most commonly presents at the lumbar and thoracolumbar levels, although it can occur anywhere in the spine. It is always progressive. The cause can either be a failure of formation of the vertebral bodies or a failure of segmentation. If the segmentation failure is purely anterior then a kyphosis results; if it is anterolaterally located, then a kyphoscoliosis results.

Kyphosis can also result from Scheuermann's disease in the thoracic spine (*see* p. 267).

Patients with congenital scoliosis and kyphosis have a high incidence (25%) of segmentation defects in the cervical spine (Winter *et al.*, 1984).

AGEING AND DEGENERATION

As individuals age, their spines undergo fairly characteristic changes. The difficulty arises when attempting to distinguish between those which are due to the 'normal' ageing process and those which are due to degeneration. The same changes may occur both in ageing and in degenerative disease of, for example, the intervertebral disc but, when degeneration is present, this may occur earlier than would be expected from normal ageing. 'Normal' age changes are considered to be those which conform to the standard in individuals of a particular age and ethnic group, so what is 'normal' in a 20-year-old spine differs from what is 'normal' in a 70-year-old spine.

Degeneration is characterized by slow, destructive changes which are not balanced by the regeneration that occurs in younger tissues (Grieve, 1981). The normal ageing process can be acclerated by increased exposure to mechanical stresses, which then give rise to degenerative changes. Which part of the motion segment is initially affected depends on the particular mechanical stresses or postures to which the spine is subjected and the integrity of the tissues themselves. However, the interdependence of the joints comprising the motion segment dictates that failure of one element, either through degeneration or trauma, tends to lead sooner or later to degenerative changes in the other elements (Andersson, 1983).

Ageing and degeneration are not necessarily synonymous and a few elderly discs may behave like younger discs when subjected to compression and torsional loads. However, the incidence of degeneration does increase with age. No correlation has been found between radiological evidence of degenerative changes in the spine and the experience of pain. Just as severe changes can be present on X-ray in the absence of pain, an individual may have intense pain of musculoskeletal origin, but a normal X-ray.

The term 'arthrosis' is used to denote degenerative changes in synovial joints, and 'spondylosis' to denote changes in the interbody joints (Figs. 9.2a,b).

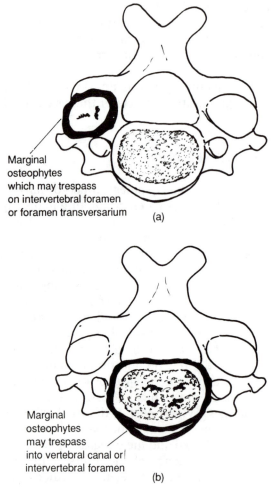

Marginal
osteophytes
which may trespass
on intervertebral foramen
or foramen transversarium
(a)

Marginal
osteophytes
may trespass
into vertebral canal or
intervertebral foramen
(b)

Fig. 9.2 Degenerative changes in the cervical spine.
(a) arthrosis of apophyseal joint; (b) spondylosis.

Changes in the Vertebral Bodies

Ageing is accompanied by loss of both trabecular and cortical bone throughout the skeleton in both sexes. The most severe degree of loss is in trabecular bone, such as that found in the vertebrae (Exton-Smith, 1983). This results in a decrease in bone strength, which is more marked in women than in men. While the structural integrity of trabecular bone is preserved with age in men but not in women, the width of the trabeculae themselves is reduced with age in men (Aaron et al., 1987).

The rate at which bone loss occurs is influenced by such factors as the menopause, reduced plasma calcitonin levels, decreased adrenal androgen production, smoking, declining calcium absorption and reduced physical exercise (Francis and Peacock, 1987). Bone mass and muscle mass are closely interrelated, and exercises play an important part in preventing bone mineral loss in postmenopausal women (Twomey and Taylor, 1985).

The height of the vertebral bodies declines in old age, principally due to the reduction in the number of transverse trabeculae which act as 'cross-braces' to the vertical trabeculae. On compressive loading, the vertical trabeculae are then less able to withstand the stresses and some of them microfracture. This is most marked below the area of nuclear pulp.

With weakening of the trabecular system, a greater proportion of the compressive load is borne by cortical bone. Consequently, the vertebral body becomes less resistant to deformation and injury. Lacking support from the underlying bone, the vertebral end plates also deform by microfracture and gradually bow into the vertebral body. This increased vertebral concavity leads to a disc convexity in old age.

Fractures may occur in the end plates at areas of reduced resistance, and they may be large enough to allow nuclear material to extrude into the vertebral body forming Schmorl's nodes, or intravertebral disc prolapses (see pp. 266–7). Their incidence is greatest in adolescence, but does not increase thereafter (Hilton et al., 1976).

Osteophytes

Osteophytes are outgrowths of healthy bone from the vertebrae. Their development is an important defence mechanism against compressive forces which exceed the capacity of the bone to resist them. They are composed of more compact, stronger bone than the rest of the vertebral body and bear a marked similarity to the capitals and bases used in architecture, which increase the resistance of pillars to compression. The vertebrae, by the formation of osteophytes, are converted into low pillars with capitals and bases.

Nathan (1962) described four successive stages in their development (Fig. 9.3).

1st degree: Isolated points of initial hyperostosis which may pass unnoticed on X-ray.

2nd degree: Bony protrusions projecting more or less horizontally from the vertebral body.

By increasing the superior and inferior surfaces of the vertebral bodies, the 1st and 2nd degree osteophytes effectively reduce the force per unit area.

3rd degree: Characteristic bird's beak shape, curving in the direction of the intervertebral disc.

4th degree: Fusion of two adjacent vertebrae.

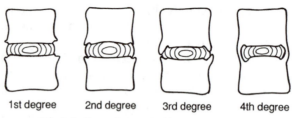

1st degree   2nd degree   3rd degree   4th degree

Fig. 9.3 Osteophytes. (After Nathan, 1962.)

A young person with normal vertebrae may develop osteophytes when the pressure on the vertebral bodies is excessive, as in heavy manual work or strenuous sports. Disc degeneration and the subsequently impaired shock-absorbing capacity of the vertebral column can also lead to their formation, as can pathological processes that weaken the vertebrae, such as osteoporosis.

In the fourth decade, most spines have osteophytes, and in the 80's, nearly all spines are affected by 3rd or 4th degree ones. They appear more where the pressure is greatest, that is in the concavities of either the normal vertebral column or one where there is a deformity such as scoliosis. In relation to the curvatures in the sagittal plane, Nathan found that the highest incidence coincided with the peaks of the spinal curves (C5, T8, L3/4), whereas the lowest incidence was where the line of gravity crossed the spine (T1, T12 and L5/S1). The incidence of anterior osteophytes was found to be greater than that of posterior osteophytes.

In the different regions of the spine, osteophytes were found to predominate in the prevertebral muscles (longus capitis and longus cervicis) in the cervical spine, in the anterior longitudinal ligament in the thoracic spine, and at the origins of the psoas muscles and crura of the diaphragm in the lumbar spine. Their formation is not a pathological reaction per se. However, they can give rise to symptoms by pressing on neural tissues, e.g. in the vertebral canal or intervertebral foramina (*see* Fig. 9.2), lumbar sympathetic ganglia, or viscera such as the oesophagus and trachea. Other factors in addition to pressure are involved, however, because symptoms can abate while the osteophytes remain.

Quite marked osteophytosis may be present without giving rise to symptoms. Depending on their size, however, osteophytes are undoubtedly associated with some degree of movement restriction. The more advanced ones may well be accompanied by pathological changes in the motion segment and this should, therefore, be taken into consideration when treating the spine.

Changes in the End Plates

At birth the end plate is part of the growth plate of the vertebral body. The disc side of the end plate is formed by fibrocartilage, the vertebral body side being the growth zone. There is a gradual reduction in the width of the growth zone up to the age of 16–20 years, after which the end plates consist of only articular cartilage, which is directly apposed to bone (Bernick and Cailliet, 1982). Collagen fibres arise from the articular cartilage and radiate into the nucleus pulposus. These fibres are independent of the anchoring fibres of the annulus and may serve to give stability to the disc. Progressive resorption and thinning of the articular cartilage occurs, with replacement by bone, so that over the age of 60 often only a thin layer of calcified cartilage separates the disc from the vertebral body. The shock-absorbing capacity of the end plates is thereby reduced. A common radiographic appearance with ageing is bulging of the lumbar end plates into the vertebral bodies (Fig. 9.4), outlined by sclerosis (Roaf, 1960).

With increasing age, it is likely that there is a decrease in the diffusion of substances through the end plates, although this has only been confirmed in rabbits. Since the cells in the disc are dependent on this route both for their supply of nutrients and the removal of waste products, closure of the end plate would be expected to lead to nutritional deficiencies as well as to a build-up of metabolic products, such as lactic acid. Thus, changes in the permeability of the end plates could be one of the causes of disc degeneration (Urban and Maroudas, 1980).

Changes in the Intervertebral Discs

In both nucleus and annulus, the fundamental change with age is the fall in the content of proteoglycans, those that persist being smaller in size. Both of these factors are largely responsible for the progressive decrease in the water-binding capacity of the nucleus. At birth, the nucleus contains 88% water; by the age of 75 this has dropped to

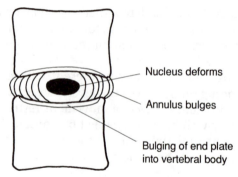

Fig. 9.4 Disc bulging.

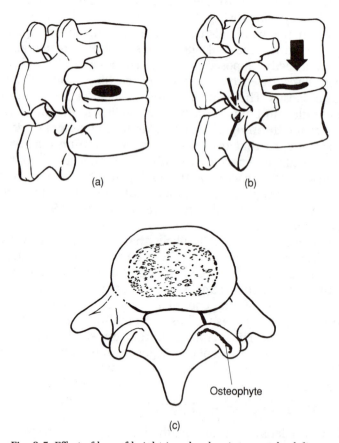

Fig. 9.5 Effect of loss of height in a lumbar intervertebral disc. (a) normal disc; (b) degenerative changes in disc leading to loss of disc height and impingement of tip of facet of apophyseal joint; (c) degenerative changes in facet of lumbar apophyseal joint (shown on one side only, but often bilateral).

65–72%, the majority of this loss occurring, however, before early adult life (Twomey and Taylor, 1985).

Most discs show signs of degeneration with ageing, and this is usually associated with some loss of disc height and bulging (*see* Figs. 9.4 and 9.5). Combined with the decrease in vertebral body height, it results in a loss of height in the spine with increasing age.

There is a gradual increase in the relative proportion of collagen in both nucleus and annulus possibly because of the loss of other components such as proteoglycans. The nature of the collagen also changes: the diameter of the collagen fibrils in the nucleus increases (Happey, 1976) and its Type II collagen resembles the Type I collagen of the annulus. Reciprocally, there is a decrease in the average fibril diameter of the annulus, resulting in less distinction between annulus and nucleus. The reduction in water content and relative increase in collagen in the nucleus affects its hydraulic properties, making it more rigid and less resilient.

If the disc becomes vascularized, which may occur through, for example, damage to the end plates, disc degeneration is accelerated. The term 'brown degeneration' is used when the nucleus becomes discoloured through the breakdown of haemoglobin. Nerve fibres then accompany the blood vessels into the disc and may serve a nociceptive function (*see* p. 79).

The concentration of elastic fibres in the annulus drops, with replacement by large fibrous inelastic bands, causing a progressive loss of elasticity.

Disc degeneration with the subsequently impaired shock-absorbing capacity of the vertebral column leads to the formation of osteophytes along the margins of the vertebral bodies (called 'lipping'). In the cervical spine, the outgrowths may include nuclear as well as annular material and, continuous at either side with the outgrowths from the joints of Luschka, form a hard, osseocartilaginous bar which projects into the spinal canal, and in severe cases compresses the cord and its meninges into a series of horizontal corrugations.

Isolated Disc Resorption

This is a condition in which a single intervertebral disc is narrowed and degenerated in an otherwise normal spine. It is caused by trauma through excessive compression which fractures the cartilage end plate, exposing the antigenic proteoglycans of the nucleus to the blood supply of the vertebral body. An autoimmune reaction is thought to result, causing disc degradation. The disc space is eventually represented by a thin slit between the vertebral bodies, filled with fibrous tissue. Vertebral bone on either side of the disc is sclerotic, and the disc is anchored around its circumference by peripheral osteophytes. Occasionally ankylosis occurs.

Incidence of Disc Degeneration

There is a strong familial predisposition to discogenic low-back pain and the etiology of degenerative disc disease is related to both genetic factors and environmental factors (Postacchini *et al.*, 1988). The incidence of disc degeneration in the spine overall is highest at the lowest two lumbar levels, particularly in the lumbosacral disc. Although this disc is the largest in the spine, there are many factors which contribute to it being more prone to degeneration. As it is a major component of the first motion segment above the sacrum, there is a longer lever arm acting on it during movements of the trunk and arms, predisposing it to more stress. Also, there is a greater degree of movement at this level, and greater shear forces acting on it with the lordotic posture in the standing position. The shape of the posterior aspect of the disc itself has also been implicated (Hickey and Hukins, 1980). This is usually flattened or rounded rather than concave and, consequently, has less annular fibres to resist flexion, lateral flexion and rotation. In addition, the planes of the apophyseal joints in the lower lumbar spine, being orientated more in the frontal plane, offer less resistance to torsional stresses than those higher in the lumbar spine, whose orientation is more in the sagittal plane.

In the cervical spine, the commonest sites of spondylosis are at the most mobile regions, namely at C5/6 and C6/7 (Bull, 1951; Mixter, 1951). In the thoracic spine, the highest incidence of spondylosis is related to its kyphotic curvature and is at T7/8 in females and T8/9 in males.

Other factors speeding disc degeneration in the spine include lack of movement (e.g. in people with a sedentary lifestyle) or excess of movement, chemical or hereditary causes. Structural factors and mechanical stresses also play an important part. Experiments have in the main been carried out on lumbar discs.

Structural Factors Influencing the Degenerative Process in the Lumbar Spine

1. *Degree of lumbar curvature*

In a study using cadaveric lumbar spines, Farfan (1973) found that the site of annular damage and Schmorl's nodes varied depending on whether the spine was flat or had a marked lordotic curve. Those with a marked lordotic curve (i.e. with a lumbosacral angle of more than 35°) had the highest incidence of (a) annular damage in the L4/5 disc, and (b) Schmorl's nodes at the L3/4 level, whereas in flat spines (with lumbosacral angles of less than 20°) the distribution of both annular damage and Schmorl's nodes was more evenly distributed over the whole of the lumbar spine. Of interest, too, was the finding that the lordotic curves showed a lesser overall incidence of Schmorl's nodes, suggesting that in these spines the discs were better able to withstand compression loads.

2. The location of the 5th lumbar vertebra in relation to the iliac crest

The location of the 5th lumbar vertebra varies in different individuals. When it is deeply seated in the pelvis, the lumbosacral disc was found to be less likely to prolapse (Farfan, 1973). In spines where the 5th lumbar vertebra was higher such that the 4th lumbar vertebra was located completely above the iliac crest, the lumbosacral disc was much more vulnerable to prolapse.

3. Local structural anomalies

a. Sacralization. In the presence of a complete or almost complete sacralization, the lumbosacral disc may show some degree of hypoplasia by its diminished vertical height, but it rarely shows radiographic evidence of degeneration and is usually stable with very limited or no movement. However, the very stability of the 5th lumbar vertebra may induce early degeneration of the L4/5 motion segment. This is probably on the basis of the reduced capacity for movement of the four-jointed lumbar spine.

b. Tropism (*see* Fig. 1.26, p. 53). One-quarter of the general population have some degree of tropism of the apophyseal joints in the lumbar spine. Depending on the degree of asymmetry, there is undoubtedly an association between tropism and the pattern of degeneration in the annulus, probably related to the failure of the joints to protect the disc from torsional injury. Joints with symmetrical facets tend to develop a symmetrical pattern of degeneration: posterior midline radial fissures in discs with a rounded posterior annulus, or bilateral posterolateral radial fissures if the joint has a flattened posterior outline. The asymmetrical interbody joint develops a unilateral posterolateral degenerative pattern. In a clinical study of consecutive patients admitted to hospital for backache and sciatica, Farfan *et al.* (1970) found that there was a high correlation between the side of sciatica and of disc protrusion with the side of the more obliquely orientated facet.

c. Spondylolysis and spondylolisthesis. The presence of a spondylolysis (defect across the pars interarticularis, without shift of the vertebral body) or a spondylolisthesis (forward slip, 'olisthesis', of a vertebral body on the one below) is thought to influence degenerative changes in the spine due to the loss of proper physiological function (Farfan, 1973). The affected motion segment is sometimes spared these secondary changes if the injury is sustained early in life, healing and growth adaptation having taken place. However, the motion segment above may then become the site at which additional stresses are transferred, leading to degenerative changes there.

It should be borne in mind that every spinal anomaly has been demonstrated in symptom-free individuals, which would indicate that the anomaly may be but one factor in the multifactorial nature of back pain.

EFFECTS OF MECHANICAL STRESSES ON THE INTERVERTEBRAL DISCS

Mechanical stresses can affect the integrity of the disc in different ways and may accelerate the normal ageing process. The changes that occur in the discs do not always follow a neat and tidy pattern, because structural as well as mechanical factors also influence the degenerative process, as outlined above.

Injuries to ligaments either precede or accompany injuries to the discs. Hyperflexion strains in the lumbar spine have been shown to damage the supraspinous and interspinous ligaments first, then the capsular ligaments and then the disc (Adams, 1980). The supraspinous and interspinous ligaments are invariably ruptured or slack in patients with a disc prolapse (Rissanen, 1960). However, flexion accompanied by lateral flexion could damage the contralateral capsular ligaments first, while not affecting the supraspinous and interspinous ligaments which lie on the axis of lateral flexion.

The first pathological changes that occur in the disc are usually circumferential tears or separations between the laminae in the outer third of the annulus (Fig. 9.6a), the yield point being at the junction of lamina with end plate. These occur mainly in the posterolateral part of the annulus and do not initially communicate with the nucleus. The snapping sounds that are sometimes heard with a sudden onset of back pain may be due to such injuries to the annulus.

The circumferential tears are commonly thought to be caused by repetitive rotation strains. Because of the orientation of the annular fibres, during axial rotation only half of them are able to resist the movement, the outer fibres being stretched more than the inner ones. In the lumbar spine, the apophyseal joints normally protect the discs from rotation beyond a few degrees and the relevance of torsion in producing damage has therefore been questioned. However, in certain circumstances, the apophyseal joints allow this 'safe degree' of rotation to be exceeded. If, for example, the cartilage lining them was thinned by 3 mm through degeneration, it was estimated that this would allow 6° of extra movement (Adams and Hutton, 1981). Also, if the apophyseal joints are more inclined towards the frontal plane, this type of facet orientation provides less resistance to torsion (see Fig. 1.25a,c, p. 51). Another factor which allows more rotation is flexion of the intervertebral joint in addition to rotation. The apophyseal joints are then less effective in resisting the rotatory component.

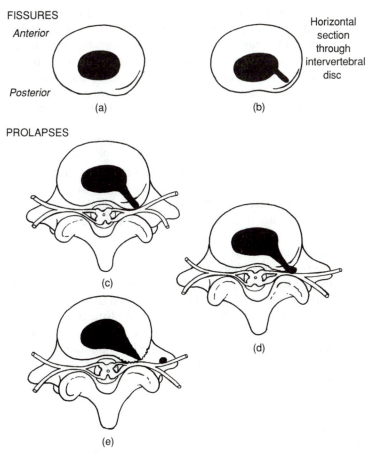

Fig. 9.6 Stages of disc prolapse. (a) circumferential annular tear; (b) posterolateral radial fissure; (c) annular protrusion; (d) nuclear extrusion; (e) sequestrated disc material.

Circumferential tears are usually evident before radial fissures appear (Fig. 9.6b). The latter are commonest in thoracic spines (Eckert and Decker, 1947). The shape of the posterior surface of the disc (*see* Fig. 2.5, p. 63) to a large extent influences the site of these radial fissures, possibly because it dictates the location of the line of maximal torsional stress (Hickey and Hukins, 1980). In discs which have a concave posterior surface, such as those in the upper lumbar spine, the line of stress radiates posterolaterally. Discs at the lower two lumbar levels most commonly have flat posterior surfaces in which the line of torsional stress radiates to the medial aspect or to the middle of the pedicle, this being the most common direction of radial fissures. Discs with rounded posterior surfaces have a stress concentration in the midline posteriorly – often seen at the lumbosacral level.

The method of formation of radial fissures has not been completely elucidated, but there are several theories. One theory considers that the circumferential tears in the annulus later become larger and coalesce to form a tear passing from the annulus into the nucleus (Kirkaldy-Willis, 1988). Farfan (1973) considers that the radial fissures commence at the nucleus and work towards the periphery to communicate with pre-existing tears. Posterolateral radial fissures have been experimentally produced (Adams and Hutton, 1982) in cadaveric lumbar discs which were fatigue compression loaded while wedged in flexion and lateral flexion. These fissures occurred as a result of creep deformation of the lamellae and they appeared on the side away from the component of lateral flexion. In clinical practice, the significance of these distortions is that it is feasible that they may give rise to symptoms if they affect the outer, innervated part of the annulus.

Once a radial fissure has formed, it creates a pathway down which nuclear material could track in certain circumstances. Prolapse and extrusion do not inevitably follow because of this, but distortion of the lamellae in this manner has been demonstrated as the early stages of a gradual disc prolapse (Fig. 9.7) (Adams and Hutton, 1985).

Once fragmentation and disruption of the disc has commenced, the nucleus and its retaining annulus become less capable of transmitting axial forces. A far greater proportion of these forces are, therefore, transmitted vertically to the end plates of the subjacent vertebra/e.

Anterior

Posterior

Fig. 9.7 Distortion of annular lamellae on repeated flexion. Repeated flexion combined with lateral flexion cause the lamellae to become more distorted in the contralateral corner of the disc. (Adapted from M.A. Adams and W.C. Hutton, 1985. Gradual disc prolapse. *Spine*, **10**, 6, 530.)

Disc Prolapse

A disc prolapse involves the displacement of nuclear material. It is most common between the age of 30–50, after which the nuclei have become more fibrotic and are less likely to be expressed as a semifluid substance. Both mechanical overload and biochemical degenerative changes are involved in its mechanics.

A prolapse can either be:

1. An annular protrusion (*see* Fig. 9.6c, p. 279) – when displaced nuclear material stretches the outer annulus, causing it to bulge outwards; the annulus is not completely ruptured.
2. A nuclear extrusion (*see* Fig. 9.6d) – when pulp escapes from the disc through a ruptured annulus.

The term 'disc herniation' is sometimes used when expelled nuclear material rests in a defect in the peripheral annulus and only partially protrudes into the vertebral canal.

Several different mechanisms may be responsible for the disc prolapsing.

1. *Gradual prolapse*

This is probably the most common cause of prolapse. The injury starts with the annular lamellae being distorted to form radial fissures. Nuclear pulp then breaks through the distorted lamellae causing the outermost lamellae, and the adhering posterior longitudinal ligament, to protrude. In the final stage, the pulp either extrudes from the mouth of the fissure or migrates behind the final barrier and emerges somewhere else.

Because of the insidious nature of events leading up to the prolapse, the 'final straw' which gives rise to the patient's signs and symptoms may be caused by a somewhat trivial event, such as picking up a pencil from the floor.

Experiments simulating what happens in life have been carried out on cadaveric lumbar discs (Adams and Hutton, 1985). These discs were fatigue-loaded in compression and flexion and underwent the trauma described above. The results suggested that prolapses could occur gradually over days or even months. Not all of the discs tested prolapsed, only those that had a soft, pulpy nucleus and a posterior annulus that was much thinner than the anterior annulus. In effect, this meant young discs at the L5/S1 and L4/5 levels. Upper lumbar discs, where the posterior annulus tends to be thicker and stronger, rarely prolapsed. Tests on older discs with pre-existing ruptures failed to demonstrate leakage of nuclear pulp. This is probably because the nucleus in these discs consists of fibrous lumps which are too large to track down a fissure, rendering them more stable.

Activities in life which could lead to a gradual disc prolapse are those involving repetitive bending and lifting, not necessarily in the fully flexed position or with maximal loads. This type of prolapse is often preceded by bouts of pain in the lumbar region which the patient passes off as 'muscular'. It is possible that one of the causes of this symptomatology is distortion of the outer annular fibres which are innervated.

2. *Sudden prolapse*

Discs can also prolapse suddenly if loading of sufficient intensity is involved, especially in flexed postures. A typical example is of a patient who describes having bent down to lift a heavy weight some distance away from his body such as a battery from a car.

This type of prolapse has been produced in the laboratory on cadaveric lumbar discs (Adams and Hutton, 1982), when they were wedged to simulate hyperflexion and lateral flexion, and compressed to a maximum that represented the likely compressive force generated by heaving lifting. Hyperflexion is flexion beyond the normal limit: about 1–6° of hyperflexion was required to produce the prolapses. The nucleus either extruded posterocentrally or on the opposite side to the component of lateral flexion where the annulus was stretched the most. The fissure through which the nuclear pulp was extruded usually occurred at the boundary between the annulus and the cartilage end plate. When the extrusion was large and central, it ruptured the posterior longitudinal ligament, whereas when they were smaller, the extrusions either formed a bulge behind the ligament (giving the impression of a bulging annulus) or were deflected sideways and appeared on one or both posterolateral margins of the disc. Adams and Hutton described their unsuccessful attempts at pushing extruded material back into the disc as 'like trying to push toothpaste back into the tube'. It was shown that the susceptibility of discs to this type of prolapse depended on age, degree of disc degeneration and spinal level. Those which were most vulnerable belonged to the 39–51 age group, had moderate degrees of disc degeneration, and were from the lower two lumbar levels.

The sudden prolapse is quite distinct from the gradual prolapse. However, a sudden prolapse can, of course, occur to a disc which is already in the various stages of a gradual prolapse.

In life, the mechanism of a sudden prolapse undoubtedly varies depending on factors such as the individual's particular anatomical structure, the position of the spine when the trauma occurs and the external forces involved. Hyperflexion of the lumbar discs can occur if the posterior ligaments are first overstretched. This does not necessarily entail high angles of flexion if, for example, the intervertebral joint is stiff. Because of the viscoelastic nature of the posterior ligaments, any prolonged period in the flexed posture will produce creep in the muscles and ligaments, and increase the normal range of flexion. The supra/interspinous ligament is usually found to be ruptured or slack in patients presenting for surgery for prolapsed disc (Newman, 1952; Rissanen, 1960) suggesting that this may be a precursor of disc injury by permitting an unacceptable degree of segmental flexion. Also, if flexion is performed quickly or is not adequately under muscular control, a joint sprain could result (Adams and Hutton, 1982).

When an individual bends to lift a weight at some distance from the body, the following series of events can be postulated. The posterior annular fibres are stretched and thinned and become the 'weak link' of the intervertebral joint. If the lumbar spine is also laterally flexed, there is further stress on the posterolateral annular fibres on the side away from this component. If the weight is heavy, the lumbar spine flexes further before the lift is executed (*see* p. 304). The force required to balance and lift the weight may be considerable, and the spinal muscles contract, compressing the vertebral column and raising the hydrostatic pressure in the nucleus. When the lumbar spine is in this position of hyperflexion combined with lateral flexion, only a moderately high compressive force is necessary to produce nuclear extrusion or annular protrusion (Adams and Hutton, 1982). The addition of rotation to flexion raises the existing level of intradiscal pressure.

Cervical disc prolapses undoubtedly differ from those which occur in the lumbar region. The cervical nucleus pulposus constitutes about 15% of the volume of a disc (Bull, 1948), and the maximum volume of nucleus which could be extruded would, if spherical, be 0.7 cm in diameter. Seldom, therefore, is the protrusion of the nucleus alone sufficient to cause compression of the spinal cord, although a lateral protrusion can easily compress the segmental nerve root. In older people, in addition to the protrusion of the nucleus, there is often osteophyte formation with or without root-sleeve fibrosis.

Effects of Compression

When the vertebral column is stressed to failure by vertical compression tests, the site of failure depends on anatomical variations and age. For example, in a middle-aged adult, a compression force may produce a wedge fracture of the vertebral body, depending on its mineral content. The same force applied to the spine of an adolescent or healthy young adult would produce vertical extrusions of the nucleus through the cartilage end plate into the vertebral bodies forming Schmorl's nodes or intravertebral disc prolapses (*see* pp. 266–7) (Porter, 1986).

Healing Process

In order for healing to occur following trauma or degeneration of an intervertebral disc, a good blood supply is necessary. The very outermost layers of a normal disc are penetrated by blood vessels and so, theoretically at least, circumferential tears could have a chance to heal. Following trauma or as a natural process of ageing, blood vessels penetrating the end plates and annulus, and fresh granulation tissue invading the nucleus, have been seen at surgery (Haley and Perry, 1950) and they provide evidence of a healing process. Initial healing by scar formation may have sufficiently different characteristics to produce a change in the mechanical behaviour of the annulus. Insufficient evidence exists of the rate of turnover of collagen in human beings, but experiments done on dogs suggest that it is likely to be extremely slow.

Following disruption of the annular fibres, the disc does not continue to leak nuclear pulp indefinitely. It has been suggested that in some patients nucleus regeneration could lead to recurrent prolapse, which may correlate with the frequent occurrence in young people of sciatica without neurological deficit (Adams and Hutton, 1985).

Sequestration

Once a mass of nuclear material has been extruded from the disc, it may become detached or sequestrated (*see* Fig. 9.6e, p. 279). Outside the confines of the retaining annulus, the nuclear material first swells and then later shrinks. The sequestrated fragment may migrate some distance from its origin, for example along a nerve root.

Compression of Neural Tissue

One of the most serious consequences of degenerative change is when neural tissue is impinged upon (1) the spinal cord or cauda equina in the spinal canal or (2) the nerve roots in the radicular canals or intervertebral foramina.

Nerve root compression

The nerve roots can be compressed along their course through the spinal canal, radicular canals, or in the intervertebral foramina. The most common cause of nerve root compression in the lumbar spine is the disc, either from bulging or from an extruded mass of nuclear material. However, the disc is by no means the only cause. Frequently, in the older spine, other culprits may be osteophytes from an apophyseal joint (*see* Fig. 9.2, p. 270), which may be combined with subluxation, a hypertrophied ligamentum flavum, an enlarged pedicle, spondylolisthesis, spinal stenosis or other pathological lesions. It is not unusual for more than one of these factors to be responsible.

Compression of a nerve root does not result in clinical signs and symptoms *per se*, as a normal nerve is able to tolerate a certain amount of deformation, especially if the process is slow, such as the growth of an osteophyte. However, it does make the root more vulnerable to trauma. If signs and symptoms do arise, they depend on which particular tissue is causing the trauma. For example, extension of the lumbar spine often relieves pain when the pathology points to an early disc lesion, but may aggravate that caused by pressure from osteophytes from an apophyseal joint.

It is doubtful that compression alone is responsible for the symptoms that follow nerve root lesions. While compression of motor fibres causes weakness or sometimes paralysis of the muscles they supply, and compression of sensory fibres causes paraesthesia and numbness in the appropriate dermatome, how it causes radicular or 'root' pain remains in dispute. Simple compression of a normal nerve root does not cause pain, just as compression of the common peroneal nerve round the head of the fibula by a too tightly fitting plaster may cause weakness in the foot, but does not give rise to pain. Some other factor is clearly responsible. Inflammation is one possibility. At surgery for a recently prolapsed intervertebral disc, the nerve root is often found to be inflamed. Repeated trauma to a nerve root rendering it fibrotic and ischaemic may result in pain when it is stretched. Vascular oedema has also been implicated in causing pressure additional to that caused by the lesion (Murphy, 1977). When a nerve root is compressed, the radicular veins which are intimately related to it are also obstructed and the resulting oedema may interfere with nerve conduction. The probability of stretching of the nerve root by a protruding disc causing sciatic pain is postulated by Farfan (1973).

Chronic inflammation with reactive fibrosis caused by repeated trauma can result in ischaemia of the nerve root. Instead of appearing red and swollen, as in acute inflammation, the nerve root now appears white and tight, and with its meninges may be embedded in fibrous tissue forming adhesions which tether the root, restricting its extensibility or mobility. In this condition of nerve root fibrosis, the nerve root and its meninges are unable to adapt freely to spinal and limb movements – in particular spinal flexion and lateral flexion (*see* p. 247) – performed passively or actively, and there may be a considerable increase in tension resulting in pain and producing at least temporary changes in the motor, sensory and autonomic function. The proximal parts of the spinal nerves themselves may also be affected by fibrotic adhesions.

Spinal cord compression

Where the spinal canal is large, the likelihood of cord compression is very much reduced. In the cervical region, the average sagittal diameter of the spinal canal is 17 mm, and in this region the average anteroposterior diameter of the cord is 10 mm. Therefore, in the average individual, gross changes in the cervical spine need to be present before cord compression is likely. Narrowing of the canal (central stenosis) through a developmental anomaly (*see* p. 267) renders the individual more likely to suffer the consequences of degenerative encroachment. In patients with myelopathy due to cervical spondylosis, the average measurement of the canal was found to be 14 mm – that is about 3 mm less than the average (Payne and Spillane, 1957).

The nucleus in the cervical spine is much smaller and nuclear protrusion alone is seldom sufficient to cause compression of the spinal cord. When this does occur, it is usually caused by a combination of osteophytes and ruptured disc.

Narrowing of the lumbar spinal canal acquired through degenerative trespass is mainly caused by osteophytic enlargement of the two inferior facets (Kirkaldy-Willis, 1988). Other causes include a prolapsed disc, lipping of the posterior aspect of the vertebral bodies, a thickened ligamentum flavum or thickening of the neural arches. Several levels may be affected. The decisive factor in the production of signs and symptoms is the available space, i.e. the relationship between the size of the canal and its contents. The cauda equina and its blood vessels are often compromised to a greater extent than individual spinal nerves.

CHANGES IN THE SYNOVIAL JOINTS

Apophyseal joints (see Figs. 9.2a; 9.5c, pp. 270, 274)

The apophyseal joints exhibit all the gross anatomical features of synovial joints elsewhere in the body, and may undergo degenerative changes characteristic of arthrosis. Although rare under the age of 30, the incidence increases with advancing age. Degenerative changes in the apophyseal joints may be primary and have been reported in the absence of disc degeneration or deformity (Lewin, 1964), but they are more commonly secondary to these factors.

Incidence of arthrosis. In the cervical spine, the incidence is highest in the upper segments, especially in the median atlanto-axial joint (Von Torklus and Gehle, 1972). Even in the presence of marked spondylosis in the lower cervical spine, the apophyseal joints here are often spared.

In the thoracic spine, the two levels showing the highest incidence of apophyseal joint arthrosis are C7/T1 and T4/5 (Shore, 1935).

In the lumbar spine, the incidence of arthrosis varies according to age (Lewin, 1964). Below the age of 45, early arthrosis is more common in the upper two lumbar segments, while after this age, the lower lumbar segments are more frequently affected.

Sustained lordotic postures such as erect standing can result in high stresses on the tips of the lumbar facets by causing them to make contact with the laminae of the subjacent vertebrae. When the lumbar spine is extended by two degrees per motion segment, as in erect standing, the apophyseal joints resist most of the shear force acting on the spine (Hutton et al., 1977) as well as about 16% of the compressive force increasing with more extension (Adams and Hutton, 1980). Prolonged pressure depresses the nutrition of the articular cartilage and chronic overloading may well cause arthrosis in these joints. Weak abdominal musculature predisposing to hyperextension could be a contributory factor in overloading the joints.

Acute injury or sprain of an apophyseal joint produces synovial effusion, histamine release, stretching or tearing of the capsule and ligaments, and bleeding. This limits the movements which are possible in the joint. With minor injuries, normal movement may be restored, but with more severe injuries some residual limitation of movement may persist.

With repetitive stresses over the years, a chronic synovial reaction becomes established and a synovial fold may project into the joint between its articular surfaces. The surface of the articular cartilage undergoes fibrillation, and becomes frayed and softened. Fragments of cartilage may break off, forming loose bodies which can lie freely in the joint or become attached to the synovial membrane. Thinning and stiffening of the subchondral bone in middle age causes a reduction in its energy-absorbing capacity, which may hasten the changes in the articular cartilage.

Later the capsule becomes lax, allowing subluxation of the joint surfaces to occur. Stresses in the capsule and periosteum result in marginal osteophytes which may encroach on the spinal canal or intervertebral foramina. Thickening or hypertrophy of the laminae may develop, which is more pronounced in the lumbar spine.

In the final stages of degeneration, there is erosion of articular cartilage from the surface with exposure of the underlying bone. Fat pads, which are mainly fibrous in the young, increase in size and become more fatty with age, acting as padding beneath the bony spurs to help to attenuate forces developed at the extremes of movement. Simultaneously, changes in the capsule occur; the dorsal capsule thickens and often areas of cartilage develop within its substance. Intra-articular adhesions passing from one articular surface to the other are not uncommon, and can vary from a single filmy strand to a dense mat, precluding all movements.

Joints of Luschka

The joints of Luschka are subject to lesions which are common to all synovial joints. Because of their close relationship to the intervertebral discs, they tend to share in the interbody joint changes. Loss of disc height increases the contact between the uncinate processes until, eventually, they are forced apart and become everted.

The effect of shearing on these joints, especially during the considerable flexion/extension movements, renders them susceptible to degenerative change, with the consequent thickening of the capsule by fibrosis and the formation of osteophytes, which may cause trespass on the nerve root and the vertebral artery. Osteophytes from the joints of Luschka may be more implicated in nerve root symptoms than those from the apophyseal joints (Boreadis and Gershon-Cohen, 1956).

Costovertebral and costotransverse joints

Studies on these joints have been relatively few, but it appears that arthrosis is on the whole less commonly found in them than in the other synovial joints in the spine. This may be related to the fact that slight movement occurs in them all the time during breathing. One study of costovertebral joints done on skeletons (Nathan *et al.*, 1964) showed an incidence of 48%, with peaks at T1, T6/7/8 and T11/12, the inferior hemifacets being affected more than the superior hemifacets.

Combined Degenerative Changes in the Spine

Degenerative changes may predominantly affect the disc in some patients, while in others they mainly affect the apophyseal joints. There is some degree of independence in these changes, at least in the initial stages. Different levels of the spine show a predisposition to either spondylosis or arthrosis. Commonly, however, the whole motion segment is eventually affected, and changes in the disc interact with those in the joints of Luschka, as well as in the apophyseal joints, albeit in varying degrees.

Loss of disc height leading to a shortening in the length of the spinal column imposes unusual mechanical strains on the synovial joints. In some patients, the apophyseal joints may be virtually 'remade' (Farfan, 1973), new articulations forming on the articular processes where there is overlap of the true facet. These new articulations are largely osteophytic, with no true articular cartilage. In severe cases of degeneration and loss of disc height, the facets may resist up to 70% of the compressive force on the spine (Adams and Hutton, 1983). Much of this abnormally high resistance is due to extra-articular impingement of the facet tips on the adjacent lamina or pedicle (*see* Fig. 9.5b, p. 274) (Dunlop *et al.*, 1984).

Shortening of the spinal column also has a marked effect on the soft tissues. Bulging of the ligamenta flava into the spinal cord causing compression on the spinal cord is seen in severe cases of degeneration. Because of its attachment to the entire undersurface of the superior lamina, but only to the upper edge of the inferior lamina, the ligament cannot bulge posteriorly away from the spinal canal. During extension movements, the upper edge of the lower lamina forces the intervening ligamenta flava downward into the spinal canal. Hypertrophy of a ligamentum flavum may occur as a response to stiffness in adjacent motion segments.

Narrowing of an intervertebral foramen (*see* Fig. 5.7, p. 176), and consequent compression of its nerve root and other contents, can be caused by many factors such as reduced disc height, a bulging or prolapsed disc, subluxation of posterior facets, a retrospondylolisthesis (backward slip) of the upper on the lower vertebra, or osteophytes projecting from the vertebral body or the apophyseal joints. Diminution of the transverse diameter of the foramen rather than its vertical diameter is more likely to affect the foramen's contents.

Distortion of the vertebral artery can occur through shortening of the vertebral column and may exacerbate the degenerative changes in the joints, or it can be displaced laterally by spondylotic changes in the vertebrae. The degree of displacement depends on the size and position of the bony prominences which arise as a result of spondylotic changes and the displacement of the artery may vary from a gentle curve to a marked distortion. Obstruction of one or other vertebral arteries may occur during movements of the cervical spine, especially rotation and extension of the head (*see* p. 152). Atheroma of the vertebral artery may also be an important factor in the production of symptoms. If the vertebral artery with the larger lumen is affected (*see* pp. 148; 153), the effects are likely to be more serious than if the smaller one is affected.

Movements become increasingly restricted and this can vary from loss of normal accessory movement to considerably reduced physiological movement. Stiffness at one level imposes strains on adjacent levels, as can be seen following fusion of one segment. A degenerative lesion previously confined to one level can later spread to involve several levels (Kirkaldy-Willis, 1988).

Stenosis of the spinal canal may occur at one or several levels. Frequently some degree of scoliosis with a rotational element is present.

Instability

Abnormal increased movement of an intervertebral joint may occur in severe disc degeneration accompanied by capsular laxity in the apophyseal joints and lack of effective muscular control. It most commonly occurs in the lumbar spine. These abnormal movements of the disc pull on the outermost annular fibres causing a spur of bone – the so-called traction spur – to develop about 1 mm away from the discal border of the vertebral body. The traction spur differs from the claw-type osteophyte which develops at the edge of the vertebral body and curves over the outer fibres of the intervertebral disc (Macnab, 1977 – *see* Fig. 9.8). The presence of a traction spur indicates that the interbody joint is, or has been at some time, unstable. Real instability should not be confused with hypermobility due to excessive laxity of ligaments, where the range of movement exceeds the normal, but is under muscular control.

When subjected to torsion, the affected disc may have increased lateral translation (2.5–10.2 mm). Another manifestation of instability is increased forward translation of a vertebra on the one below on flexion, and increased backward translation on extension. The inter-

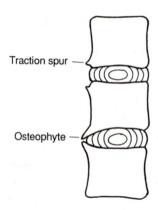

Traction spur —

Osteophyte —

Fig. 9.8 Difference between osteophyte and traction spur. (After Macnab, 1977.)

vertebral joint's ability to withstand the normal strains of movement is reduced; consequently, more stress falls on the ligamentous and joint structures. Not all degenerated joints go through this unstable phase, and it is sometimes temporary as the stiffening that eventually occurs with degeneration tends to stabilize the motion segment. Forced manipulation of joints with instability will increase the instability and it is, therefore, contraindicated. It is sometimes difficult to assess the degree and direction of abnormal movement from X-rays due to the fact that in many individuals pure movements are not possible (Farfan, 1973); also, if the paravertebral muscles are in spasm when the X-ray is taken, the movements possible will be limited.

REFERENCES

Aaron J.E., Makins N.B., Sagreiya K. (1987). The histology and microanatomy of trabecular bone loss in normal ageing men and women. *Clin. Orthop. Relat. Res.,* **215**, 260.

Adams M.A. (1980). The mechanical properties of lumbar intervertebral joints with special reference to the causes of low back pain (PhD Thesis). London: Polytechnic of Central London.

Adams M.A., Hutton W.C. (1980). The effect of posture on the role of the apophyseal joints in resisting intervertebral compressive force. *J. Bone Jt. Surg.,* **62B**, 358.

Adams M.A., Hutton W.C. (1981). The relevance of torsion to the mechanical derangement of the lumbar spine. *Spine,* **6**, 3, 241.

Adams M.A., Hutton W.C. (1982). Prolapsed intervertebral disc. A hyperflexion injury. *Spine,* **7**, 3, 184.

Adams M.A., Hutton W.C. (1983). The mechanical function of the lumbar apophyseal joints. *Spine,* **8**, 3, 327.

Adams M.A., Hutton W.C. (1985). Gradual disc prolapse. *Spine,* **10**, 6, 524.

Andersson G.B.J. (1983). The biomechanics of the posterior elements of the lumbar spine. *Spine,* **8**, 3, 326.

Bagnall K.M., Harris P.F., Jones P.R.M. (1984). A radiographic study of variations of the human fetal spine. *Anat. Rec.,* **208**, 265.

Bernick S., Cailliet R. (1982). Vertebral end-plate changes with aging of human vertebrae. *Spine*, **7**, 97.

Bogduk N., Twomey L.T. (1987). *Clinical Anatomy of the Lumbar Spine*. Edinburgh: Churchill Livingstone.

Boreadis A.G., Gershon-Cohen J. (1956). Luschka joints of the cervical spine. *Radiology*, **66**, 181.

Bradford D.S., Hensinger R.M., eds. (1985). *The Pediatric Spine*. New York: Thieme.

Brain, Lord, Wilkinson M. (1967). *Cervical Spondylosis*. London: William Heinemann Medical Books.

Brown T., Hansen R.J., Yorra A.J. (1957). Some mechanical tests on the lumbosacral spine with particular reference to the intervertebral discs. *J. Bone Jt. Surg.*, **39A**, 1135.

Bull J.W.D. (1948). Section of neurology. Discussion on rupture of the intervertebral disc in the cervical region. *Proc. R. Soc. Med.*, **41**, 513.

Bull J.W.D. (1951). *Modern Trends in Neurology*. (Feiling A., ed.) London: Butterworth.

Carpenter E.B. (1961). Normal and abnormal growth of the spine. *Clin. Orthop.*, **21**, 49.

Cyron B.M., Hutton W.C. (1980). Articular tropism and stability of the lumbar spine. *Spine*, **5**, 2, 168.

Dunlop R.B., Adams M.A., Hutton W.C. (1984). Disc space narrowing and the lumbar facet joints. *J. Bone Jt. Surg.*, **66-B**, 5, 706.

Eckert G., Decker A. (1947). Pathological studies of the intervertebral discs. *J. Bone Jt. Surg.*, **29**, 477.

Exton-Smith A.N. (1983). Metabolic Bone Disease. In *Bone and Joint Disease in the Elderly*. (Wright V., ed.) Edinburgh: Churchill Livingstone, pp. 150–166.

Farfan H.F. (1973). *Mechanical Disorders of the Low Back*. Philadelphia: Lea and Febiger.

Farfan H.F., Sullivan J.D. (1967). The relation of facet orientation to intervertebral disc failure. *Can. J. Surg.*, **10**, 179.

Farfan H.F., Cossette J.W., Robertson G.H. *et al.* (1970). The effects of torsion on the lumbar intervertebral joints: the role of torsion in the production of disc degeneration. *J. Bone Jt. Surg.*, **52-A**, 468.

Francis R.M., Peacock M. (1987). The local action of oral 1, 25 (OH)$_2$ Vitamin D3 on calcium absorption in osteoporosis. *Am. J. Clin. Nutr.*, **46**, 315.

Grieve G.P. (1981). *Common Vertebral Joint Problems*. Edinburgh: Churchill Livingstone.

Grieve G.P. (1989). *Common Vertebral Joint Problems*, 2nd edn. Edinburgh: Churchill Livingstone, p. 426.

Haley J.C., Perry J.H. (1950). Protrusions of intervertebral discs: study of their distribution, characteristics and effects on the nervous system. *Am. J. Surg.*, **80**, 394.

Happey F. (1976). A biophysical study of the human intervertebral disc. In *The Lumbar Spine and Back Pain*. (Jayson M.I.V., ed.) New York: Grune & Stratton, pp. 293–316.

Hickey D.S., Hukins D.W.L. (1980). Relation between the structure of the annulus fibrosus and the function and failure of the intervertebral disc. *Spine*, **5**, 2, 106.

Hilton R.C., Ball J., Benn B.T. (1976). Vertebral end-plate lesions (Schmorl's nodes) in the dorsolumbar spine. *Ann. Rheum. Dis.*, **35**, 127.

Hutton W.C., Stott J.R.R., Cyron B.M. (1977). Is spondylolysis a fatigue fracture? *Spine*, **2**, 202.

James J.I.P. (1976). *Scoliosis*, 2nd edn. Edinburgh: Churchill Livingstone.

Jeffreys E. (1980). *Disorders of the Cervical Spine.* London: Butterworth.

Kirkaldy-Willis W.H. (1988). *Managing Low Back Pain*, 2nd edn. Edinburgh: Churchill Livingstone.

Lewin T. (1964). *Osteoarthrosis in Lumbar Synovial Joints.* Gothenburg: Orstadius Bokryckeri Aktiebolag.

Macnab I. (1977). *Backache.* Baltimore: Williams & Wilkins, p. 4.

McMaster M.J., David C.V. (1986). Hemivertebrae as a cause of scoliosis. *J. Bone Jt. Surg.*, **68B**, 588.

McRae D.L. (1953). Bony abnormalities in the region of the foramen magnum: correlation of the anatomic and neurologic findings. *Acta Radiol.*, **40**, 335.

Mixter W.J. (1951). *Modern Trends in Neurology.* (Feiling A., ed.) London: Butterworth.

Murphy R.W. (1977). Nerve roots and spinal nerves in degenerative disk disease. *Clin. Orthop.*, **129**, 46.

Nathan H. (1962). Osteophytes of the vertebral column. *J. Bone Jt. Surg.*, **44-A**, 2, 243.

Nathan H., Weinberg H., Robin G.C. *et al.* (1964). The costovertebral joints: anatomico-clinical observations in arthritis. *Arth. Rheum.*, **7**, 228.

Newman P.H. (1952). Sprung back. *J. Bone Jt. Surg.*, **34B**, 30.

Odgers P.N.B. (1933). The lumbar and lumbosacral diarthrodial joints. *J. Anat.*, **67**, 301.

Payne E.E., Spillane J.D. (1957). The cervical spine. An anatomico-pathological study of 70 specimens (using a special technique) with particular reference to the problem of spondylosis. *Brain*, **80**, 571.

Peacock A. (1951). Observations on the prenatal development of the intervertebral disc in man. *J. Anat.*, **85**, 260.

Porter R.W. (1986). *Management of Back Pain.* Edinburgh: Churchill Livingstone.

Postacchini F., Lami R., Pugliese O. (1988). Familial predisposition to discogenic low-back pain. An epidemiologic and immunogenetic study. *Spine*, **13**, 12, 1403.

Rissanen P.M. (1960). The surgical anatomy and pathology of the supraspinous and interspinous ligaments of the lumbar spine with special reference to ligament ruptures. *Acta Orthop. Scand.* (Suppl), **46**.

Roaf R. (1960). A study of the mechanics of spinal injuries. *J. Bone Jt. Surg.*, **42B**, 4, 810.

Schmorl G., Junghanns H. (1971). *The Human Spine in Health and Disease*, 2nd edn. (USA). New York: Grune & Stratton, p. 55.

Shore L.R. (1935). On osteoarthritis in the dorsal intervertebral joints. *Br. J. Surg.*, **22**, 833.

Singh S. (1965). Variations of the superior articular facets of atlas vertebrae. *J. Anat.*, **99**, 565.

Spillane J.D., Pallis C., Jones A.M. (1957). Developmental abnormalities in the region of the foramen magnum. *Brain*, **80**, 11.

Taylor J.R. (1983). Scoliosis screening in the Kimberleys. *Med. J. Aust.*, **1**, 352.

Taylor J.R., Twomey L.T. (1984). The role of the notochord and blood vessels in vertebral column development and in the aetiology of Schmorl's nodes. In *Manual Therapy, 1, The Vertebral Column.* (Grieve G.P., ed.) Edinburgh: Churchill Livingstone.

Tredwell S.J., Smith D.F., Macleod P.J. *et al.* (1982). Cervical spine anomalies in fetal alcohol syndrome. *Spine*, **7**, 331.

Twomey L., Taylor J. (1985). Age changes in lumbar intervertebral discs. *Acta Orthop. Scand.*, **56**, 496.

Urban J., Maroudas A. (1980). The chemistry of the intervertebral disc in relation to its physiological function and requirements. *Clin. Rheum. Dis.*, **6**, 1.

Verbout A.J. (1985). The development of the vertebral column. *Adv. Anat. Embryol. Cell. Biol.*, 90.

Von Torklus D., Gehle W. (1972). *The Upper Cervical Spine.* London: Butterworth, p. 21.

Williams P.L., Warwick R., eds. (1980). *Gray's Anatomy*, 36th edn. Edinburgh: Churchill Livingstone.

Winter R.B., Moe J.H., Lonstein J.E. (1984). The incidence of Klippel-Feil syndrome in patients with congenital scoliosis and kyphosis. *Spine*, **9**, 363.

FURTHER READING

Scoles P.V., Latimer B.M., DiGiovanni B.F. *et al.* (1991). Vertebral alterations in Scheuermann's kyphosis. *Spine*, **16**, 5, 509.

10

Posture

Posture is the position assumed by the body either by means of the integrated action of muscles working to counteract the force of gravity, or when supported during muscular inactivity. Many postures are, of course, assumed during the course of 24 hours, but only those that are most frequently used are considered in this chapter.

In addition to the *intrinsic* mechanisms which influence posture, principally the muscular system, *extrinsic* factors such as the supporting surface have to be considered, as their construction plays a very important part in influencing spinal postures, which may aggravate or relieve symptoms arising from spinal pathology.

CONTROL OF POSTURE

Postures are maintained or adapted as a result of neuromuscular coordination, the appropriate muscles being innervated by means of a complex reflex mechanism. Afferent stimuli arise from a variety of sources all over the body, including the joints, ligaments, muscles, skin, the eyes and ears, and are conveyed and coordinated in the central nervous system. The efferent response is a motor one, the antigravity muscles being the principal effector organs.

The apophyseal joints in the upper cervical region have a particularly abundant supply of these receptors, and degeneration in these joints and soft tissues can lead to alterations in the discharge of afferent impulses and disturbances in the perception of posture and balance. The importance of the correct head/neck relationship on the posture of the whole spine has been highlighted by Alexander (1932).

While it is accepted that the bony structure in individuals may vary, it is less obvious that the amount of muscle activity used when performing identical tasks may also vary, and this could account for the apparent contradictions shown in different studies of muscle activity. Although some people may be able to sit comfortably and relax in many positions without a large increase in muscular activity, people who are tense show a pronounced increase in muscular activity in various postures and when performing tasks, and do not relax completely in more than a few positions (Lundervold, 1951). When the spinal muscles contract, they have a compressive effect on the intervertebral discs; consequently, muscular contractions in excess of normal requirements may well have a detrimental effect on nutrition of the discs, as this is dependent on imbibition of fluid, which occurs when the compression is reduced.

LYING POSITION

The lowest levels of back muscle activity and intradiscal pressure (see Fig. 2.8, p. 68) are found in the lying position. Patients with some (though not all) types of intervertebral disc pathology obtain relief from pain in this position. The position that the spine normally assumes varies according to several factors, such as the resilience of the surface, the build of the individual and the position of the limbs.

For example, if the surface is soft, this encourages the spine to flex more when lying supine, or extend more when lying prone, than it would on a firmer surface. Prone-lying is a position not easily tolerated by people with stiff spines or who have symptoms arising from degenerated apophyseal joints, usually because either the neck is in full rotation or the lumbar spine is at the end of its extension range; the apophyseal joints are under stress in both cases.

The build of the individual when lying on the side influences the degree of lateral flexion in the spine, e.g. a woman with a wide pelvis would tend to flex the lumbar spine laterally more than a man with a narrower one.

The position of the limbs influences spinal posture in a similar manner to that described for the sitting position (see p. 300).

STANDING POSITION

The idealized normal erect posture is one in which the line of gravity is reputed to fall in the midline between the following bilateral points:

1. The mastoid processes;
2. A point just in front of the shoulder joints;
3. The hip joints (or just behind);
4. A point just in front of the centre of the knee joints and
5. A point just in front of the ankle joints (Basmajian, 1978).

In quiet standing, assuming that the curvatures of the spine are in correct alignment, surprisingly little muscular activity is required to maintain this position, slight or moderate activity being present for only 5% of the time (Soames and Atha, 1981). Yet man's so-called antigravity muscles are strong, not so much to maintain postures such as the upright position, but more to produce the powerful movements necessary for the major changes in posture.

Economical though it may be in terms of spinal muscular energy, the idealized erect posture is not often sustained for long periods, and people often resort to standing asymmetrically, using the right and left leg alternately as the main support. They may do this in order to cope with the inadequacies of the venous and arterial circulation, or because they find a reduced lordosis, with a consequent reduction in the compressive forces on the apophyseal joints (Adams and Hutton, 1980), more comfortable, even at the expense of increasing back muscle activity. Standing with the weight supported mainly by one leg, with the other leg relaxed, increases EMG activity at L5 on the side of the weight-bearing leg (Dolan *et al.*, 1988). If the curvatures are not in correct alignment due to disease, poor posture or through congenital abnormalities such as idiopathic scoliosis, far greater muscular activity over the affected area is then required to maintain the upright posture.

It used to be thought that, in the standing position, there was a fine balance between abdominal and erector spinae activity. However, it is now known that about three times as many people exhibit slight constant or intermittent activity in erector spinae only, rather than abdominal muscle activity (Floyd and Silver, 1951). This suggests that the centre of gravity is situated slightly *anterior* to the lumbosacral disc in a significant proportion of people.

In the standing position, the pelvic girdle is tilted forwards due to tension in the anterior thigh muscles, so that the angle between the upper surface of the sacrum and the horizontal is about 50–53° (Hellems and Keates, 1971). This tilt, and compression from body weight on the lumbar spine, accentuates the lumbar lordosis (*see* p. 37) (Fig. 10.1). It can be further increased by pregnancy, obesity or by wearing high-heeled shoes.

The apophyseal joints resist most of the *shear* force acting on the spine in the erect posture (Hutton *et al.*, 1977), as well as about 16% of the *compressive* force (Adams and Hutton, 1980). The resulting stress between the articular surfaces is concentrated in the lower margins of the joint (Dunlop *et al.*, 1984).

Intervertebral disc pressures are higher than in the lying position, but usually lower than in sitting (*see* Fig. 2.8, p. 68).

SITTING POSITION

There is an increasing tendency for people to spend long hours in the sitting position, both for work and leisure purposes. Many people suffering from backache find that this position aggravates their problem. The incidence of musculo-skeletal disorders in people with administrative jobs is higher than in some industrial sectors.

Postural problems can start at an early age and an increasing number of children seem to present clinically with backache, the main cause of which points to unsatisfactory seating in schools. Undoubt-

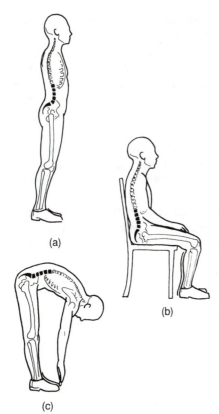

(a)

(b)

(c)

Fig. 10.1 The effects of standing, sitting and stooping on the lumbosacral curve. (a) the lumbar curve is accentuated in the standing position; (b) marked flattening of the lumbosacral curve occurs when the patient is sitting in an ordinary straight chair with trunk and thighs at a right angle; (c) note how similar is the flattened lumbar curve to that of (b). (From J.J. Keegan, 1953. Alterations of the lumbar curve related to posture and seating. *J. Bone Jt. Surg.*, **35-A**, 3, 590, with permission.)

edly, many more children suffer discomfort, but are not referred for treatment. Patterns of poor sitting posture, when started at such a young age, are difficult to improve later in life, and this emphasizes the need for chairs and tables that can be adjusted to the individual's requirements, coupled with postural education in schools.

It seems unlikely that back pain in people with predominantly sitting occupations would come from very high loads on the spine. Rather it would be reasonable to speculate that it is the static posture of sitting itself that is an important factor in back pain aggravation. People who change their positions, varying sitting with moving, have on the whole a low incidence of back pain (Magora, 1972). The reason for this may be because nutrition of the disc is dependent on movement and variation in posture. Prolonged overloading (or underloading) are factors leading to disc degeneration (Grieco, 1986). Any posture which results in sustained static muscle work induces fatigue. Therefore, when considering the optimal sitting position for a particular individual, the aim should be to reduce static muscle work to a minimum.

People's needs concerning seating vary according to the range of movement present in the spine, any pathological condition present and the requirements of the task being performed.

Intradiscal pressure is generally higher in the unsupported sitting position (*see* Fig. 2.8, p. 68) than in the standing position, largely due to psoas major, which is vigorously active as a stabilizer of the lumbar spine in this position and at the same time has a considerable compressive effect on the spine (Keagy *et al.*, 1966). Further increases or decreases in intradiscal pressure can be brought about by an alteration in either the lumbar lordosis or in the seat or backrest inclination, the lumbar support, and the chair and (if applicable) table height. In a well-designed chair, the intradiscal pressure can be lower than when standing.

The ideal sitting posture for most people is with the intervertebral joints somewhere in the *mid-range* (Fig. 10.2b), allowing freedom of movement, with balanced anterior and posterior muscles. In this

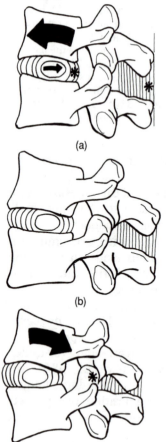

(a)

(b)

(c)

Fig. 10.2 Lumbar motion segments in different sitting positions. (a) flexion; (b) mid range; (c) extension. * = sites of stress.

position, the stress between the articular surfaces of the apophyseal joints is lower than in the standing position, and is concentrated in the middle and upper parts of the joint (Dunlop *et al.*, 1984). The joints resist the shear force, but play less part in resisting the intervertebral compressive force. However, even an 'ideal' sitting posture cannot be maintained for long periods, and it is important that the seat design permits changes in posture.

Deviating from the mid-range for *sustained* periods leads to stresses on joint and ligamentous structures. In a normal spine, sitting in a slumped posture can lead to overstretching of the posterior intervertebral ligaments and posterior annular fibres (Fig. 10.2a), and increases intradiscal pressure considerably. Myoelectric activity in the erectores spinae is nil in this posture (Floyd and Silver, 1955), which is one of the reasons why people tend to find it comfortable initially. Patients with spondylolisthesis or degenerative changes in their lumbar apophyseal joints none the less sometimes find that sitting with their lumbar spine in some degree of flexion gives them relief from pain. Sitting in *sustained hyperextension* tends to put more stress on the apophyseal joints (*see* Fig. 10.2c) and pars interarticularis.

Effect of pelvic and limb positions

The position of the head, shoulders and trunk is determined by the task to be done, especially in relation to the visual requirements.

For close work, such as reading or writing, the optimal distance for the work is approximately 30 cm from the eyes. As soon as the arms are moved forwards in front of the body, neck and shoulder muscle activity increases. In particular, a considerable increase in the activity levels of the upper thoracic and cervical spine extensors was found to be caused by arm abduction (Schuldt *et al.*, 1986), which tends to occur when working at a table which is too high.

Activities such as typing or operating a video display terminal do not impose high loads on the neck and shoulder muscles, but they cause sustained tension. This can lead to fatigue and pain, because the capacity for sustained static muscle load is very limited (Bjorksten and Jonsson, 1977). There are considerable differences in the levels of static activity in neck and shoulder muscles in different sitting postures. The slumped posture gives higher levels of activity than does the erect posture, but even lower activity levels than this have been found in subjects who sat with a slightly backward-inclined thoracolumbar spine with the cervical spine vertical, when performing light assembly work (Schuldt *et al.*, 1986). However, this position carries with it an increased risk of extreme flexion in the lower cervical spine, and if used, instruction should be given as to how to avoid extreme positions. Schuldt suggested that the backward inclination should be no more than 10–15°.

The position of the lumbar spine is also affected by the angulation of the pelvis, the position of the hips and, sometimes, the position of the knees.

When moving from a standing to an unsupported sitting position, as the hips move into flexion, tension in the hamstring and gluteal muscles rotate the pelvis backwards, taking with it the lumbar spine, which starts to flex. From X-ray examinations, Schoberth (1962) found that in the 'traditional' sitting posture, i.e. with the thighs at 90° to the trunk, this was divided on average into 60° of flexion in the hips, and 30° of flexion in the lumbar spine, 80–90% of which occurred at L4 and 5. There is a similarity between this position of the lumbar spine and bending forwards from the standing position (see Fig. 10.1 p. 297). It is not easy to maintain this 'traditional' sitting posture if the spine is unsupported, because the lumbar spine is so flexed that the tendency is for it to flex even more. Balance between the muscles anterior and posterior to the pelvis is achieved when the hip joint is in its neutral position of 45° of flexion; simultaneously, the lumbar spine assumes a neutral position which is easier to maintain.

Due to the hamstring muscles acting over both the hip and knee joint, the amount of knee extension may affect the position of the hips and, ultimately, the lumbar spine. When the knee is flexed to 90° or more, the lumbar mechanism is not very sensitive to small alterations in the position of the hip. However, it is extremely sensitive to any change in the hip flexion angle, if the knee is flexed to 70° or less (Brunswic, 1984), an increase in knee extension of 20° corresponding roughly to a 10° increase in hip flexion. This is significant for patients when the knee position is determined by, say, the location of pedals to operate machinery or drive a car, when knee flexion may vary between 10 and 70°, causing more flexion in the lumbar spine.

Intradiscal pressure increases as the lumbar lordosis decreases. Even higher pressures have been recorded when drivers change gear (Andersson et al., 1975). This is due to an increase in knee extension and, consequently, lumbar flexion when depressing the clutch pedal, coupled with movement of the leg against gravity, and possibly also additional trunk flexion with the movement of the arm.

Seat inclination

Spinal posture in the sitting position is also influenced by degree of seat inclination (Fig. 10.3). A seat which is inclined backwards encourages the lumbar spine to flex. In order to sit upright on a 5° backward-sloping seat, the lumbar spine will be flexed to 35°. If the individual is working at a desk on this type of seat, it tilts the body away from the working surface and, to position the eyes at a suitable distance from the work, he compensates for this by flexing the spine even more.

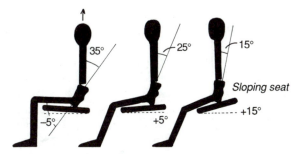

Fig. 10.3 The backward-sloping seat increases the flexion of the lumbar region. (From *Human Factors*, 1982, 24(3), 257–269, with permission of The Human Factors Society Inc.)

With increasing forward inclination of the seat, the lumbar spine moves into more extension. With a 5° forward slope, the individual can sit upright with only 25° lumbar flexion, and this can be reduced to 15° when the seat is tilted forwards 15° (Mandal, 1984). This type of seat also tilts the body closer to the working surface and is often preferred by patients who need to avoid over-flexing their spines.

Laboratory studies (Eklund and Corlett, 1987) have been carried out on workers performing an assembly task when sitting on seats with two different inclinations: a 'sit-stand' seat (i.e. with a forward inclination) and a conventional horizontal seat. The 'sit-stand' seat was found to cause substantially less loss of disc height (*see* pp. 76–7), there was a lower biomechanical load on it, less discomfort from the spine, and it encouraged a slightly less flexed spinal posture.

Backrest inclination and lumbar support (Figs. 10.4; 10.5)

A backrest is usually positioned at right angles to the horizontal or sloping backwards to varying degrees. When performing a task at a table or bench, the body weight is usually transferred forwards and the backrest is then not used. When sitting on a horizontal seat with the backrest inclined backwards, there is a decrease in myoelectric activity in the paravertebral muscles (Andersson *et al.*, 1979) because the need for them to stabilize the spine is less as it approaches the horizontal position. Correspondingly, there is a decrease in intradiscal pressure (*see* Fig. 10.4). This position is, of course, often sensibly chosen for relaxation.

A lumbar support was found to have a similar effect on myoelectric activity and intradiscal pressure when the body was inclined. Experimenting with lumbar supports ranging from -2 to $+4$ cm, the latter depth causing a lumbar lordosis which resembled that in the standing position, Andersson *et al.* (1979) found that there was a marked effect

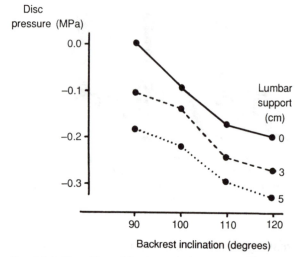

Fig. 10.4 The effect of backrest inclination and lumbar support on intradiscal pressure. (Adapted from A. Nachemson, 1976. The lumbar spine: an orthopaedic challenge. *Spine*, 1, 59–71.)

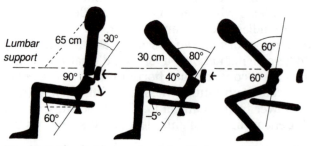

Fig. 10.5 The lumbar support is effective only when the seated person leans backward. (From *Human Factors*, 1982, 24(3), 257–269, with permission of The Human Factors Society Inc.)

on the amount of total lumbar extension, which changed from a mean of 9.7° to 46.8° as the lumbar support was increased.

Seat and table height

These need to be considered as a single unit. A seat which is too low for a particular individual will encourage a flexed sitting posture, especially when he is working at a desk. A table which is too low has the same effect. Mandal's experiments (1984) on the postures of Danish schoolchildren during a four-hour examination illustrate this clearly (Figs. 10.6; 10.7). He recommended that the chair height should be at least one-third of the individual's body height and the table at least half the body height.

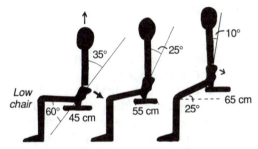

Fig. 10.6 The low chair increases the flexion of the lumbar region. (From *Human Factors*, 1982, **24(3)**, 257–269, with permission of The Human Factors Society Inc.)

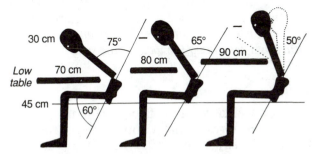

Fig. 10.7 The low table increases the flexion of the lumbar region. (From *Human Factors*, 1982, **24(3)**, 257–269, with permission of The Human Factors Society Inc.)

Arm rests

Supporting the arms on arm rests or a desk in front reduces both spinal muscular activity and intradiscal pressure, lower levels of both being recorded in writing than when typing (Andersson *et al.*, 1975).

LIFTING

The manual transport of loads is responsible for up to 30% of all industrial injuries (Hayne, 1981). It has been found that those most likely to sustain back injuries are the unprepared, unskilled, young people and those in their first year or so of a new job (Blow and Jackson, 1971; Magora, 1974). This finding highlights the importance of understanding the forces acting on the lumbar spine during lifting before giving instructions on the correct methods of lifting to uninjured workers, and following injury.

Load on the Spine in Lifting

Leverage

When the trunk moves in the sagittal plane, the intervertebral discs act as a series of fulcra of movement, the lumbosacral disc usually being referred to as the main fulcrum in the spine. The force exerted on it is the product of the weight to be lifted (which includes the weight of the trunk above the disc) and its distance from the fulcrum. The lever which has to balance and lift the weight is shorter, being provided by the back muscles. Therefore, the greater the distance of the weight from the body, in effect the heavier the weight becomes and the stronger the force required to lift it. As the weight is progressively brought closer to the body, the lever exerted by the lifted weight becomes shorter. In the initial stages of a lift, if the weight is a substantial distance from the body, the force required to lift it can be considerable. *This distance is significantly more important than the actual method of lifting in determining the load on the spine.*

Muscle activity

Prior to lifting a weight from the floor, the lumbar spine is lowered into flexion, the erectores spinae contracting eccentrically until a critical point is reached (*see* p. 130), when they become electrically silent. As flexion continues, the muscles sustain tension together with the thoracolumbar fascia and posterior ligaments. If the weight to be lifted is very heavy (over 68.4 kg), the lumbar spine is initially flexed further, when inertia has to be overcome and ground reaction forces are greatest (Fig. 10.8) (Frievalds *et al.*, 1984). The lift is then continued by the powerful hip and knee extensors, the activity of the erectores spinae being nil in the early stages. It is thought that the back muscles alone, even with maximal contraction, are unable to

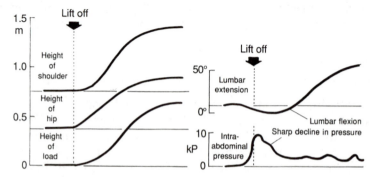

Fig. 10.8 Features of typical lift of heavy weight from floor to standing position, beginning with knees flexed. (Adapted from J.D.G. Troup, 1979. Biomechanics of the vertebral column. *Physiotherapy*, **65**, 8, 241.)

provide the power to raise the trunk at this stage and a combination of three 'back support mechanisms' come into play to enable the lift to be completed without injury to the spine (*see below*).

Later in the lift, when the back muscles do contract to extend the spine they also have a compressive effect on the vertebral column, which raises intradiscal pressure. The further away from the body the weight is, the greater is the amount of erector spinae activity required to lift it, and there is a proportionate increase in intradiscal pressure.

If a load is carried high on the back, the trunk automatically tends to lean slightly forward to prevent imbalance, causing increased activity in the lower back muscles. If, however, the load is placed low on the back, the activity of the back muscles is reduced (Carlsöö, 1964).

Sudden extra strains

A loaded spine does not have the same ability as an unloaded one to compensate for even a minor sudden extra strain (Hirsch, 1955). When not under pressure from carrying a weight, the intervertebral discs usually absorb strains, such as a fall, easily, since the demands on the elasticity of the disc are less in an individual bearing only the weight of his own body. If, on the other hand, the spine is under pressure (as in carrying a heavy weight), the disc is compressed closer to its elastic limit. A sudden extra strain such as can be caused by losing a grip on a bulky object which is difficult to hold, will cause additional compression, which may at its maximum amplitude exceed the elastic limits of the collagen system somewhere in the annulus, of the end plate, or of the attachment of the collagen to bone with the result that rupture may occur.

Back Support Mechanisms

A combination of the following mechanisms is considered to assist the back muscles in the initial phase of a lift.

1. *Intra-abdominal pressure*

Heavy weight lifting is always associated with a marked increase in intratruncal – that is, intra-abdominal and intrathoracic – pressure. This is usually brought about by a reflex contraction of the transversus abdominis muscles primarily (and, to a lesser extent, the oblique abdominal muscles), the muscles of the pelvic floor and the muscles of the larynx, which close the glottis. EMG studies have shown that the recti are inactive in lifting, avoiding additional flexion of the spine. The fluid contents in the abdominal and thoracic cavities are compressed, and this leads to a rise in pressure.

Bartelink (1957) first proposed the theory that this raised intra-abdominal pressure acted upwards on the diaphragm like a balloon (Fig. 10.9), separating the pelvis from the thoracic cage, and serving to lift or support the thorax, especially when the trunk is flexed, thereby supplementing the back muscles. Through this mechanism some of the compressive stress on the lumbar intervertebral discs may be relieved. The raised intrathoracic pressure acts to stabilize the rib cage during activities of the arms.

Pressure increases are greater when heavier loads are lifted and also when the speed of action is faster (Davis and Troup, 1964). However, raised intra-abdominal pressure (IAP) with increasing loads is not a purely linear relationship, and it is dependent on several cooperating factors, only one of which is the activity of the abdominal muscles. Studies have shown that the IAP is unrelated to training of the abdominal muscles, and that increased strength in them has not been shown to result in an increase in their activity when lifting (Hemborg *et al.*, 1983. See also 'Further reading'). It should be considered that strengthening regimes for the abdominal muscles using solely iso-metric contractions may be inadequate for training what is essentially a dynamic process of eccentric and concentric contraction.

Greater pressure increases have been demonstrated in patients with back pain than in normal subjects when lifting weights of 5–10 kg, and this was thought to emphasize their supportive role (Fairbank and O'Brien, 1979).

Generally, pressure increases are active for a very short time only. If there is a need to breathe again when lifting, the contraction of the diaphragm limits the pressure increase to the abdominal cavity and its supporting mechanism to the lumbar spine. However, it is during the initial phases of the lift that the pressures are at their highest, when spinal stress is likely to be at a maximum. As the weight is lifted closer

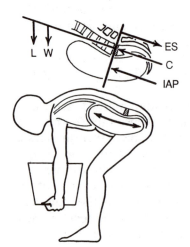

Fig. 10.9 The spine, thoracic and abdominal cavities during lifting. The force diagram indicates how the increases in intra-abdominal pressure (IAP) may relieve the intervertebral compression (C) which is equal and opposite to the tensile force in erector spinae (ES) required to raise the load (L) and the upper part of the body (W). (Adapted from J.D.G. Troup, 1979. Biomechanics of the vertebral column. *Physiotherapy*, **65**, 8, 239.)

to the body, the lever exerted by it becomes shorter, and it is then within the capacity of the back muscles to lift it.

2. *The supportive role of the thoracolumbar fascia*

Based on the anatomy of the thoracolumbar fascia (TLF) (*see* pp. 118–21), it is possible that this structure acts as a lumbar support mechanism in conjunction with the intra-abdominal pressure theory.

Contraction of the latissimus dorsi, internal oblique and transversus abdominis muscles can actively engage the TLF (McGill and Norman, 1986; Gracovetsky, 1988). Through its attachments to the posterior layer of TLF, lateral tension is transmitted upward through the deep lamina and downward through the superficial lamina. These mutually opposite vectors tend to approximate or oppose separation of the L2 and 4 and the L3 and 5 spinous processes, creating an extension, or antiflexion, moment through the lumbar spine. Tension along the transversus abdominis and internal oblique muscles is increased by the intra-abdominal pressure pushing out along the course of the muscles, which adds tension to the TLF. Gracovetsky *et al.* (1985) also described the 'hydraulic amplifier' mechanism whereby contraction of the erector spinae muscles, which are contained in a thick, inelastic envelope, causes the muscles to become engorged with blood, increasing tension throughout the TLF, thereby increasing its antiflexion moment.

3. *Passive support of ligaments*

When the lumbar spine is flexed, the posterior ligaments (in particular the supraspinous and interspinous), capsules of the apophyseal joints and TLF are tense, and are now strong enough to sustain large forces. In particular, the density of the TLF suggests that it can act as a major load-bearing structure. In the flexed position, the lumbar spine can be used passively to lift large weights. The power is provided by the hip extensors which extend the hips and tilt the pelvis backwards; provided the lumbar spine remains flexed, this power is transmitted to the thorax, rotating it posteriorly and executing the early stages of the lift.

Using the ligaments instead of active muscular contraction at this point in the lift reduces the compressive forces on the lumbar intervertebral discs: the ligaments lie posterior to the back muscles and thus have the mechanical advantage of a longer lever.

As the weight is brought progressively closer to the body, there is a transition from passive support by ligaments to active contraction of the back muscles, which are now able to balance the weight and continue with the lift. As soon as spinal extension begins, the ligaments are relaxed and their supportive role therefore ends.

Methods of Lifting

Although one lifting method alone does not suit every individual, some general rules are widely agreed upon, such as keeping the load close to the body and squat lifting if possible. Rotating or laterally flexing the spine while lifting should be avoided because, when combined with loading, these movements can damage the apophyseal joints and intervertebral discs.

The two methods commonly compared are *stoop lifting* (with the spine flexed) and *squat lifting* (with the knees flexed).

The *stoop lift* has a lower energy expenditure than the squat lift because of the greater body weight displaced vertically (Grieve, 1975; Troup, 1977) and this explains why it is often used by people who are untrained in lifting techniques.

The *squat lift* makes it possible for the subject to lift the weight from between the legs. This close proximity of the weight to the fulcrum of the lumbosacral disc means that the lever exerted by the weight is short; this is by far the most important factor in reducing both the force required to lift it and the load on the spine. If the hands have to be near to floor level in order to grasp the weight, some degree of lumbar flexion is usually necessary. One disadvantage of this type of lift is that the compressive forces across the knee joints are high. Lifting the objects from a raised platform or providing them with handles helps to reduce the load on the spine and knees.

As the squat lift involves a greater expenditure of energy, endurance for the quadriceps and gluteal muscles should be incorporated in lifting training programmes.

Much debate has centred around whether there is an optimum position of the lumbar spine – extension, neutral or flexion – to be used during lifting (Delitto *et al.*, 1987; Hart *et al.*, 1987). Gracovetsky *et al.* (1981) demonstrated that individuals will choose their own unique posture that shares the load between the thoracolumbar fascia, the posterior ligaments and the posterior annulus. This unique posture always reduces the lordosis. Experimental work done on cadaveric intervertebral discs suggests that there might be some benefit in flexing the lumbar spine in heavy lifts as the stress distribution is favourable for sustaining higher compressive loads (Hutton and Adams, 1982). By flexing the lower lumbar spine and extending the thoracic spine, the weight to be lifted can still be kept close to the body.

Clearly there is no single position that suits every individual for every lift, and a flexible approach is necessary when training unin-jured workers in lifting techniques, taking into account anthropo-metric measurements. A 'straight-back' (neutral) position (McGill and Norman, 1986) produces the greatest support; while reducing the compressive forces of an extended spine, it also reduces the ligamen-tous stress of a flexed spine. Lifting in flexion is difficult to avoid when lifting from the floor, because it is necessary to flex somewhat during this task, in which case the lift should be performed quickly. Where a slower lift is necessary, an extended lumbar spine may be preferable in order to reduce creeping of ligamentous tissue, but pretraining for strength and endurance of the extensor muscles is advisable to make it safe and effective (Scott Sullivan, 1989).

For the patient with low back pain, however, choosing one lumbar posture over another should be dependent on the type of injury and the response of injury to mechanical stress. For instance, when it is known that the ligamentous system, including the posterior annulus, has been injured, a heavy lift may be more safely carried out with the lumbar spine in neutral. Conversely, it has been suggested that a flexed posture may spare the erector spinae and multifidus excessive stress if they have been injured (Scott Sullivan, 1989). These postures should be tested and only used if they do not increase the patient's symptoms.

Repetitive Loading of the Spine

Activities such as repeated heavy lifting or digging subject the spine to fatigue compressive loading. Tyrrell *et al.* (1985) found that, following dynamic lifting, there was a measurable loss of height in the spine, in proportion to the applied load and rate, due to the expulsion of fluid from the intervertebral discs. Repetitive lifting led to greater shrinkage than did equivalent static loading, and it was concluded that lifting a 50 kg load repeatedly would induce shrinkage equal to the entire diurnal loss of stature (*see* p. 77) within 20 min (Corlett *et al.*, 1987). Loss of disc height has a clear relevance to structural geometrical changes and changed properties of the spine, such as disc bulging, end plate bulging, the stiffness of the discs, and the load on the apophyseal joints. There could also be a relation to nutritional factors of the disc.

On unloading the spine, either by a cessation of lifting or by adopting certain postures, a regain of stature occurs relatively quickly (Tyrrell *et al.*, 1985). This implies that if even short periods of unloading the spine are allowed in a heavy job, a substantial recovery can take place during these rest periods, and the total shrinkage or disc compression will be diminished.

By testing cadaveric lumbar motion segments to destruction, the effect of repetitive heavy loading of the spine has been simulated. The outcome depended on the posture used. If the motion segment was compressed and flexed, the lamellae of the annulus sometimes became distorted leading to radial fissures in the discs, which are the precursors to a gradual disc prolapse (Adams and Hutton, 1983). However, not all of the discs showed these distortions, which indicates that there are individual variations. If the motion segment was compressed and not flexed, the site of failure was in the vertebral body and end plate (Hardy *et al.*, 1958).

The response of a spine to the stresses of repetitive heavy lifting very much depend on its pre-existing condition. A spine such as that possessed by an athlete, which has been subjected to repeated strenuous activity, but not to the point of injury, will have responded to this by developing hypertrophied bone, a thicker vertebral body cortex and a more dense trabecular system, giving the vertebral body and end plate a higher resistance to failure.

Lifting Ability in Males/Females

Women are approximately 30% weaker than men of equivalent height, weight and training (Hayne, 1981), and this obviously influences their load tolerance. Guidelines have been laid down recommending maximum weights and work loads which are acceptable to industrial workers.

It has been hypothesized that women may be at a mechanical disadvantage when lifting in a stooped posture: the hip joints in women are located more anteriorly than in men, away from the line of gravity. This produces a force couple acting on the lumbosacral joint which means that, in effect, any object handled by a woman would seem approximately 15% heavier than were it handled by a man of identical stature and strength (Tichauer, 1976).

In the presence of ligamentous laxity, the risk of sacroiliac joint strain when lifting in a stooped posture is increased; this would apply to some women during menstruation or pregnancy.

PUSHING AND PULLING

The capacity of an individual for pushing and pulling depends on body weight, the posture used, the stability of the feet and the ability to transfer energy from the body to the load.

During these activities, there is an increase in intra-thoracic and intra-abdominal pressures – more so in pushing than pulling (Davis and Troup, 1964). During pushing, the recti are tense and the load on the lumbosacral disc is less than when pulling. The biomechanical explanation for this is depicted in Figs. 10.10a,b.

The *pulling* force (P_1) is directed anteriorly and increases the bending moment and erector spinae force considerably, because of the short lever arm this muscle group has with respect to the axis of rotation. Thus, the load on the disc is also increased. In *pushing*, however (Fig. 10.10a), the horizontal pushing force (Ps) is now directed posteriorly. Its bending moment is counterbalanced by the force of the recti.

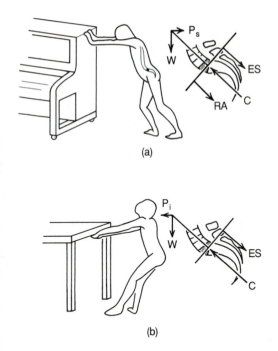

Fig. 10.10 Reaction at lumbo-sacral disc to truncal muscle activity parallel to the spinal axis. (a) *Pushing:* effect of weight of upper part of body (W) is countered by activity of erector spinae (ES), the pushing force (P_s) by rectus abdominis (RA). The sum of ES and RA is equal and opposite to the force compressing the L5/S1 disc (C). (b) *Pulling:* the pulling force P_1 is applied and the effect of W is countered by ES which is equal and opposite to C. (Adapted from J.D.G. Troup, 1979. Bio-mechanics of the vertebral col-umn. *Physiotherapy,* **65,** 8, 239.)

Because these muscles have a larger lever arm compared with the erector spinae muscles, their force is relatively less and induces a smaller increase in disc load.

EFFECTS OF LUMBOSACRAL CORSETS

Corsets are often prescribed for patients with back pain, and, in some instances, are of great value in relieving their pain. In other instances, however, patients find that they are ineffective. An under-standing of the effects of wearing corsets on spinal mobility, intradiscal pressure and muscle strength will assist in choosing the correct type of corset for the patient, to suit individual requirements.

An infinite number of lumbosacral supports is available, varying from the light elasticated type to the longer steel-braced type. Both the length of the corset and its construction will influence the effect that it has when worn. Some of the lighter corsets can be surprisingly effective in relieving pain; the reason for this is not really known, and it may simply be that they keep the area warm, with a consequent reduction in muscle spasm, or they may act as a placebo.

Mobility

The simple lumbosacral corset does not restrict movement except at the extremes of range (Van Leuven and Troup, 1969). Restricted movement in the lower thoracic and upper lumbar spine can lead to *increased* movement at the lumbosacral level. Therefore, if the aim is to immobilize an area, it is important to know the precise level of the spinal lesion before prescribing a corset for a patient. Lumsden and Morris (1968) found that lumbosacral *rotation* was very slightly restricted by corsets.

Intradiscal Pressure

A tightly-fitting corset, by compressing the abdomen and raising the intra-abdominal pressure, decreases the load on the vertebral column. In this way, intradiscal pressure is reduced by approximately 30% (Nachemson, 1964).

Muscle Activity

Subjects were found to have decreased activity in the abdominal muscles when wearing an experimentally inflated corset during lifting (Morris and Lucas, 1964). Without a support, these muscles assist during loading in increasing the intra-abdominal pressure. When the longer, non-inflated corsets were worn, they produced increases in intra-abdominal pressure during sitting; the elasticated varieties produced significant increases in intra-abdominal pressure in walking (Grew and Deane, 1982).

EMG studies have shown that activity in erectores spinae is not affected during standing and slow walking by wearing a corset, presumably because this muscle inserts much higher in the spine and, therefore, continues to work to keep the spine upright. During fast walking, however, it was found that wearing a corset *increased* muscle activity (Waters and Morris, 1970).

There is no evidence that the wearing of corsets for periods of up to 5 years in itself leads to muscle weakness (Nachemson and Lindh, 1969), although there may be a degree of physical dependence (Grew and Deane, 1982).

EFFECTS OF COLLARS

Mobility

It would appear that no splinting device has yet been devised which can completely immobilize the neck from the occipito-atlantal junction down to C7. However, many varieties of collar provide different degrees of support. This ranges from very little support provided by the soft cervical collar made from felt or foam rubber, which was found to limit only 5–10% of flexion, extension and lateral flexion and had no effect at all on rotation (Hartman *et al.*, 1975), to more effective support provided by more rigid bracing.

This does not mean that the lighter collars are ineffective; in addition to any other effects that they have, they also serve to remind the patient to avoid certain neck movements when wearing one. As with all orthoses, they should only be supplied to the patient if accompanied by instructions as to their purpose.

Orthoses which best immobilize the lower cervical spine allow the upper cervical vertebrae to move in a non-uniform manner (Fisher *et al.*, 1977). It was noted that when subjects attempted flexion of the neck against the orthosis, the upper cervical spine extended and the lower cervical spine flexed. On attempting extension against the orthosis, the upper cervical spine flexed and the lower cervical spine extended. This is particularly important when considering the supply of a collar for a patient with rheumatoid arthritis if there is excessive laxity of the transverse ligament or erosion of the odontoid peg.

Rotation in the upper cervical spine is the movement which is most difficult to restrict because conventional collars end here. The only orthosis which limits it to any degree has been found to be the halo orthosis.

The obvious conclusion to be drawn from these studies is that before an appropriate collar can be selected with the aim of restricting movement, it is important to know the spinal level which is affected.

Mechanoreceptors

Relative immobility of the upper three cervical vertebrae, and a reduction in the normal compressive force of the weight of the head, disturbs the normal pattern of afferent impulses from Type I and II mechanoreceptors in ligaments, the apophyseal joints and the joints of Luschka. These receptors subserve postural control and their importance in governing the degree of dexterity when performing intricate manual operations has been demonstrated (Wyke, 1965).

Adhesion Formation

Following trauma to the neck, e.g. in so-called 'whiplash' injuries, *excessive* immobilization in a collar leads to adhesion formation due to organization of extravasated blood and tissue fluid, shortening of contracted muscles, thickening of periarticular tissues and muscle atrophy (Mealy *et al.*, 1986).

REFERENCES

Adams M.A., Hutton W.C. (1980). The effect of posture on the role of the apophyseal joints in resisting intervertebral compressive forces. *J. Bone Jt. Surg., (Br.)*, **62-B**, 358.

Adams M.A., Hutton W.C. (1983). The effect of fatigue on the lumbar intervertebral disc. *J. Bone Jt. Surg.*, **65-B**, 2, 199.

Alexander F.M. (1932). *The Use of Self.* London: Methuen.

Andersson B.J.G., Ortengren R., Nachemson A. *et al.* (1975). The sitting posture: an electromyographic and discometric study. *Orthop. Clin. N. Am.*, **6**, 1, 105.

Andersson B.J.G., Murphy R.W., Ortengren R. *et al.* (1979). The influence of backrest inclination and lumbar support on lumbar lordosis. *Spine*, **4**, 1, 52.

Bartelink J.V. (1957). The role of abdominal pressure in relieving the pressure on the lumbar intervertebral discs. *J. Bone Jt. Surg.*, **39-B**, 4, 718.

Basmajian J.V. (1978). *Muscles Alive: Their Functions revealed by Electromyography*, 4th edn. Baltimore: Williams & Wilkins.

Bjorksten M., Jonsson B. (1977). Endurance limit of force of long-term intermittent static contractions. *Scand. J. Environ. Health*, **3**, 23.

Blow R.J., Jackson J.M. (1971). An analysis of back injuries in registered dock workers. *Proc. Roy. Soc. Med.*, **64**, 735.

Brunswic M. (1984). Ergonomics of seat design. *Physiotherapy*, **70**, 2, 40.

Carlsöö S. (1964). Influence of frontal and dorsal loads on muscle activity and on the weight distribution in the feet. *Acta Orthop. Scand.*, **34**, 299.

Corlett E.N., Eklund J.A.E., Reilly T. *et al.* (1987). Assessment of workload from measurements of stature. *Appl. Ergon.*, **18**, 1, 65.

Davis P.R., Troup J.D.G. (1964). Pressures in the trunk cavities when pulling, pushing and lifting. *Ergonomics*, **7**, 465.

Delitto R.S., Rose S.J., Apts D.W. (1987). Electromyographic analysis of two techniques for squat lifting. *Phys. Ther.*, **67**, 1329.

Dolan P., Adams M.A., Hutton W.C. (1988). Commonly adopted postures and their effect on the lumbar spine. *Spine*, **13**, 2, 197.

Dunlop R.B., Adams M.A., Hutton W.C. (1984). Disc space narrowing and the lumbar facet joints. *J. Bone Jt. Surg., (Br.)*, **66-B**, 706.

Eklund J.A.E., Corlett E.N. (1987). Evaluation of spinal loads and chair design in seated work tasks. *Clin. Biomech.*, **2**, 27.

Fairbank J.C.T., O'Brien J.P. (1979). Intra-abdominal pressure and low back pain. Paper read at Annual Meeting of International Society for the Study of the Lumbar Spine, Gothenburg, June, 1979.

Fisher S.V., Bowar J.F., Awad E.A. *et al.* (1977). Cervical orthoses – effect on cervical spine motion: roentgenographic and goniometric method of study. *Archs. Phys. Med. Rehab.*, **58**, 109.

Floyd W.F., Silver P.H.S. (1951). Function of erectores spinae in flexion of the trunk. *Lancet*, i, 133.

Floyd W.F., Silver P.H.S. (1955). The function of the erectores spinae muscles in certain movements and postures in man. *J. Physiol.*, **129**, (1), 184.

Frievalds A., Chaffin D.B., Garg A. *et al.* (1984). A dynamic biomechanical evaluation of lifting maximum acceptable loads. *J. Biomech.*, **17**, 251.

Gracovetsky S. (1988). *The Spinal Engine.* New York: Springer.

Gracovetsky S., Farfan H.F., Lamy C. (1981). The mechanism of the lumbar spine. *Spine*, 6, 249.

Gracovetsky S., Farfan H.F., Helleur C. (1985). The abdominal mechanism. *Spine*, 10, 317.

Grew N.D., Deane G. (1982). The physical effects of lumbar spine supports. *Prosth. Orthot. Int.*, 6, 2, 79.

Grieco A. (1986). Sitting posture: an old problem and a new one. *Ergonomics*, 29, 3, 345.

Grieve D.W. (1975). Dynamic characteristics of man during crouch- and stoop-lifting. In *Biomechanics IV*. (Nelson R.C., ed.) Baltimore: University Park Press, pp. 19–29.

Hardy W.G., Lissner H.R., Webster J.E. *et al.* (1958). Repeated loading tests of the lumbar spine: a preliminary report. *Surg. Forum*, IX, 690.

Hart D.L., Stobbe T.J., Jaraiedi M. (1987). Effects of lumbar posture on lifting. *Spine*, 12, 138.

Hartman J.T., Palumbo F., Jay Hill B. (1975). Cineradiography of the braced normal cervical spine. *Clin. Orthops. Rel. Res.*, 109, 97.

Hayne C.R. (1981). Manual transport of loads by women. *Physiotherapy*, 67, 8, 226.

Hellems H.K., Keates T.E. (1971). Measurement of the normal lumbosacral angle. *Am. J. Roentgenol.*, 113, 642.

Hemborg B., Moritz U., Hamberg J. *et al.* (1983). Intra-abdominal pressure and trunk muscle activity during lifting – effect of abdominal muscle training in healthy subjects. *Scand. J. Rehab. Med.*, 15, 183.

Hirsch C. (1955). The reaction of intervertebral discs to compression forces. *J. Bone Jt. Surg.*, 37-A, 6, 1188.

Hutton W.C., Adams M.A. (1982). Can the lumbar spine be crushed in heavy lifting? *Spine*, 7, 6, 586.

Hutton W.C., Stott J.R.R., Cyron B.M. (1977). Is spondylolysis a fatigue fracture? *Spine*, 2, 202.

Keagy R.D., Brumlik J., Bergan J.L. (1966). Direct electromyography of the psoas major muscle in man. *J. Bone Jt. Surg.*, 48-A, 1377.

Keegan J.J. (1953). Alterations to the lumbar curve related to posture and seating. *J. Bone Jt. Surg.*, 35, 589.

Lumsden R.M., Morris J.M. (1968). An *in-vivo* study of axial rotation and immobilisation at the lumbo-sacral joint. *J. Bone Jt. Surg.*, 50-A, 1591.

Lundervold A.J.S. (1951). *Electromyographic Investigations of Position and Manner of Working in Typewriting*. Oslo: W. Brøggers Boktrykkeri A/S.

McGill S.M., Norman R.W. (1986). Partitioning of the L4-5 dynamic moment into disc, ligamentous and muscular components during lifting. *Spine*, 11, 666.

Magora A. (1972). Investigation of the relation between low back pain and occupation, 3. Physical requirements: sitting, standing and weight lifting. *Ind. Med. Surg.*, 41, 5.

Magora A. (1974). Investigation of the relation between low back pain and occupation, 6. Medical history and symptoms. *Scand. J. Rehab. Med.*, 6, 81.

Mandal A.C. (1984). The correct height of school furniture. *Physiotherapy*, 40, 2, 48.

Mealy K., Brennan H., Fenelon G.C.C. (1986). Early mobilization of acute whiplash injuries. *Br. Med. J.*, 292, 656.

Morris J.M., Lucas D.B. (1964). Biomechanics of spinal bracing. *Arizona Med.*, **21**, 170.

Nachemson A. (1964). *In vivo* measurement of intra-discal pressure. *J. Bone Jt. Surg.*, **46-A**, 1077.

Nachemson A., Lindh M. (1969). Measurement of abdominal and back muscle strength with and without low back pain. *Scand. J. Rehab. Med.*, **1**, 60.

Schoberth H. (1962). Sitzhaltung, Sitzschaden, Sitzmobel. Berlin: Springer Verlag.

Schuldt K., Ekholm J., Harms-Ringdahl K. *et al.* (1986). Effects of changes in sitting work posture on static neck and shoulder muscle activity. *Ergonomics*, **29**, 12, 1525.

Scott Sullivan M. (1989). Back support mechanisms during manual lifting. *Phys. Ther.*, **69**, 1, 52.

Soames R.W., Atha J. (1981). The role of the antigravity musculature during quiet standing in man. *Eur. J. Appl. Physiol. Occup. Physiol.*, **47**, 159.

Tichauer E.R. (1976). Biomechanics sustains occupational safety and health. *Ind. Eng.*, **8**, 2, 46.

Troup J.D.G. (1977). Dynamic factors in the analysis of stoop and crouch lifting methods: a methodological approach to the development of safe materials handling standards. *Orthop. Clin. N. Am.*, **8**, 201.

Tyrrell A.R., Reilly T., Troup J.D.G. (1985). Circadian variation in stature and the effects of spinal loading. *Spine*, **10**, 2, 161.

Van Leuven R.M., Troup J. (1969). The instant lumbar corset. *Physiotherapy*, **55**, 499.

Waters R.L., Morris J.M. (1970). Effect of spinal supports on the electrical activity of the muscles of the trunk. *J. Bone Jt. Surg.*, **52-A**, 51.

Wyke M. (1965). Comparative analysis of proprioception in left and right arms. *Quart. J. Exp. Psychol.*, **17**, 149.

FURTHER READING

Intra-abdominal Pressure

Davis P.R., Troup J.D.G. (1964). Pressures in the trunk cavities when pulling, pushing and lifting. *Ergonomics*, **7**, 465.

Gracovetsky S., Farfan H.F. (1986). The optimum spine. *Spine*, **11**, 543.

Morris J.M., Lucas M., Bressler J. (1961). The role of the trunk in stability of the spine. *J. Bone Jt. Surg. (Am.).*, **43**, 327.

Index